Statistical First Aid

Interpretation of

Health Research Data

Statistical First Aid

Interpretation of Health Research Data

Robert P. Hirsch, Ph.D.

Master of Public Health Program
The George Washington University Medical Center
Washington, D.C.

Richard K. Riegelman, M.D., Ph.D.

Boston
BLACKWELL SCIENTIFIC PUBLICATIONS
Oxford · London · Edinburgh · Melbourne · Paris · Berlin · Vienna

Blackwell Scientific Publications

Editorial offices:
Three Cambridge Center, Cambridge,
   Massachusetts 02142, USA
Osney Mead, Oxford OX2 0EL, England
25 John Street, London, WC1N 2BL, England
23 Ainslie Place, Edinburgh, EH3 6AJ,
   Scotland
54 University Street, Carlton, Victoria 3053,
   Australia

Other editorial offices:
Arnette SA, 2 rue Casimir-Delavigne, 75006
   Paris, France
Blackwell-Wissenschaft, Meinekestrasse 4,
   D-1000 Berlin 15, Germany
Blackwell MZV, Feldgasse 13, A-1238 Wien,
   Austria

Distributors:
USA
Blackwell Scientific Publications
Three Cambridge Center
Cambridge, Massachusetts 02142
(Telephone orders: 800-759-6102)

Canada
Times Mirror Professional Publishing
5240 Finch Avenue East
Scarborough, Ontario M1S 5A2
(Telephone orders: 416-298-1588)

Australia
Blackwell Scientific Publications (Australia)
   Pty Ltd
54 University Street
Carlton, Victoria 3053
(Orders: Telephone: 03-347-0300)

Outside North America and Australia
Blackwell Scientific Publications, Ltd.
Osney Mead
Oxford OX2 0EL
England
(Orders: Telephone: 011-44-865-240201)

Typeset by Science Press
Printed and bound by The Maple-Vail Book Manufacturing Group

© 1992 Blackwell Scientific Publications
Printed in the United States of America
92 93 94 95   5 4 3 2 1

The tables in Appendix B were adapted from tables in Zar JH. *Biostatistical Analysis*. 2nd ed.
Englewood Cliffs, NJ: Prentice-Hall, Inc., 1984.

Library of Congress Cataloging-in-Publication Data

Hirsch, Robert P.
   Statistical first aid : interpretation of health research data /
Robert P. Hirsch, Richard K. Riegelman.
      p.   cm.
   Includes index.
   ISBN 0-86542-138-2
   1. Medicine—Research—Statistical methods.   2. Biometry.
I. Riegelman, Richard K.   II. Title.
R853.S7H57   1991
610'.72—dc20
                                                      90-24885
                                                      CIP

CONTENTS

PREFACE

Statistical First Aid is designed to provide clinicians and health researchers with a systematic approach to understanding the most commonly encountered statistical procedures in health research. Our goal is to help you develop an ability to select an appropriate method of analysis and to interpret the results. We do not expect that *Statistical First Aid,* or any other single book, can communicate all there is to know about statistics. We hope, however, that *Statistical First Aid* will prepare you to handle many data analysis and interpretation issues in health research. Moreover, we hope that *Statistical First Aid* will help you determine when you need to consult with a statistician and how to communicate with that statistician about your data. Thus the title *Statistical First Aid:* this book is designed as a guide to what should be done until the statistician arrives.

Our approach to statistics is an unusual one. Through our experience in teaching statistics to clinicians and health researchers, we have learned two important lessons. First, you have a strong desire to understand, not simply to memorize, statistics. Second, the traditional approaches to statistics (at least in our hands) do not facilitate understanding among clinicians and researchers who are not completely comfortable with mathematics. As a result, we have largely abandoned traditional approaches to statistics and focused on understanding methods for analyzing data without relying on mathematical explanations.

The first three chapters of *Statistical First Aid* present some of the basic principles of statistics that are common to all methods of analysis. The remaining nine chapters are organized around the logical processes used by statisticians to select statistical procedures for a particular set of data. At the beginning of each of those chapters is a flowchart summarizing the crucial decisions in selecting statistical procedures. These flowcharts are also presented together in Appendix C for easier reference after the reader is familiar with how the statistical methods work. In addition, we have provided with this book the opportunity for you to obtain, free of charge, *Stat-Aid P.L.U.S.*

(*Programmed Learning for Understanding Statistics*), a computer-assisted learning tool intended to reinforce the important concepts contained in the flowcharts.

Statisticians are experts in using the language of mathematics. Mathematics is a very useful language for describing quantitative phenomena. The major advantages that mathematical language has over English (or any other literary language) are its precise and consistent rules: you do not need to rely on the context to appreciate the meaning. To persons who speak this language, mathematics is a beautiful way to communicate ideas. Unfortunately, many of the persons who are fluent in mathematical language seem to assume that literary language automatically contains the same sort of precision. In *Statistical First Aid,* we have placed special emphasis on precise and consistent terminology. Our goal is to make our use of literary language as precise as mathematical language. To increase the precision of the terminology that we have used, we have carefully defined statistical concepts. We have sought to avoid confusion by excluding statistical terms that conflict with their meaning in nontechnical English. In addition to clarifying statistical terminology, we have also attempted to provide the reader with an understanding of the terminology that statisticians actually use.

One of our goals in teaching statistics is to rely as little as possible on mathematics. Of course, statistics is a mathematical discipline so that one cannot completely escape from encountering some equations, but *Statistical First Aid* uses other types of illustration to develop an understanding of what the mathematical equations in statistics are all about. These types of illustration include graphic representation of mathematical concepts and analogies to other aspects of health and medicine.

As you read *Statistical First Aid,* we hope to show you the conceptual unity, order, and coherence that give statistics an intellectual elegance. Our ultimate goal is to help you become comfortable enough with statistics that you come back asking for more.

Robert P. Hirsch
Richard K. Riegelman

ACKNOWLEDGMENTS

We thank our medical, public health, and graduate students and fellows from Tufts University, Harvard School of Public Health, University of Pittsburgh, The Foundation for Advanced Education in Science (NIH), and The George Washington University for teaching us how to teach statistics. Without their demands to truly understand statistics, we probably would not have developed our unusual approach to this subject. We also thank those students and colleagues who have encouraged us to write this book and who have been so patient with us during its development. We are much indebted to James Krosschell as well as the production, editorial, and marketing staff at Blackwell Scientific Publications for their encouragement, patience, and professional skills. We also are most thankful to Tom Plant for reading the manuscript and to Steve Hansen for assisting in the development of *Stat-Aid P.L.U.S.*

NOTICE

The indications and dosages of all drugs in this book have been recommended in the medical literature and conform to the practices of the general medical community. The medications described do not necessarily have specific approval by the Food and Drug Administration for use in the diseases and dosages for which they are recommended. The package insert for each drug should be consulted for use and dosage as approved by the FDA. Because standards for usage change, it is advisable to keep abreast of revised recommendations, particularly those concerning new drugs.

Statistical First Aid

Interpretation of
Health Research Data

PART ONE

Understanding Basic Principles

Health researchers' need to use statistical methods can be stated simply. We are interested in understanding health phenomena as they relate to large groups of individuals, but we cannot, for practical and financial reasons, study those large groups. Rather, we would like to develop an understanding of those phenomena by examining a subset of individuals. The purpose of statistical methods is to allow us to use observations made on a subset to understand the whole. Before we can appreciate the specific statistical methods used in health research to accomplish this goal, there are some basic principles that we need to understand. In this first part of *Statistical First Aid* we examine the building blocks that are the foundation of statistical reasoning.

When we gather a subset (called a **sample**) from a larger group (called the **population**), chance will influence how closely the subset reflects the larger group. Thus, a large part of the task in understanding the larger group based on examination of a subset is to account for the influence of chance. We think about chance in terms of probabilities of various things occurring. One of the building blocks of statistical reasoning is to understand what probabilities are, how they behave, and how they interact. In Chapter 1, we begin building the foundation for understanding statistics by learning about probabilities.

If we are to draw a subset from a larger group, we need to know how that is done. Further, we need to know what aspects of the larger group we will address by examining the subset. In Chapter 2, we examine the basic principles of sampling and the properties of the data collected in a sample. Those data form particular patterns (called **distributions**) in the larger group which need to be described based on observations in the subset. Generally, just a few summary numbers (called **parameters**) are required to characterize the pattern in the larger group. We will discover the nature of those summary numbers and how they relate to the role of chance in selecting individuals from the larger group.

In Chapter 3, we complete our foundation for understanding the basic principles of statistical reasoning by investigating two important processes: estimation and inference. The purpose of estimation is to make our best guess at the value of the summary numbers describing the pattern of data in the larger group based on observations in the subset. There are two types of guesses that we will encounter. The first is a specific value for a summary number that represents our best guess (called a **point estimate** or **statistic**). The second is an interval of numbers (called an **interval estimate**) that allows us to take into account the role of chance in drawing the subset from the larger group. Another way to take into account this role of chance, which we also examine in this chapter, is by hypothesizing the value of the summary number and testing the validity of that hypothesis using the observations in the subset (a process called **statistical inference**).

Once we have developed an understanding of these basic principles, we will be ready to learn about specific statistical methods that are commonly used in the analysis of health research data. As you learn about those specific methods in the last three parts of *Statistical First Aid,* you will find that we use these basic principles over and over again. Thus, full appreciation of the last three parts of this book relies on a firm understanding of the material in the first part. Because Part I builds a foundation on which the rest of this text relies, you should be comfortable with the principles discussed in the next three chapters before going on to Part II. To aid you in reaching that level of comfort we have used a variety of approaches. We think that you will discover in Part I that you need not be a mathematician to truly understand statistics.

CHAPTER 1

Probability

You cannot get away from it, whether in health research or in clinical practice: we are constantly confronted with probabilities. We cannot be absolutely certain that a drug that has efficacy in a clinical trial will work on any particular patient, nor can we be certain that factors that appear to be risks for a disease in one group of subjects would appear to be part of the etiology of that disease if another group were examined. Therefore, it is important for the clinician and the health researcher to be comfortable with probabilities and how they behave.

A **probability** is a mathematical expression of how many times we can expect something *actually* to happen compared to the number of times it is *possible* for it to happen. For example, we might think of the probability that a patient presenting with a sore throat has streptococcal pharyngitis. If that probability is 0.10, that means that we can expect 10 patients to actually have streptococcal pharyngitis out of every 100 patients seen with a sore throat.

In statistical terminology, how many times something happens is called its **frequency** and that "something" is called an **event.** When using the concepts of probability, we can observe that an event has one of only two **states** or conditions: it either occurs or it does not occur. In the previous example, the event was streptococcal pharyngitis. The opportunities for an event to occur are called **observations.**[1] In our example, the patients seen with sore throats are our observations.

A probability is calculated as the frequency with which a particular event occurs divided by the number of observations. The resulting probability is a **proportion.** In this case, the denominator of the proportion contains the number of times that the event occurs plus the number of times that the event does not occur. In general, a

---

[1]Statisticians also refer to the opportunity for an event to occur as a **trial.** Since a trial, in health research terminology, is used to refer to a clinical experiment, we will use the term "observation" exclusively instead of "trial" to refer to this component of a probability.

proportion is a frequency divided by another frequency that includes the first frequency. In other words, the numerator is a subset of the denominator.

Example 1.1   In 1985, there were 3,760,561 live births in the United States. Of those live births, 7,521 infants died of sudden infant death syndrome in the first year of life. What is the probability of dying of sudden infant death syndrome in the first year of life?

In this example, the event is dying of sudden infant death syndrome in the first year of life and the observations are live births. Thus, the probability of an infant dying of sudden infant death is equal to:

$$\frac{7,521}{3,760,561} = 0.002$$

That probability can be interpreted to mean that, if we considered 10,000 live births, we would expect to observe 20 cases of sudden infant death syndrome.

Thus, we see how probabilities are calculated from a collection of observations. We have also seen how the interpretation of a probability calculated from one collection of observations might be applied to another collection of observations. For instance, in Example 1.1 we interpreted the probability of an infant dying of sudden infant death syndrome by estimating that we would expect 20 such deaths if we followed 10,000 infants through their first year of life. That estimation was made by multiplying the probability times 10,000, the number of observations in the new collection of live births.

Another circumstance to which we apply probabilities is especially important to the clinician: that is the estimation of the chance of an event occurring in a single observation. For example, we might wish to estimate the probability that a particular patient with a sore throat has streptococcal pharyngitis. In this application, "chance" is considered a synonym for probability. Often, when that synonym is used, probability is expressed as a percentage, such as a 10% chance of streptococcal pharyngitis. Technically, a percentage is an expression of a **relative frequency** rather than of probability, but the two are so closely related (relative frequency is equal to probability times 100%) that the distinction is of little importance.

Regardless of whether probabilities are applied to individuals or to groups, they have the same basic properties. For example, all probabilities lie within the range of 0 to 1. A probability of *0* indicates that the event in question is *impossible*. A probability of *1* indicates that the event is *certain*.

Earlier, we said that an event can have two states: Either it occurs or it does not occur. The probabilities that we have calculated so far have been for the event occurring. The situation in which an event *does not occur* is called the **complement** of the event. Having an etiology *other than* a streptococcal infection associated with a sore throat is the complement of having streptococcal pharyngitis. The sum of the probability of an event and the probability of its complement is always equal to one, reflecting our certainty that an event will either happen or not happen. Therefore, we can calculate the probability of the complement of an event by subtracting the probability of the event from one. The probability that a patient with a sore throat does not have streptococcal pharyngitis as the etiology is equal to $1 - 0.10 = 0.90$.

Relationships between a probability and its complement can be presented in mathematical language. The probability of an event is symbolized in mathematical language as $p(A)$ where A stands for the name of the event (such as streptococcal pharyngitis). The complement of an event is represented by placing a bar above the name of the event. Therefore, the probability of the complement of event A (such as the probability that a patient *does not* have streptococcal pharyngitis) is $p(\overline{A})$, and it is related to the probability of the event occurring as follows:

$$p(\overline{A}) = 1 - p(A) \tag{1.1}$$

where

$p(A)$ = probability of event A occurring

$p(\overline{A})$ = probability of event A not occurring

Example 1.2 What is the probability that an infant born in the United States in 1985 would not die due to sudden infant death during the first year of life?

Not dying from sudden infant death is the complement of dying from sudden infant death. Therefore, the probability of that complement is:

$$p(\overline{\text{SIDS}}) = 1 - p(\text{SIDS}) = 1 - 0.002 = 0.998$$

Note that, in Example 1.2, the complement of dying of sudden infant death syndrome is *not* the probability of surviving the first year of life, but rather it is the probability of not dying of sudden infant death syndrome during the first year of life. Surviving the first year of life has as its complement dying of any cause during that period. An event and its complement must include all possible states. In statistical terminology, we say that any collection of events that includes all possibilities is **collectively exhaustive.**

Another characteristic of probabilities associated with ultimate or immediate causes of death is that they refer to events that are usually considered to be **mutually exclusive.** That is to say, mortality data is compiled in such a way that each death is associated with one and only one immediate cause.[2] Therefore, from the point of view of death certificates and, therefore, mortality statistics, the probability of an individual dying due to, say, atherosclerosis and carcinoma of the lung is zero. In contrast to causes of mortality, types of morbidity are not considered to be mutually exclusive. For

---

[2] The US Standard Certificate of Death lists only one immediate cause of death. Other, contributory causes might also be listed that are thought to have precipitated the immediate cause.

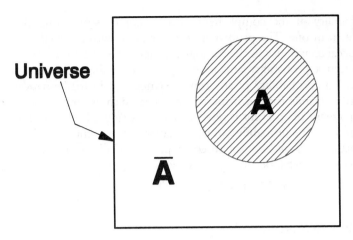

FIGURE 1.1 An example of a Venn diagram. The rectangular area, called the universe, represents all possible events. The circular area represents the occurrence of event A. The part of the rectangular area not in the circle represents event A not occurring, called the complement of event A, symbolized by $\overline{A}$. The size of the circle relative to the size of the rectangle corresponds to the number of observations with event A relative to all observations.

example, it is possible to have morbidity associated with both atherosclerosis and carcinoma of the lung.

VENN DIAGRAMS

There are two ways in which we can examine probabilities associated with events. The first approach is mathematical, as examined in Equation 1.1 above. The second approach is diagrammatic. In the diagrammatic approach, we use the *area* within a diagram or figure to represent a relative frequency.

In a commonly used diagrammatic approach, we draw a rectangular area to represent all possible events related to the event(s) of interest. This collection of all possible events is called the **universe.** If, for example, we were interested in causes of death, the universe would include any cause of death. Since the universe contains all possible events (i.e., it is collectively exhaustive), there is a probability of one that an observation will be included in the universe. In this approach, we use areas to depict frequencies relative to the universe. To make comparison of areas as easy as possible, we define the total area within the rectangle symbolizing the universe to be equal to one. To represent each event of interest, we draw a figure, most often a circle, within the rectangular area. To depict the relationship between frequency and area, the circle representing the frequency of an event is drawn so that its area relative to the area of the rectangle is equal to the probability of that event. Such an illustration is known as a **Venn diagram.** Figure 1.1 illustrates a Venn diagram for an event called A.

Example 1.3 Draw a Venn diagram to represent the probability of death due to sudden infant death syndrome within the first year of life presented in Example 1.1.

In Example 1.1, we looked at sudden infant death syndrome relative to all live births. Therefore, the rectangle in our Venn diagram will represent all live births. Next, we draw a very small circle that has an area equal to 0.002 relative to the area of the rectangle. The area of that circle relative to the area of the entire rectangle signifies the proportion of all live births that result in sudden infant death syndrome mortality. The area within the rectangle but outside the circle represents the complement of a death due to sudden infant death syndrome (a live birth that does not result in sudden infant death mortality). The area within the rectangle but outside the circle is equal to $1 - 0.002 = 0.998$ relative to the area of the rectangle.

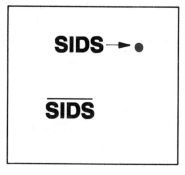

Thus, Venn diagrams allow us to examine pictorially the relationship between an event and the universe of events that are addressed by probabilities. The components of Venn diagrams can be used further to demonstrate how those probabilities are calculated. For example, the probability of event A is calculated by dividing the number of times event A occurs by the total number of observations. Using the diagrammatic approach, Figure 1.2 illustrates that calculation as the division of the area associated with event A by the total area in a Venn diagram.

$$p(A) = \frac{\text{(A)}}{\text{(rectangle)}}$$

FIGURE 1.2 A diagrammatic representation of the probability of event A using elements from a Venn diagram. Those observations in which event A occurs are represented by the circular area in the numerator. All possible observations are represented by the rectangular area (the universe) in the denominator.

Venn diagrams are especially useful when examining relationships among events. For example, consider the Venn diagram in Figure 1.3. In that Venn diagram, we have drawn event C to be mutually exclusive of both events A and B. The Venn diagram shows us that event C is mutually exclusive by having no point (or observation) within the rectangle that is included both in the circle representing event C and in the circles representing either events A or B. On the other hand, we have drawn events A and B not to be mutually exclusive of each other, which is symbolized by depicting overlapping circles for events A and B. The collectively exhaustive set of events includes events A, B, and C, as well as the remainder of the rectangular area that is not part of one of those circles (the complement of events A, B, and C).

COMBINATIONS OF EVENTS

INTERSECTIONS   For events that are not mutually exclusive, it is often of interest to determine the probability that two or more of those events will occur together. For example, we might be interested in the probability that patients who smoke have elevated diastolic blood pressure (two contributory causes of coronary heart disease). In statistical terminology, we are interested in the **intersection** of high diastolic blood pressure and smoking.

Let us first investigate what is meant by an intersection of events using the diagrammatic approach. If we reexamine events A and B in Figure 1.3, we can see that where the circles representing those events overlap, both events occur. This area of overlap is the intersection of the two events. The probability of the intersection, or of both events A and B occurring, is equal to the area of overlap relative to the

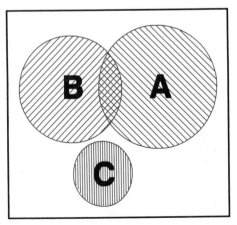

FIGURE 1.3 A Venn diagram illustrating the relationships among three events: A, B, and C. Event C is mutually exclusive of events A and B, but events A and B are not mutually exclusive of each other.

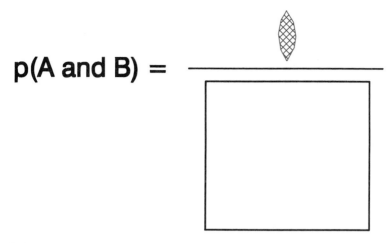

FIGURE 1.4 A diagrammatic illustration of the probability of the intersection between events A and B. The area in which both events A and B occur (see Figure 1.3) is in the numerator. The universe is in the denominator.

area of the rectangle symbolizing all possible observations. Diagrammatically, this probability can be illustrated as in Figure 1.4.

In practice, the probability of an intersection between events is easier to determine mathematically than it is diagrammatically. Before we can determine the probability of an intersection mathematically, however, we must consider another characteristic of sets of events: **independence.** Two (or more) events are said to be independent of one another if the probability of one event occurring is the same regardless of whether the other event(s) has occurred or if that event(s) has not occurred. For example, consider cigarette smoking and drinking coffee. The probability that someone drinks coffee is *not* independent of the probability that he or she smokes cigarettes since a greater proportion of cigarette smokers tend to drink coffee than do nonsmokers. Elevated diastolic blood pressure and cigarette smoking, however, might well be independent. If they are independent, that would imply that the probability that an individual has elevated diastolic blood pressure is the same whether he or she does or does not smoke cigarettes.

If a set of events is independent, the probability of their intersection is found by multiplying together the probabilities for each event:

$$p(A \text{ and } B \text{ and } C) = p(A) \cdot p(B) \cdot p(C) \tag{1.2}$$

where A, B, and C = three independent events.

Equation 1.2 describes what is sometimes called the **multiplication rule of probability theory.**

Example 1.4 In a particular community of 10,000 persons, 2,000 are known to have elevated diastolic blood pressure (defined as a pressure greater than 110 mm Hg). It is also known that half of the people in that community smoke cigarettes. Assuming that elevated diastolic blood pressure and smoking are independent events, what is the probability that any particular member of that community will have elevated diastolic blood pressure and be a cigarette smoker?

First, let us calculate the probabilities of the two events without regard to each other. The probability of any person in this community having elevated diastolic blood pressure is:

$$p(\text{DBP} > 110) = \frac{2,000}{10,000} = 0.2$$

The probability of any person in the community being a cigarette smoker is:

$$p(\text{SMOKER}) = \frac{1}{2} = 0.5$$

Next, we calculate the probability that an individual in the community is both a cigarette smoker and has elevated diastolic blood pressure by multiplying the probabilities of those two events:

$$p(\text{DBP} > 110 \text{ and SMOKER}) = 0.2 \cdot 0.5 = 0.1$$

In other words, if diastolic blood pressure and smoking are independent, one-tenth of the individuals in the community (or 1,000 persons) should be cigarette smokers who have elevated diastolic blood pressure.

Diagrammatically, we could represent the relationship between cigarette smoking and elevated diastolic blood pressure as two overlapping circles: one with an area of 0.2 (diastolic blood pressure) and the other with an area of 0.5 (smoking). The area of overlap should be one-tenth of the total area of the Venn diagram.

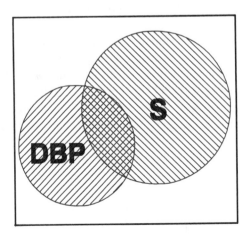

Then, we could illustrate the probability of having elevated diastolic blood pressure and being a cigarette smoker diagrammatically as follows:

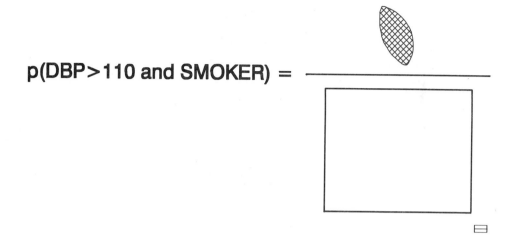

$$p(DBP>110 \text{ and } SMOKER) = \frac{}{}$$

If we are interested in an intersection of events that we are unable to assume are independent, we can still calculate their intersection. We cannot, however, simply multiply the probabilities of the events as we did in Equation 1.2. Rather, we must use **conditional** probabilities to calculate the intersection, as opposed to the **unconditional** probabilities that we have used so far. A conditional probability expresses the chance that a particular event will occur *under the condition* that another event(s) has occurred or will occur.

Symbolically, conditional probabilities are represented in the form $p(A|B)$. The event(s) represented by the letter to the left of the vertical bar is called the **conditional event.** The entire expression represents the probability of this conditional event occurring. The event(s) represented by the letter to the right of the bar is called the **conditioning event.** The conditioning event B defines limitations or conditions under which we are interested in the probability of the conditional event A occurring. Thus, $p(A|B)$ states the probability of event A occurring given the occurrence of the conditioning event B. In other words, $p(A|B)$ is the probability of A occurring given that B occurs.

To understand conditional probabilities, let us first use the diagrammatic approach. Reconsider the Venn diagram in Figure 1.3 that shows relationships between three hypothetical events: A, B, and C. If we were interested in the probability of event A occurring given that event B occurs $[p(A|B)]$, the first thing we would do is to confine our interest to portions of the Venn diagram in which the conditioning event has occurred: namely, the area within the circle representing event B (see Figure 1.5). Notice that the occurrence of event A within that circle (cross-hatched area) is the same as the intersection between events A and B.

The calculation of the probability of event A occurring given that event B occurs can be represented diagrammatically as shown in Figure 1.6. Compare the diagrammatic illustration of calculating the probability of event A occurring conditional on event B occurring with the calculation of the unconditional probability of event A

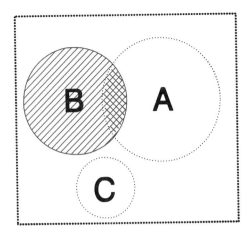

FIGURE 1.5 A Venn diagram illustrating the conditional relationships of events *A* and *C* to event *B*. Our interest is confined to the colored area in which event *B* occurs. The cross-hatched area represents event *A* occurring given that event *B* occurs. There is no area that represents event *C* occurring given that event *B* occurs (i.e., events *B* and *C* cannot occur together in a single observation).

examined previously (Figure 1.2). The important difference between these two probabilities is the information in their denominators. *The unconditional probability contains the universe of all possible observations (the rectangular area) in its denominator, while the conditional probability contains only those observations in which event B occurs in its denominator.* That distinction is what defines the difference between conditional and unconditional probabilities. The numerators of those two probabilities also differ. The numerator of the unconditional probability contains all of event *A*. The conditional probability, on the other hand, contains only that part of event *A* that is included in the denominator of the conditional probability (i.e., the part of the circle representing event *A* that overlaps the circle representing event *B*).

From the diagrammatic representation of a conditional probability, we might anticipate the mathematical approach to its calculation. Mathematically, we calculate conditional probabilities by dividing the probability that both events will occur

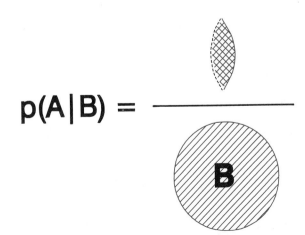

FIGURE 1.6 A diagrammatic representation of the probability of event *A* occurring conditional on event *B* occurring. The area representing the occurrence of both events *A* and *B* in Figure 1.5 is in the numerator. The area representing the occurrence of event *B* is in the denominator.

together (the probability of the intersection) by the probability of the conditioning event occurring:

$$p(A|B) = \frac{p(A \text{ and } B)}{p(B)} \tag{1.3}$$

where $p(A|B)$ = probability of event A given that event B occurs.

Example 1.5 In Example 1.4, we found that, in a community in which one-half of the members smoke cigarettes, the probability that an individual has elevated diastolic blood pressure and is a cigarette smoker is 0.1. From that information, calculate the probability that an individual has elevated diastolic blood pressure given that the person is a cigarette smoker.

We are told that the probability of the intersection between elevated diastolic blood pressure and cigarette smoking is 0.1 and the unconditional probability of smoking is 0.5. Using Equation 1.3, we then can calculate the probability of elevated diastolic blood pressure conditional on an individual being a cigarette smoker:

$$p(\text{DBP} > 110 | \text{SMOKER}) = \frac{p(\text{DBP} > 110 \text{ and SMOKER})}{p(\text{SMOKER})} = \frac{0.1}{0.5} = 0.2$$

Diagrammatically, we can represent that conditional probability as follows:

$$\textbf{p(DBP>110|SMOKER)} = \underline{\hspace{5cm}}$$

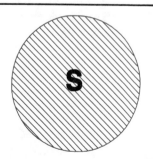

As we said before, calculating the probability of the intersection of events that are not independent relies on conditional probabilities. To see how the probability of intersection is calculated, we need to perform a little algebra to rearrange Equation 1.3. If we multiply both sides of Equation 1.3 by $p(B)$, we get Equation 1.4.

Both sides of Equation 1.3 multiplied by $p(B)$:

$$p(B) \cdot p(A|B) = \frac{p(A \text{ and } B)}{p(B)} \cdot p(B)$$

Canceling $p(B)$ on the right and interchanging the left and right sides gives us:

$$p(A \text{ and } B) = p(B) \cdot p(A|B) \tag{1.4}$$

In Equation 1.2, we calculated the probability of the intersection of three independent events by multiplying together their unconditional probabilities. To calculate the probability of the intersection of more than two events that are not assumed to be independent, we use conditional probabilities in much the same way. There is one added complexity, however. In an equation to calculate the probability of the intersection of events that are not independent, the probabilities can be considered in any order. However, having chosen the order, each subsequent conditional probability must be calculated based on the condition that *all* of the previously listed events have occurred. For example, we could calculate the probability of the intersection of three events (*A, B,* and *C*) without assuming independence among those events as follows:

$$p(A \text{ and } B \text{ and } C) = p(A) \cdot p(B|A) \cdot p(C|AB) \tag{1.5}$$

where $p(C|AB)$ = probability of event C given that both events A and B have occurred.

The order in which probabilities are listed in the calculation of the probability of an intersection does not matter. For example, we would obtain the same answer as in Equation 1.5 if we multiplied $p(C) \cdot p(B|C) \cdot p(A|CB)$. The order in which the events are listed in that calculation depends only on the information available to us.

Example 1.6   The community described in Example 1.4 was composed of 10,000 persons, half of whom smoked cigarettes and 20% of whom had elevated diastolic blood pressure levels. Let us now assume that, of the 2,000 persons with elevated diastolic blood pressure, 1,500 are cigarette smokers and 500 are nonsmokers. Based on this information, what is the probability that any particular person is both a smoker and has elevated diastolic blood pressure?

In Example 1.4, we assumed that cigarette smoking and elevated diastolic blood pressure were independent events. Recall that if two events are independent, then the probability of one event is the same regardless of whether or not the other event occurs. The assumption that cigarette smoking and elevated diastolic blood pressure are independent is tantamount to saying that the relative frequency of cigarette smoking should be the same (i.e., 50% in this example) among persons with elevated diastolic blood pressure compared to those without elevated diastolic blood pressure. Now, we are told that 1,500 (or 75%) of the 2,000 individuals with elevated diastolic blood pressure smoke cigarettes. Since the overall relative frequency of cigarette smoking in the community is 50%, the probability of an individual with elevated diastolic blood pressure being a cigarette smoker must be higher than the probability of an individual without elevated diastolic blood pressure being a smoker. Therefore, in this example, we find that cigarette smoking and elevated diastolic blood pressure are *not* independent events.

Now, we want to calculate the probability of an individual in this community being both a cigarette smoker and having elevated diastolic blood pressure. The easiest and most direct way to answer this question is to divide the number of individuals who both smoke cigarettes and have elevated diastolic blood pressure by the total number in the community (1,500/

10,000 = 0.15). But, to illustrate the use of conditional probabilities in calculating the probability of the intersection between two events, let us solve this problem in a less direct way.

First, we will calculate the probability of elevated diastolic blood pressure given that a person is a cigarette smoker, based on the information provided in this example. To reflect the conditional nature of this probability, we divide the number of persons with elevated diastolic blood pressure levels who smoke cigarettes by the total number of cigarette smokers in the community:

$$p(\text{DBP} > 110|\text{SMOKER}) = \frac{1,500}{5,000} = 0.3$$

Then, let us use that conditional probability to calculate the probability of the intersection between smoking and diastolic blood pressure. Using the relationship in Equation 1.4:

$$p(\text{DBP} > 110 \text{ and SMOKER}) = p(\text{SMOKER}) \cdot p(\text{DBP} > 110|\text{SMOKER})$$
$$= 0.5 \cdot 0.3 = 0.15$$

By now, you should have the impression that independence between events is an important property that influences how we think about and calculate probabilities of events. Although we have defined independence and provided some examples, we have not explicitly discussed how we can determine whether or not two events are, in fact, independent. To discover some clues that can be used as criteria to make the distinction between independence and lack of independence, let us compare the results we obtained in Examples 1.4 and 1.5. In Example 1.4, we assumed that cigarette smoking and elevated diastolic blood pressure were independent events and found that the unconditional probability of having elevated diastolic blood pressure was 0.2. In Example 1.5, still assuming independence, we found that the conditional probability of elevated diastolic blood pressure among cigarette smokers was also 0.2. Thus, the unconditional and the conditional probabilities were equal. In general, a good way to determine if two events are independent is to compare their unconditional and conditional probabilities. By definition, *events are independent if, and only if, their unconditional probabilities are equal to their conditional probabilities.*

UNIONS   Thus far, we have considered a combination of events in which both occur (intersection) or in which the probability of one event is dependent on the occurrence of another (conditional probabilities). One more combination of events is often of interest: the **union** of events, by which we mean the case in which at least one of two or more events occurs. For example, the union of elevated diastolic blood pressure and cigarette smoking refers to individuals who have elevated diastolic blood pressure *and/or* smoke cigarettes.

Calculation of the union of two or more events is easiest if the events are mutually exclusive (i.e., there is no possibility of two of the events occurring in the same observation). Recall our previous example of immediate causes of death as mutually exclusive events. When events are mutually exclusive, the probability that one of the

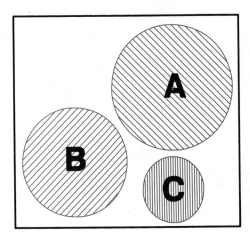

FIGURE 1.7 A Venn diagram for three mutually exclusive events: *A*, *B*, and *C*. Mutually exclusive events are represented by circular areas that do not overlap.

events will occur is equal to the sum of probabilities for each of the events.

$$p(A \text{ or } B \text{ or } C) = p(A) + p(B) + p(C) \qquad (1.6)$$

This is often called the **addition rule of probability theory.**[3]

The reason for requiring that the probabilities be mutually exclusive in order to apply Equation 1.6 becomes clear if we use Venn diagrams to investigate unions of events. First, let us examine Figure 1.7, which is a Venn diagram of three mutually exclusive events.

Since the union of events means that at least one of the events occurs, any point within the circles representing events *A*, *B*, or *C* would satisfy the union. Therefore, we can depict the probability of the union of *A*, *B*, or *C* from components of the Venn diagram by adding the areas defined by those three events and dividing by all possible observations (Figure 1.8).

Now, let us consider the problem encountered when the events are *not* mutually exclusive. In that case, circles representing events in the Venn diagram would overlap to indicate that it is possible for more than one event to occur in the same observation. Lack of mutual exclusion for all three events is illustrated in the Venn diagram in Figure 1.9.

To satisfy the union of events that are not mutually exclusive, a point in the Venn diagram representing an observation would have to fall within one of the circles. This is the same as for mutually exclusive events. When the events overlap (intersect),

---

[3]Now that we know the addition rule we can, with a little algebra, see why the probability of the complement of an event is equal to one minus the probability of the event (Equation 1.1). Since the complement of an event includes all possible occurrences other than the event, it is certain (i.e., it has a probability of one) that either the event or its complement will occur. Therefore, the probability of the union of an event and its complement, $p(A \text{ or } \overline{A})$, is equal to one:

$$p(A) + p(\overline{A}) = 1$$

Subtracting $p(A)$ from both sides of the equation, we get Equation 1.1:

$$p(\overline{A}) = 1 - p(A)$$

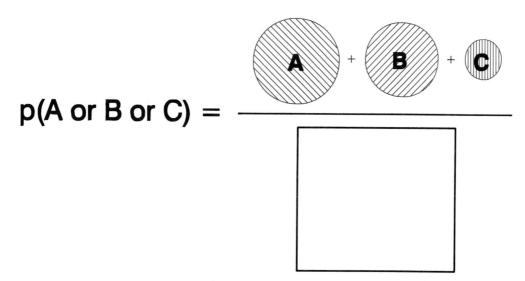

$$p(A \text{ or } B \text{ or } C) =$$

FIGURE 1.8 A diagrammatic representation of the union of mutually exclusive events *A, B,* and *C*. The numerator contains the sum of the areas representing the events in the union. The denominator contains the universe.

however, some points would fall within two or more of the circles simultaneously. Thus, if we were simply to add the areas corresponding to the three events, those areas of intersection would contribute to the sum more than once. The result, in that case, would be that the sum would overestimate the area associated with *A, B,* or *C*. Again, this result can be illustrated by creating equations from the components of the Venn diagram (Figure 1.10).

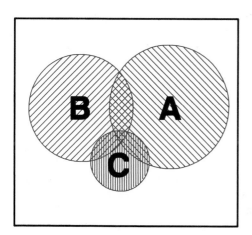

FIGURE 1.9 A Venn diagram for three events (*A, B,* and *C*) that are not mutually exclusive. We know that the events are not mutually exclusive because the circular areas overlap.

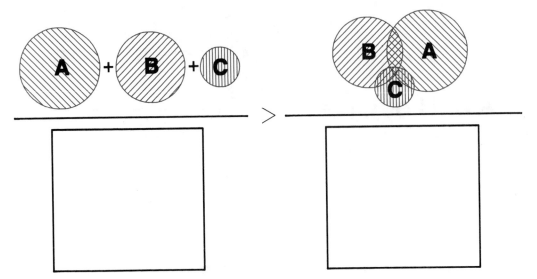

FIGURE 1.10 A diagrammatic illustration of the relationship between the union of three mutually exclusive events (on the left) compared to three events that are not mutually exclusive (on the right).

Since the problem in calculating the probability of the union of events that are not mutually exclusive is that we are counting areas of intersection more than once, the solution is to subtract these areas of intersection. If three events all intersect each other, such as in the previous Venn diagram, simply subtracting the areas of intersection creates a new problem. The problem arises because the area representing the intersection of all three events is no longer taken into account. This occurs because we have subtracted it from each of the three areas. To solve that problem, we add back in the area representing the intersection of all three events.

We calculate the probability of a union of events by adding the probabilities of the individual events and taking into account their intersections if the events are not mutually exclusive. Equation 1.7 shows the calculation for the union of three events that are not mutually exclusive.

$$p(A \text{ or } B \text{ or } C) = p(A) + p(B) + p(C) - p(A \text{ and } B) - p(A \text{ and } C) \tag{1.7}$$
$$- p(B \text{ and } C) + p(A \text{ and } B \text{ and } C)$$

Example 1.7 In Example 1.4, we considered a community in which 20% of the members had elevated diastolic blood pressure and 50% smoked cigarettes. If we assume that elevated diastolic blood pressure and cigarette smoking are independent, then, as we found in Example 1.4, 10% of the members of this community both smoke and have elevated diastolic blood pressure. If that assumption of independence of diastolic blood pressure and smoking is correct, what is the probability that a particular individual has at least one of those risk factors (i.e., smokes cigarettes and/or has elevated diastolic blood pressure)?

The first realization from this example is that smoking cigarettes and having elevated diastolic blood pressure are not mutually exclusive events. There are two statements in this example that tell us that. Perhaps the more obvious statement is that a probability of the intersection of those two events is equal to 10% and is, therefore, not equal to zero. By definition, events that are mutually exclusive have a zero probability of occurring together. The second statement is that we are assuming that the events are independent. Events *cannot* be both mutually exclusive and independent. Being mutually exclusive, in fact, is an extreme of a lack of independence.

Note. Recall that the definition of independence is that conditional and unconditional probabilities are equal. If two events are mutually exclusive, then the probability of either of the events being conditional on the other is equal to zero. Thus, conditional and unconditional probabilities of those events cannot be equal unless the unconditional probabilities of those events are equal to zero.

To answer a problem such as this, it is useful to organize what we know. Three probabilities are provided in this problem. They are:

$$p(DBP > 110) = 0.2$$
$$p(SMOKER) = 0.5$$
$$p(DBP > 110 \text{ and } SMOKER) = 0.1$$

Using that information, we can calculate the probability of the union of cigarette smoking and elevated diastolic blood pressure by adding the probability of having elevated diastolic blood pressure to the probability of smoking cigarettes (addition rule of probability). Since elevated diastolic blood pressure and smoking are not mutually exclusive events, we need to take into account in our calculation the intersection of those two events by subtracting the probability of the intersection.

$$p(DBP > 110 \text{ or } SMOKER) = p(DBP > 110) + p(SMOKER)$$
$$- p(DBP > 110 \text{ and } SMOKER)$$
$$= 0.2 + 0.5 - 0.1 = 0.6$$

|| SUMMARY

In this chapter, we have learned some basic properties of probabilities. First, we learned that a probability is a mathematical expression of how many times we can expect an event to happen compared to the number of observations or times it is possible for it to happen. Probabilities can be applied to groups to estimate the number of events we would expect to observe or to individuals to estimate the probability that an individual will experience the event. In statistical terminology, the opposite of an event occurring is called the complement of the event. The complement of an event is symbolized by placing a bar over the symbol for the event. The probability of the complement of an event is found by subtracting the probability of the event from one:

$$p(\overline{A}) = 1 - p(A) \tag{1.1}$$

When we speak of probabilities of events, we can think of two types of probabilities. The first is the probability of the event without regard to the occurrence of any other events. This is known as an unconditional probability. Alternatively, we can consider the probability of an event under the condition that another event or events have occurred. This is known as a conditional probability. For independent events, conditional and unconditional probabilities are equal.

Conditional probabilities are important when we are calculating the probability of two or more events occurring together. That is known as the probability of the intersection of events. To calculate the probability of the intersection of events, we multiply the probabilities of the individual events, using what is known as the multiplication rule of probability theory.

$$p(A \text{ and } B \text{ and } C) = p(A) \cdot p(B|A) \cdot p(C|AB) \tag{1.5}$$

The probability of one or more of a group of events occurring is called the probability of the union of the events. That probability is found by adding the probabilities together, using what is known as the addition rule of probability theory. If the events are not mutually exclusive (i.e., more than one of the events can occur in the same observation), calculating the probability of the union of the events must take into account the probabilities of intersections among the events:

$$p(A \text{ or } B \text{ or } C) = p(A) + p(B) + p(C) - p(A \text{ and } B) - p(A \text{ and } C) \tag{1.7}$$
$$- p(B \text{ and } C) + p(A \text{ and } B \text{ and } C)$$

||| PRACTICE PROBLEMS

1.1 In the Collaborative Perinatal Project (Heinonen et al., 1977), 50,282 pregnant women were followed to completion of their pregnancies. Among the offspring of those women, 3,248 congenital malformations were observed. Based on those observations, what is the probability that a pregnancy will result in a congenital malformation?

1.2 Each year, about 5% of the people in a particular community die with heart disease listed as the immediate cause of death on their certificates of death, and about 1% die with respiratory disease listed as the immediate cause. What is the probability that a particular person in that community will *not* die during the next year with either heart disease or respiratory disease as their immediate cause of death?

1.3 In a Venn diagram, indicate the area corresponding to the probability computed in Problem 1.2.

1.4 In a study of smoking and alcohol consumption, it was found that 5% of the persons studied smoked but did not consume alcohol, 45% consumed alcohol but did not smoke, 35% both smoked and consumed alcohol, and 15% neither smoked nor consumed alcohol. Among people in that study, is smoking independent of consuming alcohol?

CHAPTER 2

Populations and Samples

The need for statistics in health research stems from the fact that we can make measurements and observations on only a subset of the individuals for whom we would like to draw conclusions or make estimations. For example, we might wish to examine the relationship between cigarette smoking and elevated diastolic blood pressure. In Example 1.4, we considered a community of 10,000 persons in which we observed 2,000 persons with elevated diastolic blood pressure and 5,000 persons who smoke cigarettes. In practice, we would not examine all 10,000 members of this community. Rather, we would most likely draw conclusions about the relationship between smoking and diastolic hypertension by making measurements on a few hundred individuals from that community. Even if we were able to make measurements on all existing persons in the community, we might expect our conclusions about that particular community to be applicable to persons in similar communities or to persons who will be members of that community in the future. Thus, we attempt in health research to draw conclusions about the nature of the whole by examining only a portion.

In statistical terminology, we call the whole a **population** and the portion examined a **sample.** The use of the term "population" in this context might, at first, be misleading. Most often, when we think of a population, we imagine a group of persons defined, for example, by some geopolitical criterion (such as the community in Example 1.4). For example, we might think of the population of the Chicago metropolitan area. In statistics, however, population has a broader definition. A population in statistical terminology refers to the collection of all possible measurements (or data[1]) that could be used to address the study question. In the case of our study of cigarette smoking and elevated diastolic blood pressure, the data that make up

---

[1]The term "data" refers to anything that could possibly be observed or measured. Data that are actually measured or observed in a sample are called measurements or observations. Thus, both the population and the sample contain data, while only samples can contain measurements or observations.

the population are the frequencies of smoking and diastolic hypertension among all possible community members now and in the future.

The purpose of obtaining a sample, therefore, is to allow us to estimate or infer the nature of the population without being able to observe (i.e., measure data from) the entire population. In our example, we wish to estimate the probabilities of smoking and diastolic hypertension in the community without examining all 10,000 community members. To make estimates or draw inferences, statistical procedures assume that the sample is representative of the population. That is to say, it is assumed that only chance could cause the composition of the sample to differ from the composition of the population in all aspects other than the quantity of data contained in each. There are many ways in which a representative sample can be drawn from a population, but all depend on some **random sampling** component. Random sampling means that only chance determines whether or not a particular datum in the population will be part of the sample. Without such a sample, one must be concerned about **bias** (a systematic tendency in one particular direction). Bias is a problem for which statistical procedures can be of little help.

Populations are defined, for statistical procedures, as containing all possible measurements that could be used to address the study question. Thus, a population can be characterized in part by the data that it contains. To think about populations further, we need to examine the nature of data encountered in health research.

TYPES OF DATA

To understand statistical procedures, we need to distinguish among three different types of data: continuous, ordinal, and nominal. **Continuous** data are characterized by having an infinite number of evenly spaced potential values between any two values. For example, ages of persons are measured using continuous data. We know that ages are continuous data since between any two ages are an unlimited number of possible ages measured in infinitely small units of time.

This characteristic is not true of **ordinal** data. With ordinal data, we can choose two values from a limited number of possible values between which no other values are possible. For instance, the number of children in a family is ordinal. There are a limited number of possible values for number of children, and it is not possible to find a family that includes more than two but less than three children. Furthermore, it is not necessary for the values of ordinal data to be evenly spaced as are continuous data. A commonly encountered type of ordinal data in health research is stage of disease. We cannot say that the distance between stages I and II is the same as the distance between stages II and III. We do know, however, that those stages imply some order to the severity of disease. That is to say, stage II is more advanced than stage I but less advanced than stage III.

With **nominal** data, we cannot establish such an order. Race is an example of nominal data. We can observe that a person is Asian, black, white, etc., but we cannot establish any ordering of those possible values. Like ordinal data, nominal data contain a finite number of possible values. Because of this limitation, we say that ordinal and nominal data are **discrete** types of data.

We recognize that these definitions of types of data are, in practice, theoretical rather than real. Age, for example, is *theoretically* continuous since we can imagine time measured in infinitely small units, but we do not usually measure age in time units smaller than days. Thus, the way we measure age, or any other continuous data, forces us to have a limited number of values between two of which no other potential values exist. If we measure age by recording birth date, it is not possible for us to distinguish the ages among persons born on the same day. For statistical purposes, however, we can still think of age as continuous data. The practical definition of continuous data requires that they include a large (rather than infinite) number of evenly spaced values.

What about data that are theoretically ordinal but have a large number of evenly spaced values, such as the number of hairs on a person's head? No matter how we measure the number of hairs, it is impossible to find a head with a number between 999,999 and 1,000,000. This truly represents ordinal data, but it is not different, in practice, from data that are theoretically continuous. For statistical purposes, we can consider any data with a large number of evenly spaced values to be virtually continuous, even if they are theoretically ordinal.

As part of the process of research, the researcher records data. Those data, however, are not necessarily used in statistical analyses in the same form that they are recorded. Statisticians think of the collection of measurements that is used in a statistical procedure a little bit differently from the collection of measurements that is recorded by the researcher. Rather than data, the statistician thinks about **variables.** Variables represent the data in a form that will allow statistical analysis. For continuous or ordinal data, corresponding variables represent those measurements just as they were observed. Thus, there is a one-to-one correspondence between continuous or ordinal data recorded by the researcher and continuous or nominal variables analyzed by the statistician.

Nominal data, however, are often not directly translatable into variables. For most statistical procedures, nominal variables are limited to dichotomous (yes/no) classification indicating presence or absence of a condition. Nominal data with only two categories, such as gender, can be represented by one nominal variable. Here, we might use a nominal variable indicating the presence or absence of, say, being female. For nominal data consisting of more than two categories, on the other hand, more than one variable is needed to represent these data. Let us consider race as a characteristic that we measure with four categories: black, Asian, white, and other. In this case, we need to create three variables to represent race. The first variable might indicate the presence or absence of being black; the second variable might indicate the presence or absence of being Asian; and the third variable might indicate the presence or absence of being white. Notice that we do not need a fourth variable to indicate the presence or absence of being a member of a race included in the category called "other," for anyone who is not black, Asian, or white *must* be a member of one of the other races. In general, if nominal data contains k categories of a characteristic, then $k - 1$ nominal variables will be used in statistical procedures to represent that characteristic.

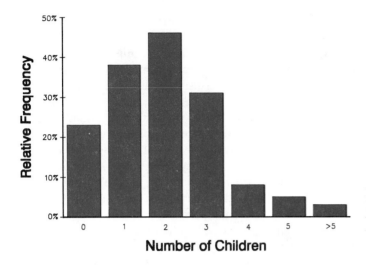

FIGURE 2.1 An example of a bar graph. Bar graphs are used to pictorially represent distributions of discrete data such as ordinal or nominal data.

DISTRIBUTIONS OF DATA

Earlier in this chapter, we said that a sample is the portion of a population for which we actually make observations or measurements. The purpose of those measurements on the sample is to enable us to make some statement about the population. That statement usually involves estimation of or inference about the population's **distribution.** By the population's distribution, we mean the frequencies or relative frequencies (probabilities) with which various data values occur in the population.[2] To understand populations further, we need to understand distributions. Distributions can be presented graphically or as mathematical equations. Graphical representations are useful in helping us get an overall feeling for distributions.

As we said earlier, ordinal and nominal data are both discrete. That is to say, even theoretically, only a limited number of values are possible. We can examine the distribution of discrete data graphically with a **bar graph.** Figure 2.1 shows a bar graph for the number of children in a family (ordinal data). Along the abscissa (*x*-axis), we find the value that the bar represents. Along the ordinate (*y*-axis), a bar graph can display the frequency, relative frequency, or probability of the values of the data in the population. Notice that the bars in a bar graph are drawn so that they do not touch each other. We present discrete data in this way to remind ourselves that no values are possible between the values defining each of the bars.

As stated earlier, data can be considered continuous if they consist of a large number of evenly spaced values. We used age as an example of continuous data. Another example is systolic blood pressure. One way to present continuous data

[2] Note here that the term "distribution," as it is used in statistics, differs somewhat from how it is used in everyday language. In the latter case, it is often synonymous with the range or spread of data. In statistics, we are referring to the frequency with which *each* of the data values occur.

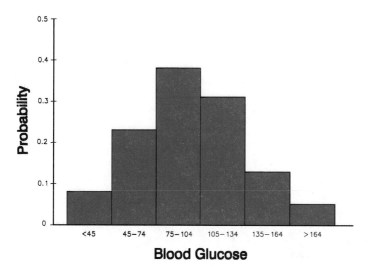

FIGURE 2.2 An example of a histogram. Histograms are used to represent continuous data pictorially. Notice that, unlike bar graphs (Figure 2.1), the bars in a histogram touch each other.

graphically is with a **histogram.** A histogram is similar to the bar graph used with discrete data except that each bar in a histogram represents an interval of possible values rather than a single value. If the intervals differ among the bars in a histogram, the width of the bars should also differ to reflect the interval represented by each bar.[3] To remind us that data in a histogram are continuous, bars in histograms are drawn so that they touch. Figure 2.2 shows an example of a histogram. An alternative graphical presentation of continuous data is the **frequency polygon,** in which bar midpoints are connected with a line. Figure 2.3 shows an example of a frequency polygon.

As the bars in a histogram are made to represent smaller and smaller intervals, the corresponding frequency polygon becomes more and more a smooth line. If we made the width of the bars to correspond to the width of the interval that a bar represents, the relative area within a bar would be a representation of the probability of a value being observed in that interval. What is the limit of how narrow those histogram bars might become? Since there are an infinite number of values possible for continuous data, we could make those bars infinitely narrow. How much area is contained in an infinitely narrow bar? An infinitely narrow bar has an area virtually equal to zero. Does that mean that the probability of observing any particular value with continuous data is virtually equal to zero? Yes, it does!

If this seems incongruous, let us offer an analogy. We know that the distance traveled by an automobile is equal to its velocity multiplied by the time during which distance is being measured (all three variables represent continuous data). If that time interval were made smaller and smaller, the distance traveled would also become less. If we made the time interval infinitely small, the distance traveled would be virtually zero

---

[3]In Figure 2.2, the widths of the bars are the same, indicating that the intervals represented by the bars are the same. The first and last bars, however, have open-ended intervals (<45 and >164). The bars for these intervals have been drawn with widths equal to the other bars.

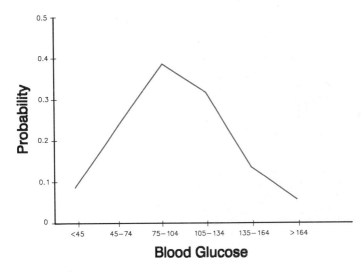

FIGURE 2.3 An example of a frequency polygon. A frequency polygon is another way to represent a distribution of continuous data pictorially. It is drawn by connecting the midpoints of the bars in a histogram.

even though the automobile has a positive velocity![4] Thus, in this analogy and in determining probabilities for continuous variables, we can determine values for intervals, but not for single points within an interval.

With discrete data, **probability distribution functions** can be used to describe mathematically[5] the probability for any particular outcome in the population. We can also describe distributions of continuous data mathematically, but they are distinct from probability distribution functions in that they can only be used to calculate probabilities by integrating ("summing") the function over an interval of values. To emphasize this distinction, statisticians refer to the mathematical descriptions of continuous data as **probability density functions.**

The most commonly considered probability density function in statistics is the mathematical description of data that has a **Gaussian (or "normal") distribution.** More than 300 years ago, mathematicians noticed that frequency polygons of continuous data frequently had a symmetric, "bell-shaped" distribution, with data near the middle of the distribution occurring most frequently and data toward the extremes of the distribution occurring more and more rarely as values became more extreme. Figure 2.4 shows a graphical representation of a Gaussian distribution[6] of systolic blood pressure data for a hypothetical population.

---

[4]If you are experiencing the firing of some old neural pathways as you consider this characteristic of continuous data, it is probably because the distance–time–velocity analogy reminds you of your college calculus instructor's introduction to integration. If you are not experiencing this phenomenon, do not panic, for all you need to remember about calculus is that integration is the way we sum an infinite number of infinitely small areas.

[5]Mathematicians use the term "describe" in reference to a distribution to mean that a mathematical formula can be presented in such a way that, when values are assigned to the parameters of that formula, it will allow calculation of any or all points within the distribution.

[6]Although it is not possible to show in a graphical representation, a Gaussian distribution theoretically includes all values from $-\infty$ to $+\infty$.

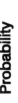

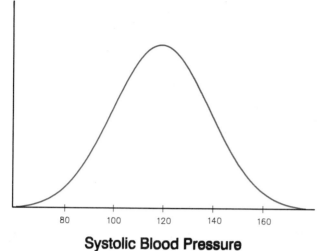

Systolic Blood Pressure

FIGURE 2.4 A frequency polygon of a Gaussian distribution of systolic blood pressure for a hypothetical population. This symmetric, bell-shaped curve is the most commonly assumed distribution in statistical procedures.

As we mentioned earlier, a graphical representation of a population's distribution is useful in helping us to get an overall feeling for a distribution. Unfortunately, distributions contain so much information that they are too unwieldy for analytical purposes in health research. Rather than make estimates or draw conclusions about an entire population's distribution, we begin analysis by assuming that the distribution of the population from which our sample was drawn belongs to a family[7] of known distributions. In health research, there are two families of distributions that we consider almost exclusively: Gaussian and binomial. The distributions in the Gaussian family are appropriate for populations of continuous data. The distributions in the binomial family are appropriate for populations of nominal data.

For now, we will be concerned only with distributions related to the Gaussian family. The "parent" of the Gaussian family is the Gaussian distribution we have just discussed and examined in Figure 2.4. Although the Gaussian distribution is used for populations of continuous data, we will see that many statistical procedures for ordinal or nominal data use methods that approximate a Gaussian distribution. Understanding the Gaussian distribution, therefore, is essential to understanding most statistical procedures.

Even after we have selected a family of distributions that we will assume best fits our population's data, it is necessary to identify a particular distribution within that family. At first, this might seem a difficult task, for each family of distributions contains an infinite number of separate distributions. Fortunately, a particular distribution can be identified by very few numeric values called **parameters.** To identify a particular Gaussian distribution, we need to determine only two parameters: (1) a measure of the central location of the distribution, and (2) a measure of the variation of data within the distribution.

[7]Statisticians refer to populations' distributions that have similar basic mathematical formulas as a family of distributions.

MEASURES OF LOCATION

Measures of location indicate where data in a distribution occur (or are "centered") on a continuum of possible values. The most commonly used measure of location is the **mean** (μ). It is one of the two parameters of Gaussian distributions. Figure 2.5 shows Gaussian distributions that differ in the values of their means.

If asked to define a mean of a population, you would probably be forced to rely on a mathematical definition. Specifically, you would most likely suggest that a population's mean is the sum of all data values divided by the number of data in the population:

$$\mu = \frac{\Sigma\, Y_i}{N} \tag{2.1}$$

where

μ = population's mean
Y_i = the ith data value in a series of data values
$\Sigma\, Y_i$ = sum (Σ) of all data values in the population
N = number of data values in the population

To understand, in nonmathematical terms, what a mean is, imagine finding the center of gravity of a bar (as you might have done in an introductory college physics course). That center of gravity of the bar corresponds to the location of the mean of a distribution. The mean is the point in a distribution at which the distribution "balances" (that is, there is an equal "weight" of data above and below the mean).

The change in the mean produced by adding data at various points within a distribution is analogous to adding weights at various points along a balanced bar. If we add a weight to that bar at the center of gravity, the center of gravity would not

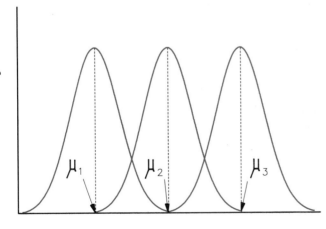

FIGURE 2.5 Gaussian distributions with different locations of data values. The location of each distribution is specified by the mean (μ) of the distribution.

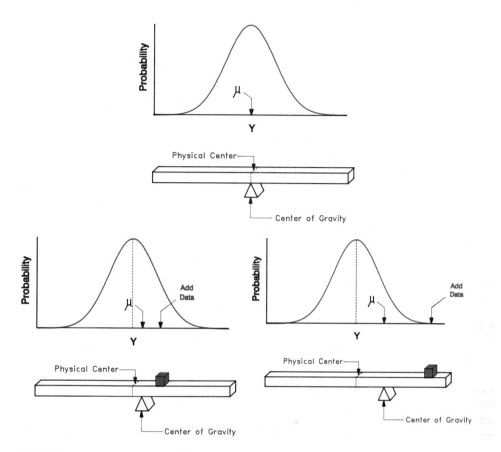

FIGURE 2.6 The analogy of adding weights to a bar to illustrate the effects of adding data at various distances from the mean on the value of the mean. The further from the balance point a weight is added to a bar, the more the balance point must be moved. Similarly, the further from the mean data are added, the more the mean moves.

change its location. The same is true for the mean of a distribution of data; we can add or subtract data that have the same value as the mean without changing the mean. Adding data at any other point along a distribution, however, will cause the mean to move toward the value of the data added. The further the added data are from the mean, the further the mean will move. Again, the analogy of the balanced bar with the mean represented by the center of gravity provides an illustration of this effect. If weights were added to that bar at points that were various distances from the center of gravity, we would see the center of gravity move further from its original position for those weights that were added at a further distance from the original position. This principle is illustrated in Figure 2.6.

Although the mean of a distribution of continuous data has properties that are attractive to the statistician (this parameter is used in the mathematical description of the Gaussian distribution), the mean's tendency to be affected by extreme data values can be worrisome. One way to decrease concern about extreme data values is to consider an alternative to the mean as a measure of the center of a distribution. One such alternative is the **median.** The median is the *physical* center (rather than the center of gravity) of a distribution for which half the data are greater and half are less. Extreme data values cause the median to move in the direction of the extreme values, but to no greater degree than for values close to the median.

In addition to being a measure of the location of a distribution in its own right, the median can be thought of as a **resistant** (i.e., not influenced by extreme values that might be of questionable validity) estimate of the mean of a distribution. For a symmetric distribution (e.g., the Gaussian distribution), the mean and the median have identical values. When a sample contains extreme values that occur infrequently in the population being sampled, the sample median will be a better estimate of the population mean than would the mean of the sample observations.

Example 2.1 Suppose we have a population of 15 patients for whom we have measured blood urea nitrogen (BUN) with the following results:

Patient	BUN (mg/dl)
JK	8.2
TG	8.7
RW	9.3
EF	9.5
PS	10.8
LC	11.4
KP	11.9
WB	13.6
RD	14.1
CW	15.7
AH	16.2
PO	16.8
YH	17.3
VB	18.8
MS	19.0
Total	201.3

Calculate the mean and the median for those data.

Next, suppose that, instead of 19.0 mg/dl for patient MS, we actually found a BUN equal to 25.0 mg/dl. How does that change affect the mean and the median?

Note. We are generally interested in populations with much greater numbers of data elements than 15. Rather, 15 values is more the number we would expect in a sample than in a population. For now, however, we want to imagine a very small population to examine some principles. We will consider these same principles using samples in Chapter 3.

To calculate the mean BUN for this population, we use Equation 2.1:

$$\mu = \frac{\Sigma \, \Upsilon_i}{N} = \frac{201.3}{15} = 13.42 \text{ mg/dl}$$

The median BUN can be found by determining the value for which half of the data are greater and half are smaller. This task is easier if the data are arrayed in numeric order. That has been done for us in the preceding table. Since 7 patients have BUN values less than 13.6 mg/dl and 7 patients have BUN values greater than 13.6 mg/dl, 13.6 mg/dl is the median BUN value.

Note. When we have an odd number of data values, one of those data values is equal to the median. When we have an even number of data values, we find the median by taking a value halfway in between the two middle values.

Now, let us see what happens when we change patient MS's BUN value from 19.0 mg/dl to 25.0 mg/dl. In calculating the mean, we notice that the sum of the BUN measurements now equals 207.3 mg/dl instead of 201.3 mg/dl. Thus, the mean changes from 13.42 mg/dl to 13.82 mg/dl:

$$\mu = \frac{\Sigma \, \Upsilon_i}{N} = \frac{207.3}{15} = 13.82 \text{ mg/dl}$$

The median BUN, on the other hand, remains equal to 13.6 mg/dl. Seven patients still have BUN values less than 13.6 mg/dl and 7 patients still have BUN values greater than 13.6 mg/dl even though we have changed the BUN measurement for patient MS. This demonstrates how the mean, more than the median, is affected by extreme data values.

Another measure of location that is even more resistant to the influence of extreme data is the **mode.** This is the data value that is observed most frequently (i.e., the peak of a distribution). The mode is completely unaffected by extreme data values.[8] In a Gaussian distribution (and any other symmetric, unimodal distribution), the mode has the same value as the mean and the median. Figure 2.7 shows the location of the mean, median, and mode for symmetric and asymmetric distributions.

---

[8]There are, however, some shortcomings of the mode as a measure of the location of a distribution. First, determination of the mode uses very little of the information contained in a set of data values since, to make that determination, we need only to establish the relative frequencies of those data values. Second, with samples of continuous data, ranges of values must be defined (as in construction of a histogram) to estimate the mode. How those ranges are defined is dependent on the nature of the sample and the choice of the researcher, yet different definitions can result in different estimates of the mode from a single set of data values. Third, distributions of some sorts of data may not have a definable mode. At the extreme, for example, is a uniform distribution in which all possible data values are of equal frequency.

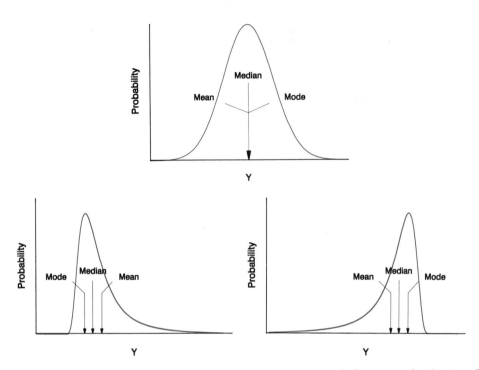

FIGURE 2.7 The relative positions of the mean, median, and mode for various distributions. For symmetric distributions like the Gaussian distribution, the mean, median, and mode are all equal to the same value. For asymmetric distributions, the mean is closest to the longer "tail" of the distribution.

MEASURES OF VARIATION

For data from a Gaussian distribution, even after the location of a distribution has been specified accurately by calculating the mean, an infinite number of possible distributions exist with that same mean. Those distributions differ in how much the data vary from the mean (see Figure 2.8).

As with location, there are a number of ways in which we might express the variation or dispersion of data within a distribution. One way we might consider measuring the variation in a distribution is by determining how much, on the average, data values differ from the mean (the usual location measure chosen for a Gaussian distribution). Calculation of that **mean deviation** would then be as follows:

$$\frac{\Sigma \, (Y_i - \mu)}{N} \tag{2.2}$$

The mean deviation has one drawback that unfortunately is rather important. The result of the calculation in Equation 2.2 is always zero! This is true, of course, because, by definition, there is always an equal "weight" of data above and below the mean. Therefore, the sum in the numerator of Equation 2.2 will contain an equal magnitude of positive and negative values, causing the total to equal zero.

One way to keep Equation 2.2 from equalling zero is to ignore the negative signs for data values below the mean and sum the absolute values of the differences between the mean and each of the data values. That **mean *absolute* deviation** would then be:

$$\frac{\Sigma \, |\Upsilon_i - \mu|}{N} \tag{2.3}$$

There are, in fact, some (older) statistical procedures that use the mean absolute deviation to measure the spread of a distribution, especially with the median as the measure of the location of that distribution.

An alternative way to keep the numerator of Equation 2.2 from adding up to zero is to sum the squared differences between the mean and the data (called the **sum of squares**). That **mean *squared* deviation** is calculated as in Equation 2.4:

$$\sigma^2 = \frac{\Sigma \, (\Upsilon_i - \mu)^2}{N} \tag{2.4}$$

That mean squared deviation is more commonly known as the **variance** (σ^2) of a distribution. The variance is the parameter of the Gaussian distribution that indicates the variation of the data values. The square root of the variance is called the **standard deviation** (σ). The standard deviation, rather than the variance, is often used to express variation in a Gaussian distribution because it has the same units as the mean (the variance has those units squared).

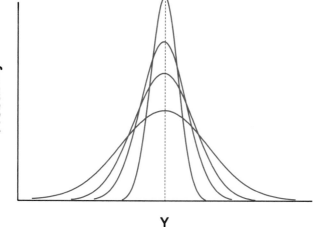

FIGURE 2.8 Gaussian distributions with different degrees of variation of data values. Each distribution has a different amount of variation from the same mean value.

Example 2.2 Using the data in Example 2.1, calculate the standard deviation of BUN measurements among patients in the population.

First, we calculate the sum of squares for BUN measurements. This is easiest to do in a table such as the following:

Patient	BUN (mg/dl)	$\Sigma \, (\Upsilon_i - \mu)$	$\Sigma \, (\Upsilon_i - \mu)^2$
JK	8.2	−5.22	27.25
TG	8.7	−4.72	22.28
RW	9.3	−4.12	16.97
EF	9.5	−3.92	15.37
PS	10.8	−2.62	6.86
LC	11.4	−2.02	4.08
KP	11.9	−1.52	2.31
WB	13.6	0.18	0.03
RD	14.1	0.68	0.46
CW	15.7	2.28	5.20
AH	16.2	2.78	7.73
PO	16.8	3.38	11.42
YH	17.3	3.88	15.05
VB	18.8	5.38	28.94
MS	19.0	5.58	31.14
Total	201.3	0.00	195.10

Notice that, as we suggested earlier, the sum of the deviations between data values and their mean is equal to zero. Squaring those deviations, however, results in a nonzero sum.

Now, we are ready to calculate the variance for this population. Using Equation 2.4:

$$\sigma^2 = \frac{\Sigma \, (\Upsilon_i - \mu)^2}{N} = \frac{195.10}{15} = 13.01$$

The standard deviation is the square root of the variance. Thus, for this population, the standard deviation is:

$$\sigma = \sqrt{\frac{\Sigma \, (\Upsilon_i - \mu)^2}{N}} = \sqrt{\frac{195.10}{15}} = \sqrt{13.01} = 3.61$$

In addition to its importance to statistical procedures (by its relationship to the Gaussian distribution), the standard deviation is a sensible way to quantify how much, "on the average," data in a distribution vary from the mean. The mean plus or minus ($\pm$) one standard deviation defines an interval of data values in a Gaussian distribution that includes about two-thirds of all the population's data values. Within the interval of the mean ± 2 standard deviations lie approximately 95% of the population's data values. Nearly all (about 99.7%) of the population's data values from a Gaussian distribution occur in the interval of the mean ± 3 standard deviations.

So far, we have only considered variation in data relative to some specific point in a distribution (specifically, to the mean). This is a reasonable approach, but it is not the only one possible. For example, one measure of variation that is completely independent of any measure of location is the **range**.[9] To determine the range of a distribution, one simply subtracts the lowest from the highest value. When we try to estimate the population's range from our sample's observations, however, we encounter an important problem. For distributions (like the Gaussian distribution) in which extreme values occur rarely, even moderately sized samples are unlikely to include those extreme values. Further, the more observations that are made in a sample, the more we expect to observe values close to those extremes. Therefore, a sample's estimate of the population's range depends not only on the population's actual range, but also on how many observations are made in the sample.

A measure of variation that is rarely used, yet has some attractive properties, is the **interquartile range.** To determine the interquartile range, the distribution is first divided in half by determining the median. Then, the median of each half is used to separate the entire distribution into four equal parts or quartiles. The interquartile range is the distance between the extremes of the middle two quartiles (thus, describing the middle half of the distribution). When estimating a population's value from a sample's observations, the interquartile range has an advantage over the range of extremes in that we do not have to assume that our sample contains extreme and very rare data values from the population. Thus, the interquartile range is not as influenced by the number of observations in a sample as is the simple range of extremes.

Another advantage of the interquartile range is that it can be used as a *resistant estimator* (i.e., it is not greatly affected by unusual observations) of the population's standard deviation. Recall from our discussion above that the mean ± 1 standard deviation (i.e., an interval equal to two standard deviations centered around the mean) is equal to two-thirds of the population's data values. The interquartile range includes one-half of the population's data values. Therefore, a little bit of algebra tells us that two-thirds of the interquartile range is equal to the standard deviation of a Gaussian distribution.

---

[9]Range has two meanings in statistics. Here, it is used to refer to the distance between the most extreme data values. It is also used more generically to refer to the distance between any two values. We will use the term "interval" to convey the generic concept.

STANDARD NORMAL DISTRIBUTION

As mentioned above, probability density functions of continuous variables are used to calculate the probability of observing data within an interval of data values. That is accomplished by using calculus to determine the integral of the mathematical expression of the Gaussian distribution for the interval of values. That integral tells us the area under the distribution for that interval. The area under the entire distribution is equal to one. Therefore, the area under any portion of the distribution is the same as the probability of observing a value within that interval.

Most of us would like to avoid determining integrals. It would be most convenient if those integrals were available in tables, but as long as the parameters of the Gaussian distribution can have any of an infinite number of values, an infinite number of tables would be required. To avoid having to use calculus to calculate the probability associated with an interval of values of interest, it is possible to convert that interval to a standard scale that has a particular mean and a particular standard deviation. For that standard scale, if we choose zero for the mean ($\mu = 0$) and one for the standard deviation of the distribution ($\sigma = 1$), we have a particular Gaussian distribution known as the **standard normal distribution.** Conversion of data from other Gaussian distributions to the standard normal distribution results in a value known as a **standard normal deviate** (denoted by z). Calculation of a standard normal deviate is straightforward. To convert data from any distribution to a distribution with a mean of zero, we need only subtract the value of μ for the distribution of data from the data value (Y_i) that we would like to convert (i.e., $Y_i - \mu$). To convert the spread of a distribution to one, we divide the converted mean by the σ for that distribution.

$$z = \frac{Y_i - \mu}{\sigma} \tag{2.5}$$

Table B.1 in Appendix B gives us probabilities associated with various standard normal deviates. Table B.1 lists the probabilities of randomly drawing a particular standard normal deviate value or a value further from the mean (the mean is equal to zero in the standard normal distribution) than that particular standard normal deviate. We will take a closer look at the standard normal distribution and standard normal deviates in Chapter 3. For now, let us see how they can be used to calculate probabilities in Example 2.3.

Example 2.3   Consider a population in which systolic blood pressure has a Gaussian distribution with $\mu = 120$ mm Hg and $\sigma = 20$ mm Hg. What is the probability that an individual, selected at random, will have a systolic blood pressure between 90 and 150 mm Hg?

Using Equation 2.5, we find that the standard normal deviates associated with 90 and 150 mm Hg are:

$$z_{90} = \frac{90 - 120}{20} = -1.50$$

$$z_{150} = \frac{150 - 120}{20} = +1.50$$

From Table B.1, we find $z = 1.50$ associated with an area of 0.0668. Therefore, the probability of observing a value of 150 mm Hg or greater is 0.0668. Since the standard normal distribution is symmetric with its center at zero, $z = -1.50$ is also associated with an area of 0.0668. That tells us that the probability of observing a systolic blood pressure less than or equal to 90 mm Hg is 0.0668 in this population. Since the Gaussian distribution represents all possible values of systolic blood pressure (i.e., like any probability distribution, it is collectively exhaustive[10]), we can use the "addition rule" to determine the probability of observing a value between 90 and 150:

$$p\,(90 < \Upsilon < 150) = 1.0000 - (0.0668 + 0.0668) = 0.8664$$

Graphically, the area corresponding to the probability of interest is the shaded area in the following figure:

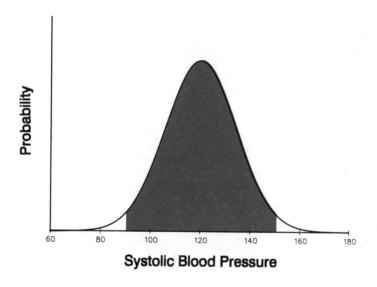

SUMMARY

One of the basic principles of statistics is that research involves observation of a subset of a large group of interest. That subset is called a sample, while the large group is called a population. For all statistical procedures, it is assumed that the sample is representative of the population. This is accomplished by a variety of methods, all of which include a random sampling component.

Populations are made up of data that can be of three types. Continuous data are characterized, in practice, as having a large number of values that must be evenly spaced. Ordinal data have a limited number of values that need not be evenly spaced. Nominal data are different

[10]Recall from Chapter 1 that a collection of events that includes all possible events is said to be collectively exhaustive.

from the other two types in that they cannot be ordered one above another. Like ordinal data, nominal data have a limited number of values.

In statistical procedures, variables are used. Variables represent data. Each continuous or ordinal variable represents a single collection of continuous or ordinal data. Each nominal variable can have only two possible categories. Thus, several nominal variables must be used to represent nominal data such as race that have more than two possible categories.

Samples are used to make statements about the distribution of data in populations. A distribution tells us how frequently various data values occur. The description of a distribution can be graphical, using a bar graph for ordinal or nominal data or a histogram or frequency polygon for continuous data. Graphical representations of populations' distributions are useful for getting an overall feeling for a population's data, but mathematical descriptions of populations' distributions are used for statistical analyses.

To describe a population's distribution mathematically, we assume a particular form for the distribution and then specify the values of the particular distribution's parameters. The Gaussian distribution is the most commonly assumed form for statistical purposes. The parameters of a Gaussian distribution are the mean (a measure of the location of the distribution)

$$\mu = \frac{\Sigma \, \Upsilon_i}{N} \tag{2.1}$$

and the variance (a measure of the dispersion of the distribution).

$$\sigma^2 = \frac{\Sigma \, (\Upsilon_i - \mu)^2}{N} \tag{2.4}$$

The square root of the variance is called the standard deviation.

Other measures of location include the median and the mode. For a Gaussian distribution, the mean, median, and mode are all equal to the same value. Other measures of dispersion include the range and the interquartile range.

Mathematical description of a population's distribution can be used to determine the probability of observing certain intervals of data. This can be done most conveniently by converting the distribution to a standard scale that is described in statistical tables. The standard for a Gaussian distribution is called the standard normal distribution. A data value converted to the standard normal scale is known as a standard normal deviate. Values are converted to standard normal deviates by subtracting the mean and dividing by the standard deviation:

$$z = \frac{\Upsilon_i - \mu}{\sigma} \tag{2.5}$$

The standard normal distribution has a mean of zero and a standard deviation of one. Probabilities of observing data values equal to or greater than (i.e., further from the mean) a standard normal deviate value can be found in a statistical table such as Table B.1. Since the standard normal distribution is symmetric with a mean of zero, the probability of observing values of $-z$ or less is the same as the probability of observing z or greater.   ▤

‖‖ PRACTICE PROBLEMS

2.1 Indicate the type of data contained in each of the following:
   a)   Diagnosis of diabetes
   b)   Time since diagnosis

c) Level of education
d) Place of birth
e) Visual acuity
f) Family income

2.2 Fasting blood glucose levels were measured on a population of 20 patients. The following results were obtained:

Patient	Glucose (mg/dl)
WM	78.8
EL	70.2
RP	68.4
TI	63.3
YJ	95.8
ON	92.1
PB	87.7
AH	82.0
SH	76.6
DV	78.9
FG	65.4
GT	72.7
HR	82.9
JF	92.7
KC	86.3
LD	75.3
CE	73.6
BW	80.7
NS	73.5
MA	76.9

Construct a histogram in which each bar represents an interval of 5 mg/dl, starting with a bar for 60–64 mg/dl.

2.3 Calculate the mean, median, mode, variance, and standard deviation for the data presented in Problem 2.2.

2.4 Assume that we are seeing patients in a population with a mean blood iron level of 95 μg/dl and a variance of 625 $(\mu g/dl)^2$. If the distribution of data in the population is Gaussian, what is the probability that a patient selected at random would have a blood iron level equal to or greater than 145 μg/dl?

CHAPTER 3

Estimation and Inference

As suggested in Chapter 2, we rarely, if ever, observe an entire population. Rather, we examine a sample obtained from a population and attempt to make statements about the population. Those statements are of two general types. The first type includes statements about the magnitude of the numerical values calculated from the sample's observations. These numerical values are used to estimate corresponding values in the population (i.e., the parameters of the population's distribution). In the second type of statement, we use observations from a sample to make inferences (i.e., test hypotheses) about the population which has been sampled. Let us first consider the task of estimation of the population's values.

ESTIMATION OF THE POPULATION'S PARAMETERS

In performing estimation, our goal is to use observations in a sample from a population to make our best guess about the true values of the parameters of that population. To distinguish an actual parameter of the population from an estimate derived from a sample, we call the estimate obtained from a sample a **statistic** rather than a parameter. We further distinguish between statistics and parameters in the symbols used in mathematical descriptions. For the most part, a population's parameters are symbolized with Greek letters, while a sample's statistics are assigned English letters. One exception is the symbol for the number of observations, for which a capital N refers to a population and a lowercase n to a sample. Therefore, the statistic that estimates the population's mean is defined as:

$$\overline{Y} = \frac{\sum Y_i}{n} \tag{3.1}$$

where

$\overline{Y}$ = sample's estimate of the population's mean (pronounced "Y bar")

n = the number of observations in the sample (i.e., the sample's size)

and the sample's estimate of the population's variance is:

$$s^2 = \frac{\sum (Y_i - \overline{Y})^2}{n - 1} \tag{3.2}$$

where s^2 = sample's estimate of the population's variance.

In Equation 3.2, the sum of the deviations of a samples' observations from the sample's mean is divided by $n - 1$ rather than n, as might be anticipated from Equation 2.4. The reason for subtracting one from the number of observations in the sample is that *samples' estimates of a population's variance are biased.* By **bias,** we imply that an estimate is incorrect in a predictable direction (as opposed to "imprecise," which implies likely to be incorrect, but the direction of error is not predictable). In the case of the sample's estimate of the variance of data in the population, if we divided the sum of deviations from the sample's mean by the number of observations in the sample, we expect, on the average, to underestimate the variance of data in the population.

Let us take a moment to understand why sample's estimates of the variance of data in the population would be biased if we did not divide by $n - 1$. The population's data that contribute the most to the variance of data in the population are the extreme values. Looking at Equation 3.2, we can appreciate that the further a data value is from the mean, the greater will be its squared deviation from the mean and the greater will be the estimate of the variance of data in the population. In a sample, those extreme data values are not likely to be included since their occurrence in the population is unusual or rare (see Figure 2.4).[1] Further, the likelihood of an extreme value being included among the sample's observations decreases as the size of the sample decreases.[2] Thus, the numerator of Equation 3.2 is, on the average, too small, and the degree to which it is too small is greatest for small samples.

To solve this problem, we need to increase the numerator of Equation 3.2 or decrease its denominator. Either correction will have the effect of increasing the sample's estimate of the variance of data in the population. In Equation 3.2, we see why statisticians tell us to increase our estimate of the population variance obtained from a sample's observations by subtracting one from the denominator. Subtracting one from the sample's size has the effect of increasing the sample's estimate of the variance of data in the population. We can also see that the increase in the sample's estimate of that variance is greater for small samples than it is for large samples. What is

---

[1] This bias does not affect the sample's estimate of the population's mean since missing extreme data values above and below the population's mean cancels any directional effect. Since deviations from the mean are squared in calculation of the variance, the effects of missing extreme values above and below the mean do not cancel.

[2] The addition rule of probability theory (see Chapter 1) tells us that the more times that we look for something rare, the greater our chance of finding it.

more difficult to understand is why subtracting one from the sample's size is the appropriate correction (i.e., why not subtract two or some other number?). Actually, reducing the sample's size by one is a correction that results from mathematical examination of statistical theory. It is not a perfect correction, but a perfect correction is very difficult and really unnecessary.

We refer to the sample's estimates of the population's mean and the variance of data in Equations 3.1 and 3.2 as **point estimates** because they suggest a single value or "point" for a population's parameter. Since we have made those estimates from a sample that is only one of many (often assumed to be infinite) possible samples from the population, we cannot be certain that our particular sample has resulted in estimates that are correct. If we were able to examine each possible sample (of one particular size) from a population, we would find a collection of estimates for both the population's mean and variance of data that have distributions of their own. These distributions are called **distributions of estimates** or **sampling distributions.**

Since understanding the distribution of estimates from samples is an important concept that will allow us to appreciate why the practice of statistics works the way that it does, let us take some time to make the concept clear. We can think about two different kinds of distributions that relate to a particular population. The first is the kind with which we are most familiar: that is the population's distribution of *data*. If that population's distribution of data is a Gaussian distribution, then we can describe it mathematically by using two parameters: its mean and its variance. Now, we are ready to think about a second type of distribution related to that same population. The second type is the distribution of the estimates of a population's parameter that results from taking all possible samples of a particular size. Thus, we can think about two kinds of distributions in a population: a distribution of data and distributions of samples' estimates of the parameters describing the distribution of data.

A distribution of estimates of a population's paramater from all possible samples of a certain size can be described mathematically by its own set of parameters.[3] The distribution of estimates from samples that is used most often in health research statistics is the distribution of samples' means. Because it is an important concept, let us take a detailed look at the distribution of samples' means and the parameters that describe mathematically that distribution of samples' means.

You might have been wondering why statisticians are so enamored with the Gaussian distribution and the mean as the parameter of primary interest. The reason is the way in which means from samples are distributed. *Regardless of how data in a population are distributed, means calculated from samples' observations tend to have a Gaussian distribution.* Further, that tendency increases as the number of observations in each of the samples increases (Figure 3.1). This principle, known as the **central limit theorem,** allows us to apply statistical procedures that assume a Gaussian distribution

[3]Remember that the term "parameter" refers to numerical values that describe a population's distribution. We now know that there are two types of distributions that relate to a particular population: one is the distribution of data and the other is the distribution of estimates from samples of a particular size. Thus, we use "parameter" to refer to the numerical values that describe either of those distributions in the population.

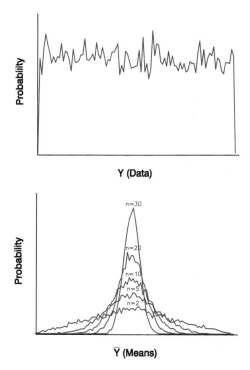

Y (Data)

Ȳ (Means)

FIGURE 3.1 Demonstration of how distributions of samples' means tend to have a Gaussian distribution even though the data from which the samples were drawn do not have a Gaussian distribution. The first graph (top) shows a distribution of data in a population that does not have a Gaussian distribution. As the size of each of the samples taken from that population increases, the distributions of the samples' estimates of the mean become more and more similar to a Gaussian distribution (graph on the bottom). This is an illustration of the central limit theorem.

to a sample's mean with the assurance that the assumption of a Gaussian distribution has been satisfied (at least when the size of a sample is sufficient).

Since means from all possible samples of a given size tend to have a Gaussian distribution, the distribution of means obtained from all possible samples of a given size can be specified by its own mean and variance (or standard deviation). The mean of that distribution (the "mean of means") is exactly equal to the mean of the distribution of data in the population:

$$\mu_{\bar{Y}} = \frac{\sum \bar{Y}_i}{N_s} = \frac{\sum Y_i}{N} = \mu \tag{3.3}$$

where

$\mu_{\bar{Y}}$ = mean of all possible samples' means

N_s = number of all possible samples of given size

N = number of individuals (data elements) in the population

Now, let us think about the dispersion of the distribution of means estimated from all possible samples of a given size. First, we might anticipate that the dispersion among the samples' means is influenced by the dispersion in the population's data from which samples are drawn. In fact, there is a direct relationship between the dispersion of the population's data and the dispersion of means from all possible samples. That is to say, as the dispersion in the population's data increases, so does the dispersion of means from all possible samples. Even so, the distribution of means from all possible samples is somewhat less dispersed than the distribution of the population's data. This lesser dispersion occurs because, for samples with sizes greater than one, extreme data contributing to the calculation of each sample's mean are "buffered" by less extreme data. In other words, if a sample contains an observation that is extremely large relative to the population's mean, chances are that the remaining data in the sample will not be so extreme. Further, this buffering effect will increase as the size of the sample increases. The more observations that we make in each sample, the greater the chance that extreme observations will be combined not only with less extreme observations, but also with observations that are similarly extreme in an opposite direction.

Thus, the dispersion of the distribution of means from all possible samples of a given size follows two principles: It increases as the dispersion of the distribution of data in the population increases, and it decreases as the size of each of the samples increases. The simplest way to express those influences mathematically is to divide the variance of data in the population by the sample's size (Equation 3.4).

$$\sigma_{\overline{Y}}^2 = \frac{\sigma^2}{n} \tag{3.4}$$

where
$\sigma_{\overline{Y}}^2$ = variance of distribution of means
σ^2 = variance of the data
n = number of observations in the sample

Dividing the variance of the population's data by the number of observations in the sample produces the variance of the distribution of means from all possible samples of that particular size. The variance of the distribution of means estimated from samples is exactly analogous to the variance of the distribution of data in the population. Figure 3.2 shows the relationship between those distributions.

The square root of the variance of the distribution of samples' means is the standard deviation of that distribution, but it is most often called the **standard error** (SE) to help us distinguish it from the standard deviation of the distribution of data.[4] The term "standard error" is also used more generally in statistics to refer to the standard deviation of the distribution of estimates of any parameter derived from all possible samples of a given size.

---

[4]Let us examine the standard error further by considering distributions of samples of extreme sizes. The smallest sample we can imagine is a sample containing only a single observation. We can see that, if we allow n to be equal to one in Equation 3.4, the variance of the distribution of samples' means is equal to the variance of the population's distribution of data. This is a sensible result, for a sample of size one is, in fact, no different from a single datum. At the other extreme, let us consider a sample's size that is equal to the population's size. In this case, Equation 3.4 equals zero. This also makes sense, for the mean of samples that include all members of the population will always be equal to the population's mean (and, thus, has no variance).

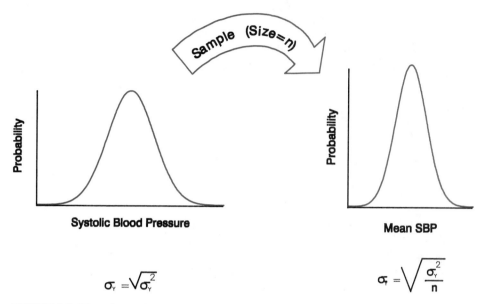

FIGURE 3.2 The relationship between the distribution of data in the population and the distribution of estimates of the mean obtained from all possible samples of a given size. The two distributions' means are equal to the same value, but the dispersion of the distribution of estimates of the mean obtained from samples is less than the dispersion of the distribution of data. Appearing below each distribution is the mathematical formula for the standard deviation of that distribution.

The observations in the single sample that we actually obtain is used to estimate the values of the parameters of *both types of distributions* representing the population. Table 3.1 summarizes how a sample's observations are used to derive those estimates of the population's parameters.

In practice, we do not observe the entire distribution of data values in the population, nor do we observe the entire distribution of estimates from all possible samples. In fact, we generally observe only a single sample from which we must estimate the population's parameters. Our best guess or estimate of the value of the population's mean is the mean of the single sample that we observe. This estimate has a greater probability of being equal to the population's mean than does any other value. How sure can we be that the sample's mean is exactly equal to the population's mean? To answer that question, let us recall our discussion about the probability of observing any particular value from a distribution of continuous data. That probability was virtually equal to zero. Since the samples' means also have a continuous distribution, we must conclude that the probability of observing a particular sample's mean exactly equal to the population's mean is virtually zero (although it is our best estimate!).

It is possible for us to calculate an estimate of the population's mean from our sample that has a probability considerably greater than zero, but to do this, we must

TABLE 3.1 Comparison of a population's parameters and a sample's estimates of those parameters. In each of the tables, the left-hand column shows how we (theoretically) would calculate the population's parameters if we could observe the entire population. The right-hand column shows how we calculate estimates of those parameters from a sample's observations. The first table lists parameters (and their estimates) of the distribution of data. The second table lists parameters (and their estimates) of the distribution of means estimated from all possible samples of a given size.

Distribution of Data

Population's Parameters	Sample's Estimates
Mean of Data	Sample's Mean
$$\mu = \frac{\Sigma Y_i}{N}$$	$$\overline{Y} = \frac{\Sigma Y_i}{n}$$
Variance of Data	Sample's Variance
$$\sigma^2 = \frac{\Sigma\,(Y_i - \mu)^2}{N}$$	$$s^2 = \frac{\Sigma\,(Y_i - \overline{Y})^2}{n - 1}$$
Standard Deviation	Sample's Standard Deviation
$$\sigma = \sqrt{\sigma^2} = \sqrt{\frac{\Sigma\,(Y_i - \mu)^2}{N}}$$	$$s = \sqrt{s^2} = \sqrt{\frac{\Sigma\,(Y_i - \overline{Y})^2}{n - 1}}$$

Distribution of Samples' Means

Population's Parameters	Sample's Estimates
Mean of Means	Sample's Mean
$$\mu_{\overline{Y}} = \frac{\Sigma\,\overline{Y}_i}{N_s} = \frac{\Sigma\,Y_i}{N}$$	$$\overline{Y} = \frac{\Sigma\,Y_i}{n}$$
Variance of Means	Sample's Variance of Means
$$\sigma_{\overline{Y}}^2 = \frac{\sigma^2}{n} = \frac{\dfrac{\Sigma(Y_i - \mu)^2}{N}}{n}$$	$$s_{\overline{Y}}^2 = \frac{s^2}{n} = \frac{\dfrac{\Sigma\,(Y_i - \overline{Y})^2}{n - 1}}{n}$$
Standard Error	Sample's Standard Error
$$\sigma_{\overline{Y}} = SE = \sqrt{\sigma_{\overline{Y}}^2} = \sqrt{\frac{\dfrac{\Sigma\,(Y_i - \mu)^2}{N}}{n}}$$	$$s_{\overline{Y}} = SE = \sqrt{s_{\overline{Y}}^2} = \sqrt{\frac{\dfrac{\Sigma\,(Y_i - \overline{Y})^2}{n - 1}}{n}}$$

use an interval of estimates rather than a single estimate.[5] It might be desirable, therefore, to calculate an interval of values with a defined probability of containing the population's mean rather than a point estimate. Such an interval of values is called an **interval estimate** or a **confidence interval.** The most commonly used interval estimate is a 95% confidence interval. With that estimate, we say that we are 95% "confident" that the mean (or other numerical value being estimated) of the distribution of data in the population from which we have obtained our sample is included in the interval.

To understand how an interval estimate is constructed, let us take another look at the distribution of all possible samples' means. As we did with a Gaussian distribution of data, we can convert the Gaussian distribution of samples' means to a standard normal distribution (Equation 3.5). As we discussed in Chapter 2, working with the standard normal distribution makes our task of considering probabilities much easier since we do not have to worry about integrating formulas for Gaussian distributions (Table B.1 does that for a standard normal distribution).

$$z = \frac{\overline{Y} - \mu_{\overline{Y}}}{\text{SE}} \tag{3.5}$$

where
 SE = standard error = $\sqrt{\sigma^2/n}$
 $\overline{Y}$ = a particular sample's mean
 $\mu_{\overline{Y}}$ = the mean of all possible samples' means

Thus, Equation 3.5 is an example of conversion of a single mean from the distribution of estimates of the mean from all possible samples (of a given size) to a standard scale. This equation is very similar to Equation 2.5, which was used to convert a single data value from the distribution of data to a standard scale. The difference between these two equations is in the parameters we use to make the conversion. Equation 2.5 converted a single data value to a standard normal deviate by subtracting the mean of the distribution of data and dividing by the standard deviation of the distribution of data. Equation 3.5 converts a single sample's estimate of the mean to a standard normal deviate by subtracting the mean of the distribution of estimates of the mean (i.e., the mean of means) and dividing by the standard deviation of the distribution of estimates of the mean (i.e., the standard error). Since the mean of the distribution of data and the mean of means are numerically equal to each other, the real difference between Equations 2.5 and 3.5 is in the standard deviations used in the conversion to the standard normal scale.

Another distinction between Equations 2.5 and 3.5 is in the numbers that are converted to a standard scale (i.e., a datum versus an estimate of the mean). In taking the influence of chance into account, statistical methods most often address how chance influences a particular sample's estimate rather than a single data value.

---

[5]Recall from our discussion of continuous distributions (Chapter 2) that nonzero probabilities can be determined by integrating intervals of values. This is done for us in Table B.1 for the standard normal distribution.

Therefore, most of the statistical methods we will encounter in health research address the distribution of estimates from all possible samples and involve conversion of a sample's estimate to a standard scale using a method similar to the one shown in Equation 3.5.

Now that we understand how a particular sample's mean can be converted to a standard normal deviate, let us consider how we can use Table B.1 to calculate intervals around the population's mean within which we can expect the sample's means to occur. Suppose we wish to define an interval containing 95% of all possible samples' means. In other words, we want to determine the interval within which lie 95% of all possible estimates of the mean once they have been converted to the standard normal scale. This is indicated by the shaded area in Figure 3.3.

To find the interval indicated in Figure 3.3, we begin by finding the standard normal deviate (from Table B.1) that corresponds to one-half the complement of 0.95. Recall from Chapter 1 that the complement of a probability is equal to one minus that probability. We use the complement of 0.95 because Table B.1 provides us with probabilities of obtaining a standard normal deviate *equal to or more extreme than* the one observed. In other words, Table B.1 gives us the probability of a **tail** of the standard normal distribution (this probability is called α). We find one-half the complement ($\alpha/2$) rather than the entire complement because we want to have an interval that is symmetric around the population's mean. Therefore, we must divide the complement evenly between the two tails of the distribution.

The complement of 0.95 is 0.05. One-half of 0.05 is equal to 0.025. From Table B.1, we find that the standard normal deviate corresponding to a probability of 0.025 is 1.96. That is to say, we expect to find samples' means that, on the standard normal scale, are in the interval -1.96 to $+1.96$ in 95% of samples from our population.

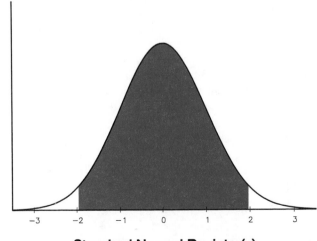

FIGURE 3.3 Portion of the standard normal distribution corresponding to 95% of the area of that distribution symmetric about the mean. The shaded area includes 95% of all possible values of the standard normal deviate.

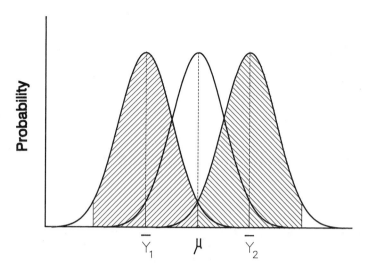

FIGURE 3.4 Relationship between a 95% interval around the population's mean (μ) and 95% intervals around samples' means ($\overline{Y}_1$ and $\overline{Y}_2$). The distribution in the center is the (theoretical) distribution of estimates of the mean from all possible samples of a given size. The shaded areas of the other two distributions indicate 95% confidence intervals calculated from two possible samples' means at the extremes of the 95% interval around the population's mean. Notice that the intervals around the two possible samples' means have, as one of their limits, the population's mean.

Unfortunately, this is not quite what we want to do. We have defined an interval around the population's mean within which 95% of the samples' means will occur. In practice, we do not know the value of the population's mean, but rather, we know the value of a sample's mean from which we would like to estimate the population's mean. Fortunately, we can perform the same sort of procedure on a sample's mean that we did on the population's mean (specifying an interval equal to the sample's mean converted to a standard normal deviate ± 1.96). Then we can see that 95% of all possible samples' means (namely, those in the shaded portion of Figure 3.3) will have the population's mean included in their interval. This is demonstrated in Figure 3.4.

We can simplify calculation of an interval estimate for the population's mean by solving Equation 3.5 for μ:

$$\mu = \overline{Y} + (z_\alpha \cdot \text{SE}) \qquad (3.6)$$

where z_α = standard normal deviate corresponding to an area of α in the standard normal distribution (Table B.1).

Equation 3.6 can be used to calculate what is known as a **one-tailed confidence interval.** This is different from the interval we just examined. Initially we were assuming that a sample's mean could be greater or less than the population's mean. In a one-tailed confidence interval, we specify on which side of the population's mean the sample's mean occurs. Thus, in a one-tailed confidence interval, the entire complement of the degree of confidence with which we would like to estimate the population's mean is contained in one, rather than two, tail of the standard normal distribution. That probability will be in the upper tail if a positive value of z is used and in the lower tail if a negative value of z is used. Thus, we use the standard normal distribution to determine only one limit of a one-tailed confidence interval. The other limit is assumed to be equal to infinity (or negative infinity).

More often, we are interested in estimating an interval for the population's mean without assuming which direction the sample's mean occurs relative to the population's mean (as in Figure 3.4). In that case, we want to calculate a **two-tailed confidence interval.** For a two-tailed confidence interval, we divide the complement of our $(1 - \alpha)\%$ confidence interval between both tails of that distribution. To calculate a two-tailed confidence interval, we determine the lower limit by subtracting the product of the standard normal deviate (corresponding to an area of $\alpha/2$) times the standard error from the sample's mean. The upper limit is found by adding that product to the sample's mean.

$$\mu = \overline{Y} \pm (z_{\alpha/2} \cdot SE) \tag{3.7}$$

where $z_{\alpha/2}$ = standard normal deviate corresponding to an area of $\alpha/2$ in the standard normal distribution (Table B.1).

Example 3.1   Suppose that we are interested in estimating the mean diastolic blood pressure in a population of patients diagnosed as hypertensive. We randomly select 11 patients, for whom we record diastolic blood pressure. Given the following results, determine point and interval (99%, two-tailed) estimates for that population's mean.

Patient	Diastolic BP
HR	96
FW	114
RG	125
IH	105
VW	97
HL	96
ZH	131
CW	117
TD	107
ER	111
EM	123

First, we calculate the sample's mean as our point estimate for the population's mean (from Equation 3.1):

$$\overline{Y} = \frac{\sum Y_i}{n} = \frac{96 + 114 + \cdots + 123}{11} = \frac{1{,}222}{11} = 111.1 \text{ mm Hg}$$

Next, we determine the squared deviation of each observation from that sample's mean:

Patient	Υ_i	$\Upsilon_i - \overline{\Upsilon}$	$(\Upsilon_i - \overline{\Upsilon})^2$
HR	96	−15.1	227.74
FW	114	2.9	8.46
RG	125	13.9	193.46
IH	105	−6.1	37.10
VW	97	−14.1	198.55
HL	96	−15.1	227.74
ZH	131	19.9	396.37
CW	117	5.9	34.92
TD	107	−4.1	16.74
ER	111	−0.1	0.01
EM	123	11.9	141.83
Total	1,222	0.0	1,482.91

Then, we calculate from the sample's observations our estimate of the variance of data in the population (using Equation 3.2):

$$s^2 = \frac{\sum (\Upsilon_i - \overline{\Upsilon})^2}{n - 1} = \frac{1,482.91}{11 - 1} = 148.291 \text{ mm Hg}^2$$

That estimate of the variance of data in the population is then used to calculate the standard deviation of the distribution of all possible samples' means (i.e., the standard error):

$$SE = \sqrt{s^2/n} = \sqrt{148.291/11} = \sqrt{13.481} = 3.67 \text{ mm Hg}$$

Next, we consult Table B.1 to determine the standard normal deviate that corresponds to an area of 0.01 (0.005 in each "tail"). In doing that, we find that an area of 0.0051 corresponds to a z-value of 2.57 and an area of 0.0049 corresponds to a z-value of 2.58. We will "split the difference" and use 2.575.[6] Now, we can use Equation 3.7 to determine a two-tailed, 99% confidence interval for the population's mean:

$$\mu = \overline{\Upsilon} \pm (z_{0.005} \cdot SE) = 111.1 \pm (2.575 \cdot 3.67) = 101.6, 120.5 \text{ mm Hg}$$

INFERENCE

In addition to estimating a population's parameters, it is often of interest to draw and test inferences (hypotheses) about the population's parameters, based on observations

[6] This procedure is known as linear interpolation. It is appropriate for finding values not included in most statistical tables.

made in a sample. This process is called **statistical inference** (also called statistical significance testing or statistical hypothesis testing). In statistical inference, we define two states for the parameter of interest (e.g., the population's mean). The first is known as the **null state.** The null state is described by the **null hypothesis** (H_0). In the null hypothesis, the population's parameter is hypothesized to be equal to a *specific* value. Most often, that specific value reflects a hypothesized state of nature in which all things are unrelated.[7] For example, a null hypothesis applicable to a clinical study of an antihypertensive agent might be that the mean of the difference in diastolic blood pressure with and without that agent is equal to zero (i.e., diastolic blood pressure is unrelated to treatment).

The second state, known as the **alternative state,** is described by the **alternative hypothesis**[8] (H_A). The alternative hypothesis is often much more general than the null hypothesis in that it defines an *interval* of possible values for the parameter. There are two types of alternative hypotheses. The more common is the **two-tailed alternative hypothesis** in which all possible values for the parameter of interest, excluding the null state, are included. In the example of the antihypertensive agent described above, a two-tailed alternative hypothesis would be that the mean of differences in diastolic blood pressure is not equal to zero. Less often, we consider a **one-tailed alternative hypothesis,** in which the parameter is assumed to deviate from the null state in only one direction. For example, if we were willing to assume that it is impossible for the antihypertensive agent to cause an increase in diastolic blood pressure, we might consider an alternative state in which the mean of differences in that measurement could only reflect lower blood pressures during treatment. The decision as to which sort of alternative hypothesis is applicable must be made *without* knowledge of the particular sample's observations. This lack of knowledge is assured if the alternative hypothesis is stated formally prior to data collection.

Of the two hypotheses, the null hypothesis is the more important to us in the process of statistical inference. It is the null hypothesis that is actually tested. This procedure requires that we assume at the beginning that the null hypothesis is correct. Then we determine the probability of obtaining the sample we actually have observed if that assumption is true. In the example of an antihypertensive agent, we would first imagine that the mean of differences in diastolic blood pressure in the population is equal to zero. Then we would ask ourselves how likely it would be to obtain a sample with a mean of differences in diastolic blood pressure as large as or larger than the one observed if the mean of those differences in the population is equal to zero.

If, under the assumption that the null hypothesis is true, the probability of obtaining a sample like the one actually observed is small, we reject the assumption

[7]Statisticians refer to this state of nature in which all things are unrelated as the state of **parsimony.** The most parsimonious condition for a population's parameter is one in which that parameter is equal to the same value regardless of any other factors.

[8]The alternative hypothesis is sometimes referred to as the "study hypothesis" since it usually reflects what the researcher believes is true. Here, we will use "alternative hypothesis" since it is the term used by statisticians and more accurately identifies the role of this hypothesis in statistical inference. As we will see, the alternative hypothesis is chosen by default if we believe that the null hypothesis is not true.

that the null hypothesis is true. In that case, we reject the null hypothesis and conclude by elimination that the alternative hypothesis is true.[9]

Alternatively, if the probability of getting the sample we have observed is not small (assuming that the null hypothesis is true), then we fail to reject the assumption that the null hypothesis is true. We do not, however, conclude that the null is, indeed, true. This distinction between failing to reject and accepting the null hypothesis is an important, but perhaps difficult to appreciate, distinction. It has, however, a parallel in the process of disease screening. Under the conditions usually encountered in health research, statistical inference is like looking for occult blood in a single stool sample. If blood is found, then the assumption that the patient does not have colon cancer (parallel to the null hypothesis) is in doubt. We would consider it to be a rare (although not impossible) occurrence to find blood in the stool of a healthy patient and we would reject the idea that the patient tested is healthy (parallel to rejecting the null hypothesis). If, on the other hand, no blood is found in the stool, we would not be so quick to accept the assumption that the patient does not have colon cancer (parallel to accepting the null hypothesis). It is not unusual for a single stool sample to be free of occult blood, even from a patient with colon cancer.

So, we reject the null hypothesis when the probability of obtaining our sample would be small if the null hypothesis were true, and we fail to reject the null hypothesis if that probability is not small. Now, we must ask ourselves: "How small is small?" How small the probability of obtaining the observed data needs to be before we reject the null hypothesis depends on how willing we are to make a mistake by rejecting a null hypothesis that truly reflects the population that was sampled. This type of mistake is called a **Type I error.** In our example of occult blood in a stool sample, a Type I error would be analogous to concluding that the patient has colon cancer when, in fact, he does not. In statistical inference, the probability of making a Type I error is called α (Equation 3.8). If, assuming the null hypothesis is true, the probability of getting the sample we have observed is less than α, then we reject the idea that the null hypothesis is true.

$$p \, (\text{committing Type I error}) = \alpha = p \, (\text{reject } H_0 | H_0 \text{ true}) \qquad (3.8)$$

The probability of committing a Type I error (α) is set by the researcher and is traditionally chosen to be 0.05.[10] That is to say, statistical inference is usually performed with a 5% chance of rejecting a true null hypothesis. An investigator is free to choose an α equal to some value other than 0.05, but that choice should be justified.

Actually, there are two types of errors that can be made during the process of statistical inference. The first type is the Type I error we have just discussed. The second type is called a **Type II error.** The probability of making a Type II error is called β (Equation 3.9). The probability of the complement of making a Type II error

---

[9]When the null hypothesis is rejected, the result is commonly referred to as being "statistically significant."

[10]This choice of 0.05 is not entirely arbitrary. Rather, choosing $\alpha = 0.05$ provides a good balance between Type I and Type II error rates for the most usual types of samples encountered in health research.

$(1 - \beta)$ is known as the **power** of a statistical procedure. A Type II error results when the null hypothesis is not rejected when, in fact, it is not a true reflection of the population that was sampled. Statistical power is the ability of a procedure to avoid a Type II error or, in other words, to reject a null hypothesis that is not true. In the example of occult blood in a stool sample, a Type II error is parallel to concluding that the patient does not have colon cancer when, in fact, he does. The power of a statistical procedure would, then, be similar to the ability to detect a case of colon cancer:

$$p\,(\text{committing Type II error}) = \beta = p\,(\text{accept } H_0 | H_0 \text{ false})$$
$$= p\,(\text{accept } H_0 | H_A \text{ true})$$

(3.9)

If we imagine a distribution with a parameter equal to the value hypothesized by the null hypothesis (called the **null distribution**), we can determine an interval of values for estimates obtained from samples for which we will reject the null hypothesis. This interval of values is called the **rejection region** since observation of a sample's estimate within that interval results in rejection of the null hypothesis. If we are unable to specify in what direction the sample's estimate will deviate from the value specified in the null hypothesis (i.e., we have a two-tailed alternative hypothesis), the rejection region will be equally divided between the two tails of the null distribution. Each tail represents a probability of $\alpha/2$ (Figure 3.5).

FIGURE 3.5 The Type I error probability (α) split between the two tails of the null distribution for estimation of the mean, as is done when a two-tailed alternative hypothesis is considered. The rejection region (shaded) is made up of values in both tails and accounts for α% of all possible values ($\alpha/2$% in each tail).

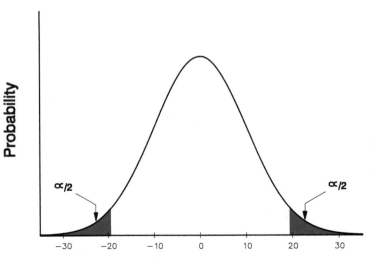

Mean Difference in Diastolic Blood Pressure

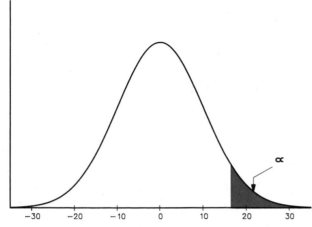

Mean Difference in Diastolic Blood Pressure

FIGURE 3.6 The Type I error probability (α) in one tail of the null distribution for estimates of the mean, as is done when a one-tailed alternative hypothesis is considered. The rejection region (shaded) is made up of values in only one tail.

If samples' estimates are assumed to be able to deviate in only one direction from the null state (i.e., a one-tailed alternative hypothesis), then the entire rejection region (representing a probability of α) is in one tail of the null distribution (Figure 3.6).

To examine the Type II error, we would have to imagine a population with a parameter equal to a value specified by the alternative hypothesis. This is more difficult than imagining a population described by the null hypothesis. The reason for this difficulty is that the alternative hypothesis does not specify a single value for a population's parameter. Rather, the alternative hypothesis suggests a wide interval of possible values.

Now we can see why statistical inference tests only the null hypothesis. This is because the null hypothesis mathematically describes the only well-defined value in the statistical inference process. Since the alternative hypothesis describes a vaguely defined interval of values, we cannot test its validity with a known probability of making an error as we can for the null hypothesis. We cannot, therefore, reject the alternative hypothesis. Rather, we can accept, by elimination, the alternative hypothesis as true only if we are willing to reject the correctness of the null hypothesis. Thus, in statistical inference, we are stuck with one of two possible conclusions. We can reject the null hypothesis (and accept, by elimination, the alternative hypothesis) if our sample's observations would be sufficiently rare should the null hypothesis be true. Alternatively, we can fail to reject (i.e., fail to draw a conclusion about) the null hypothesis if our sample's observations would not be sufficiently rare if the null hypothesis were true. Without a well-defined alternative state, we cannot calculate the probability of making a mistake if we were to reject the alternative hypothesis and accept the null hypothesis as being true. Therefore, we avoid drawing that conclusion. A test of statistical inference that fails to reject the null hypothesis should be considered to be inconclusive.

Even though we cannot know the exact value of β for a particular test of inference, we do know the things that affect that probability.[11] Our chance of making a Type II error will always increase when the variance of the relevant distribution increases. Since the distribution that we use in statistical inference is the distribution of estimates from all possible samples, we should keep the variance of the distribution of those estimates small to minimize β. If we reexamine Equation 3.4, we can see that there are two ways to decrease the variance of the distribution of estimates of the mean. One way is by decreasing the variance of the distribution of data. This is often not under our control. Another way to decrease the variance of the distribution of estimates of the mean, however, is to increase the size of the samples (i.e., the number of observations in each sample). This is under our control as we design studies. Also, we will see in subsequent sections of *Statistical First Aid* that another way to influence β to some degree is by our choice of which statistical procedure we use to analyze our sample's observations.

In spite of this limitation of statistical inference, tests of inference are very commonly used in health research. Thus, we should understand how they work. To conduct a test of inference, it is necessary to calculate the probability of obtaining the estimate calculated from the sample's observations (or a more extreme estimate), assuming that the null hypothesis is true. As we did in interval estimation, we use the standard normal distribution to simplify that calculation. In conversion of a sample's mean to the standard normal scale, we use the value of the mean specified in the null hypothesis as the population's mean. Then Equation 3.5 becomes:

$$z = \frac{\overline{Y} - \mu_0}{\text{SE}}$$
(3.10)

where

μ_0 = population's mean in the null state
$\overline{Y}$ = observed sample's mean
SE = standard error

Example 3.2   Consider a clinical study of an antihypertensive agent. Suppose in this study that we randomly select 11 hypertensive patients and randomize each patient to receive either a placebo followed by the antihypertensive agent or the antihypertensive agent followed by a placebo, each for a specified period of time. At the end of each treatment period, we measure diastolic blood pressure. Subtracting each patient's pressure on the antihypertensive agent

---

[11]If we are willing to make certain guesses about the actual values of parameters in the population, we can calculate β. This principle is employed in estimation of a sample size that will be required in a planned study. The details of estimation of a required sample's size will not be discussed in *Statistical First Aid*.

from the pressure on placebo, we make the following observations:

Patient	Difference
HR	7
FW	14
RG	27
IH	5
VW	2
HL	1
ZH	31
CW	19
TD	9
ER	9
EM	21

Test the null hypothesis that the population from which this sample was derived has a mean of differences in diastolic blood pressure equal to zero.

First, we must determine whether our alternative hypothesis should be one- or two-tailed and decide what risk of a Type I error we are willing to endure. Those decisions must be made before collecting the sample. Let us assume that we do not have sufficient reason to believe that it would be impossible to observe an increase in diastolic blood pressure under treatment. Therefore, we shall consider a two-tailed alternative hypothesis. Further, let us adopt the usual convention of allowing a 5% chance of committing a Type I error. From Table B.1, we find that the rejection region corresponding to 0.025 in each tail includes values of $z = \pm 1.96$ or beyond. In other words, if our sample's mean, converted to a standard normal deviate, is equal to or greater than $+1.96$ or equal to or less than -1.96, we will reject the null hypothesis. Now, we are ready to examine our observations.

From our sample, the estimate of the population's mean is:

$$\overline{Y} = \frac{\sum Y_i}{n} = \frac{7 + 14 + \cdots + 21}{11} = \frac{145}{11} = 13.2 \text{ mm Hg}$$

The sample's estimate of the population's variance of the distribution of data is:

$$s^2 = \frac{\sum (Y_i - \overline{Y})^2}{n-1} = \frac{-6.2^2 + 0.8^2 + \cdots + 7.8^2}{11 - 1} = \frac{1017.636}{10} = 101.764 \text{ mm Hg}^2$$

Next, from the sample's estimate of the variance of data in the population and the sample's size, we determine the standard error:

$$SE = \sqrt{\frac{s^2}{n}} = \sqrt{\frac{101.764}{11}} = \sqrt{9.25} = 3.04 \text{ mm Hg}$$

Finally, we convert our sample's estimate of the population's mean to the standard normal scale.

To do this, we assume that the null hypothesis, which says that the mean of the differences is equal to zero in the population, is true.

$$z = \frac{\overline{Y} - \mu_0}{SE} = \frac{13.2 - 0}{3.04} = 4.33$$

Since 4.33 is more extreme than 1.96, we reject the null hypothesis, accepting, by elimination, the alternative hypothesis which says that the antihypertensive agent changes the diastolic blood pressure.

P-VALUES

Thus far, we have considered inference only as a method to make a dichotomous (either/or) decision about the population from which a sample was derived. That decision is whether to reject or not to reject the null hypothesis. It is also common, however, to see the **P-value** presented in the health research literature as a quantitative indication of how comfortable we are in making that dichotomous decision. Therefore, to understand how to interpret the results of statistical inference, we must understand how to determine and use P-values.

A P-value is a probability that is very closely related to α. Recall that α is the probability of making a Type I error (rejecting a true null hypothesis). The value of α is selected by the researcher before the sample's data are examined. The P-value, however, is determined after analysis of the sample's data. Basically, the P-value is the smallest value of α that could have been selected by the researcher while still rejecting the null hypothesis based on the sample observed. Thus, the P-value is the actual probability of obtaining the observed sample or a more extreme sample if the null hypothesis makes a true statement about the population that was sampled.

Let us first take a moment to see how P-values are determined, and then we will examine their interpretation more closely. There are two basic methods for calculating P-values. To get "exact" P-values, we must use calculus and the mathematical formula for the appropriate statistical distribution. Most statistical programs for computers will do this for us. Alternatively, we can use statistical tables to determine "approximate" P-values. Those P-values are expressed as intervals within which the exact P-value lies. To see how this is done, take a look at Example 3.3.

Example 3.3 In Example 3.2 we tested the null hypothesis that the population's mean of differences in diastolic blood pressure between a placebo and an antihypertensive agent is equal to zero. The value of α for that test was set at 0.05. In a sample of 11 patients, a mean of those differences equal to 13.2 mm Hg was observed. Converted to the standard normal scale, that mean of the differences is equal to 4.33. Since an α of 0.05 corresponds to a standard normal deviate of 1.96, and 4.33 is greater than 1.96, we rejected the null hypothesis. Now, let us determine a P-value for this hypothesis test.

To find an approximate P-value, we consult Table B.1. The largest standard normal deviate in that table is 3.89, associated with a one-tailed probability of 0.0001. Since 4.33 is larger than

3.89, we know that 4.33 corresponds to a one-tailed probability less than 0.0001. We cannot tell from the table how much less, so we say that the two-tailed P-value is less than 2×0.0001 or 0.0002 ($P < 0.0002$). That implies that we could have done this test of inference with an α equal to some value less than 0.0002 and still have rejected the null hypothesis.

To find an exact P-value, we would need to perform some calculus or use a computer program. If we did that, we would find a two-tailed probability of approximately 0.00002 corresponding to a standard normal deviate of 4.33. That implies that we could have performed this test of inference with an α equal to 0.00002 and been just barely able to reject the null hypothesis.

It is important for us to realize that a P-value is *not* the probability that the null hypothesis is true. This is a common error in interpreting the results of statistical analysis. The P-value is a conditional probability. Specifically, it is the probability that we could have obtained a sample's estimate as far or further from the population's parameter specified in the null hypothesis if the null hypothesis were true. If that sounds complicated to you, you are right: the actual quantitative value of a P-value is complicated to interpret. Therefore, it is best that we restrict our use of P-values in statistical inference to making a decision about the validity of the null hypothesis and not attempt to use them to express the degree to which the null hypothesis is likely to be correct or incorrect. To make such dichotomous decisions is rather straightforward. To use P-values in making dichotomous decisions about the null hypothesis, we can compare the P-value to our chosen α. If the P-value is equal to or less than the chosen α, we reject the null hypothesis and accept, by elimination, the alternative hypothesis.

RELATIONSHIP BETWEEN ESTIMATION AND INFERENCE

In recent years, it has been suggested that health researchers should be interested only in estimation and leave inference to those involved in making decisions about health care. Although there has been an increase in the use of estimation in the health literature, inference remains the more frequent approach to research data. Therefore, whether you are a health researcher or practitioner interested in understanding relationships between exposure and outcome or a clinician making decisions about patient care, it is important that you be able to make translations between estimation and inference.

Actually, the relationship between estimation and inference is a very close one. Recall that we obtained the formula for calculation of a confidence interval by a simple algebraic rearrangement of the formula for calculating a standard normal deviate (see Equation 3.6). This implies that translations between estimation and inference should be correspondingly simple.

The simpler translation is from estimation to inference because inference contains much less information than does estimation (inference involves only a dichotomous decision about the null hypothesis). If we have a confidence interval and would like to test a particular null hypothesis, we need only determine whether or not the value of the parameter stated in the null hypothesis (i.e., the null value) is included in the confidence interval. If it is, we do not reject that null hypothesis. If the null value is outside the confidence interval, we reject the null hypothesis.[12] There are two restrictions to this process, however. First, the α of the null hypothesis test must be the same as the α used in constructing the confidence interval. For example, only a 95% confidence interval can be used for inference with a 5% chance of making a Type I error. Second, the type of alternative hypothesis being considered in inference is determined by the number of "tails" in the confidence interval. Only a two-tailed confidence interval can be used to consider a two-tailed alternative hypothesis.

Example 3.4 In Example 3.1, we found the 99% two-tailed confidence interval for the mean diastolic blood pressure to be from 101.6 to 120.5 mm Hg. Test the null hypothesis that the mean diastolic blood pressure in the population from which this sample was taken is actually equal to 110 mm Hg.

There are two ways to approach this problem. One way would be to use the data in Example 3.1 to calculate a standard normal deviate and then compare that standard normal deviate to values in Table B.1. Now that we know the relationship between confidence intervals and tests of inference, however, we can take an easier approach. In this approach, we simply notice that the null value (110 mm Hg) is contained within the interval from 101.6 to 120.5. Thus, we are unable to reject the null hypothesis. It is important to notice that our inference allowed only a 1% chance of making a Type I error since we used a 99% confidence interval.

To make a conversion from a test of inference to an interval estimate, we need to have enough information at our disposal to solve either Equation 3.6 (one-tailed confidence interval) or Equation 3.7 (two-tailed confidence interval). Two things are needed: the point estimate and the **test statistic** (e.g., the z-value that represents the observed mean of differences) calculated in the test of inference. Then, we can make a conversion from a test of inference to an interval estimate by calculating a two-tailed **test-based confidence interval** for the mean as follows:

$$\mu = \overline{Y} \cdot \left(1 \pm \frac{z_{\alpha/2}}{z} \right) \tag{3.11}$$

where

$z_{\alpha/2}$ = standard normal deviate corresponding to a probability of $\alpha/2$ in the standard normal distribution (Table B.1)

z = standard normal deviate obtained in test of inference

---

[12]If the null value is exactly equal to one of the limits of the confidence interval, we would reject the null hypothesis. This corresponds to getting a P-value exactly equal to α, in which case we reject the null hypothesis.

Example 3.5   In Example 3.2, we tested the null hypothesis that the difference in diastolic blood pressure is equal to zero in patients who are given a placebo at one time and an antihypertensive agent at another time. In a sample of 11 patients, the mean of differences was found to be equal to 13.2 mm Hg. That mean of differences converted to the standard normal scale was determined to be 4.33. Let us now calculate a 95% two-tailed confidence interval for the mean of differences.

From Table B.1, we find that a standard normal deviate with an area of 0.025 in each tail is equal to 1.96. Then, using Equation 3.11:

$$\mu = \overline{Y} \cdot \left(1 \pm \frac{z_{\alpha/2}}{z}\right) = 13.2 \cdot \left(1 \pm \frac{1.96}{4.33}\right) = 7.2, 19.2 \text{ mm Hg}$$

Thus, we can be 95% confident that the population's mean of differences occurs within the interval from 7.2 to 19.2 mm Hg. This test-based confidence interval gives us exactly the same interval estimate for the mean of differences in diastolic blood pressure that we would have obtained using Equation 3.7. ▭

SUMMARY

All statistical procedures can be said to address one of two processes: estimation or inference. In estimation, those procedures help us to make our best guesses at the values of a population's parameters, based on a sample's observations. In statistical inference, those procedures help us compare our sample's estimate to what we would have expected to observe if our hypothesis about the value of the population's parameter were correct.

There are two types of estimates of a population's parameters that we might calculate from a sample. The first is called a point estimate. It is our single best guess at the value of a population's parameter. Since the probability that the population's parameter is exactly equal to the point estimate is very low, we often choose to calculate an interval estimate (also called a confidence interval): an interval of values calculated from a sample within which we have a specified (most frequently 95%) degree of confidence that the population's parameter is included.

The point estimate of the population's mean is the mean of the sample's observations, which is calculated in the same way that the mean of the population is calculated. The point estimate of the population's variance of the distribution of data, however, is not calculated from the sample's observations in the same way that it is calculated from the population's data. If we were to use the same formula to calculate the point estimate of the variance of data in the population, our estimate would be biased. Specifically, such a point estimate would consistently underestimate the population's variance of data. To correct for that bias, we subtract one from the sample's size in the denominator of the equation to calculate the point estimate of the variance of data in the population (Equation 3.2):

$$s^2 = \frac{\sum (Y_i - \overline{Y})^2}{n - 1} \tag{3.2}$$

In this chapter, we discovered that there are two types of distributions in any population. One is the distribution of data that we discussed in the previous chapter. The other is a distribution of all possible estimates of a parameter of the distribution of data. To understand interval estimates (and inference), it is necessary to first understand this distribution of estimates obtained from samples. A distribution of estimates contains the estimates of a particular parameter of the distribution of data in the population from all possible samples that are a given size. Like distributions of data, distributions of estimates can be described mathematically by their type of distribution (e.g., Gaussian) and the values of their parameters.

The population's parameter that we are most often interested in estimating is a measure of location such as the mean. If we take all possible samples of a given size and estimate the population's mean from each sample, we find that those estimates of the population's mean tend to have a Gaussian distribution even if the population's distribution of data is not a Gaussian distribution. We further find that this tendency increases as the size of each sample increases. This important principle in statistics is called the central limit theorem.

Since the distribution of all possible samples' means tends to be a Gaussian distribution, we can identify a particular distribution by specifying its mean and variance (or standard deviation). The mean of the distribution containing all possible estimates of the mean obtained from samples of a given size is equal to the mean of the distribution containing all the data in the population. Therefore, we calculate both means in the same way, regardless of which distribution we are addressing. The variance of the distribution containing all possible estimates of the mean, on the other hand, is not the same as the variance of the distribution containing all the data in the population. Rather, the variance of the distribution of means estimated from samples is less than the variance of the distribution of the data; how much less depends on the size of the samples. Distributions of all possible means estimated from large samples have smaller variances (less dispersion) than do distributions of all possible means estimated from small samples. The variance of the theoretical distribution of all possible estimates of the mean is found by dividing the variance of the distribution of data by the size of the samples (Equation 3.4).

$$\sigma_{\bar{Y}}^2 = \frac{\sigma^2}{n} \tag{3.4}$$

Interval estimates are also based on the distribution of estimates from all possible samples. An interval estimate can either be one-tailed or two-tailed. Calculation of a one-tailed interval estimate presupposes that we are interested in deviations from the point estimate in only one direction. A two-tailed interval estimate makes no such presupposition and results in an interval that is symmetric around the point estimate of the population's mean.

Statistical inference is also based on the distribution of estimates from all possible samples. To begin the process of inference, we erect two hypotheses: the null hypothesis and the alternative hypothesis. The null hypothesis states that the population's parameter being examined (e.g., the mean) is equal to a specific value (usually zero for differences). The alternative hypothesis states that the population's parameter is equal to an interval of values. If the interval of values specified in the alternative hypothesis contains all values other than the value specified in the null hypothesis, the alternative hypothesis is two-tailed. If the interval of values in the alternative hypothesis includes only values above (or only below) the point estimate, then the alternative hypothesis is one-tailed. Testing the validity of a hypothesis in statistics requires the assumption of a specific value. Thus, it is the null hypothesis that is actually tested.

The next step in statistical inference is to decide what probability of making an error by concluding that a true null hypothesis is not true we will tolerate. This mistake in inference is called a Type I error. The probability of making a Type I error is called α. Another mistake that we could make is to conclude that a false null hypothesis is true. This is called a Type II error. The probability of making a Type II error is called β, and the probability of avoiding a Type II error (the complement of making a Type II error) is called the power of a statistical procedure.

The probability of making a Type I error (α) is determined by the researcher and is conventionally chosen to be equal to 0.05. The probability of making a Type II error (β) cannot, in practice, be determined since it is a function of the vague alternative state rather than the specific null state. This inability to know the value of β forces us to decide to reject the null hypothesis or not to reject the null hypothesis. It would not be appropriate to decide to accept the null hypothesis when we do not know the chance we are taking that such a decision would be incorrect.

The process of statistical inference involves calculating the probability of obtaining a sample like the one observed or one more extreme if the null hypothesis were true. Calculation of that probability involves conversion of the point estimate obtained from the sample (the sample's mean) to a standard scale. If the calculated probability is equal to or less than the chosen value of α (usually 0.05), we reject the null hypothesis and accept, by elimination, the alternative hypothesis. If the calculated probability is greater than the chosen value of α, we do not reject the null hypothesis. The calculated probability is called a P-value. P-values are *not* a direct reflection of the probability that the null hypothesis is true.

Both interval estimation and statistical inference are based on the distribution consisting of estimates (e.g., of the mean) obtained from all possible samples. This is not all that these two processes have in common. Inference can be performed using an interval estimate by observing whether or not the null value for the population's parameter is included in the interval. The results of inference can be used to calculate a test-based confidence interval.

||| PRACTICE PROBLEMS

3.1 In Problem 2.3, we calculated the variance and standard deviation of the distribution of data for fasting blood glucose levels in a "population" made up of 20 patients. Now, let us assume that those 20 patients represent a random sample from a much larger population of fasting blood glucose values. Compare the estimate of the variance and standard deviation of data in the population obtained using these 20 patients as a sample to the results obtained in Problem 2.3 using them as the entire population.

3.2 In a population, the variance of the distribution of data for serum uric acid level is 1.21 mg%^{2}. In a sample of 16 persons from that population, we calculate a mean of 4.2 mg%. Provide an estimate of the population's mean in which you are 95% confident that the true value of the population's mean is included.

3.3 The population from which the sample in Problem 3.2 was derived is believed to have a mean serum uric acid level of 4.8 mg%. Allowing a 5% chance of making a Type I error, test that hypothesis (using the sample's mean and population's variance presented in Problem 3.2). As an alternative hypothesis, consider that the mean is not equal to 4.8 mg% in the population.

3.4 In a clinical study of a drug thought to lower serum cholesterol levels, eight patients known to be hypercholesterolemic had serum cholesterol levels (mg/dl) determined before and after a 30-day regimen on this drug. The following measurements were observed:

Patient	Before	After
1	281	269
2	259	245
3	272	271
4	264	248
5	253	229
6	297	276
7	312	289
8	275	260

Determine a point estimate for the mean of differences in serum cholesterol in the population. Test the null hypothesis (taking a 1% chance of rejecting a true null hypothesis) that the population's mean of differences in serum cholesterol levels is equal to zero. Assume that you have reason to believe that it is impossible for the drug to increase serum cholesterol levels.

PART TWO

Understanding Univariable Analysis

In Part I, we examined the basic principles underlying the field of statistics, including the basic operations of estimation and inference. Now, we are ready to investigate the methods that are used to analyze data encountered in health research and address estimation and inference. To demonstrate how those methods of analysis are selected for a particular set of data, we have organized the parts and chapters in the remainder of *Statistical First Aid* to reflect how the statistician thinks about data. Flowchart 1 outlines this organization. When you are ready to analyze your own data or interpret the results of someone else's analysis, you can use this flowchart to find the chapter that discusses the statistical procedure that is most often applicable. Before you do that, however, there is one more thing about variables that we need to examine.

FLOWCHART 1 The organization of the remaining chapters in *Statistical First Aid*.

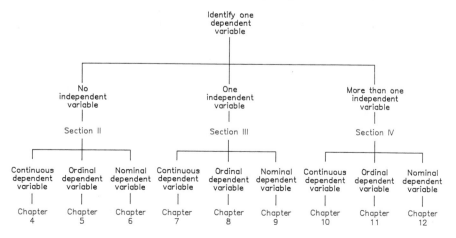

In the previous chapter, we looked at types of variables defined by the type of data that they represent. Now, we will define variables further on the basis of their function in analysis. Variables can serve one of two functions in a statistical analysis. The first function is to be the variable of primary interest to the researcher. This is the variable for which estimates are to be made or inferences are to be drawn. We call the variable of primary interest the **dependent variable.** For example, let us say that we are interested in the effect of some intervention on serum lipid levels. Here, it is of primary interest to estimate or draw conclusions about serum lipid levels; therefore, the dependent variable should be some measure of the lipid level.

Most often in health research, a single analysis will involve only one dependent variable. If a set of research observations includes more than one variable of primary interest, the usual approach is to conduct more than one analysis, each involving one of the variables of primary interest as the dependent variable. For instance, if we have several different measurements of serum lipids (e.g., high-density lipoprotein, low-density lipoprotein, total cholesterol), the usual approach to analyzing these observations would be to examine each of the serum lipid measurements in a separate statistical analysis.[1]

The second function of variables in statistical analysis is to specify conditions under which estimates of or inferences about the dependent variable will be made. Variables that serve this function are known as **independent variables.** In our example of a study of an intervention affecting serum lipid levels, an independent variable would be an indicator of whether or not a particular subject received the intervention. In other words, we are interested in comparing serum lipid levels between persons who received and persons who did not receive the intervention. Therefore, the independent variable indicating the presence or absence of the intervention defines the conditions under which we wish to examine the dependent variable. Other independent variables in this example might represent age and gender if we want to take into account (or control for) their effect on serum lipid levels.

You have probably noticed that the remaining parts of *Statistical First Aid* are identified by the number of variables we wish to analyze. Every analysis must include a dependent variable. Thus, in Part Two, where we are interested in analyzing a single variable, that single variable must be a dependent variable and there must not be any independent variables. Methods used to examine sets of observations containing a dependent variable and no independent variables are known as **univariable** methods. In Part Three, we discuss **bivariable** methods in which one dependent variable and one independent variable are considered. Part Four addresses **multivariable** methods used to analyze one dependent variable and more than one independent variable.[2]

You will notice that each part contains three chapters that correspond to the three types of data described earlier. Those three chapters in each of the remaining three parts

---

[1] Procedures for analyzing a single dependent variable are collectively called **univariate** methods. Statistical procedures that involve more than one dependent variable are collectively called **multivariate** methods. Multivariate methods are rarely encountered in health research literature except those areas of research that overlap social or behavioral sciences. For the most part, multivariate methods will not be discussed in *Statistical First Aid* except in those instances in which the methods are direct extensions of common univariate procedures.

[2] Notice a subtle distinction in terminology here. Multi*variable* methods are appropriate for three or more variables, while multi*variate* methods are appropriate for more than one dependent variable. The root "variable" refers to the number of variables without regard to their function. The root "variate" refers only to the number of dependent variables. A very common source of confusion in statistical terminology in health literature is to refer to a statistical procedure that examines one dependent variable and more than one independent variable as a multivariate, rather than a multivariable procedure.

of *Statistical First Aid* focus on the type of data represented by the dependent variable in a set of observations. In selecting an analytic approach, the statistician determines the number of variables, identifies dependent and independent variables, and classifies the type of data contained in the dependent variable.

Each chapter in the remaining sections also begins with a flowchart, which is an extension of Flowchart 1. These flowcharts will help you to choose a particular method of analysis for a set of data. They summarize the issues to consider in choosing a statistical procedure. In each chapter, you will find a discussion of how to evaluate those issues.

Following any branch of the flowchart to its end will reveal the name of a statistical procedure printed in red and underlined. That procedure is the one that is appropriate for either interval estimation or statistical inference on the corresponding data set. Interval estimation is generally based on the same or a very similar procedure (in Chapter 3, we learned that estimation and inference are closely related processes). In the remainder of *Statistical First Aid,* we will discuss these procedures primarily from the point of view of statistical inference. By that choice, we do not mean to imply that inference is the only, or even the better, way to evaluate a data set. It is, however, the more commonly encountered approach. In most applications, interval estimation can be performed by first using an inference approach and then using the result of inference to obtain a test-based confidence interval as we presented in Chapter 3 (Equation 3.11).

Thus, as we investigate specific statistical procedures in the remaining chapters of *Statistical First Aid,* we also will be following the logical process used by statisticians to select a procedure to analyze a set of research observations. To keep from losing sight of the forest as you read, we suggest that you take a moment to examine the flowcharts at the beginning of each chapter and think about how the procedures to be discussed fit into the entire scheme. This will help you to understand why particular procedures are used to analyze particular sets of data as well as understand how to interpret the results of a particular method of analysis.

CHAPTER 4

Continuous Dependent Variables

In Chapter 2, we learned that continuous data are most often assumed to come from a Gaussian distribution, which can be described by two parameters: the mean (μ) and the variance (σ^2). Although estimation and inference for continuous data can involve either parameter, most often we are concerned with the mean.[1] In Chapter 3, we examined a procedure for estimation and inference for the mean when we have a single dependent variable. Specifically, that procedure involved conversion of a sample's estimate of the population's mean to the standard normal scale by subtracting the population's mean ($\mu_{\overline{Y}}$) from the sample's mean ($\overline{Y}$) and dividing by the standard error (SE). This is a very straightforward procedure. Unfortunately, it is a little bit too simple to be entirely accurate.

To understand why the method described in Chapter 3 is not appropriate, let us take a moment to review what it is that we are doing when we perform statistical

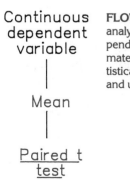

Continuous
dependent
variable

|

Mean

|

Paired t
test

FLOWCHART 2 Univariable analysis of a continuous dependent variable. Point estimates are indicated in red. Statistical procedures are in red and underlined.

---

[1]In *Statistical First Aid*, we will restrict our interest to null hypotheses that address measures of location.

procedures on a mean observed in a sample. The sample that we have observed is only one of many possible samples of that size that we could have obtained from the population. Therefore, the mean that we have calculated from our sample is only one of many possible means. We assume that chance, and only chance, determines which of the possible means we have observed. Regardless of whether we are interested in estimation or inference, the purpose of the statistical procedure that we apply to our sample's observations is to take this influence of chance into account.

The method of converting a sample's mean to the standard normal scale appropriately reflects the influence of chance on a sample's mean, but it overlooks another effect of chance. To see this other effect, let us reexamine the method we use to convert the sample's mean to the standard normal scale. From Equation 3.5:

$$z = \frac{\overline{Y} - \mu_{\overline{Y}}}{\text{SE}} \tag{4.1}$$

Recall that the standard error (SE) is calculated from the variance of data in the population (σ^2) and the sample's size. Specifically, the standard error is the square root of the variance of the distribution of all possible estimates of the mean ($\sigma_{\overline{Y}}^2$) calculated in Equation 3.4 and again in Equation 4.2:

$$\text{SE} = \sqrt{\sigma_{\overline{Y}}^2} = \sqrt{\frac{\sigma^2}{n}} \tag{4.2}$$

Thus, to calculate the standard error exactly, we must know the variance of data in the population. Since we cannot observe the entire population, we cannot know that variance exactly. Rather, we estimate the value of the variance of data in the population from the sample. Recall that calculation from Equation 3.2:

$$s^2 = \frac{\Sigma(Y_i - \overline{Y})^2}{n - 1} \tag{4.3}$$

As we said previously, conversion of the sample's mean to the standard normal scale takes into account the effect of chance in estimating the population's mean. However, it is also important for us to realize that chance influences our estimate of the variance of data in the population as well. The value calculated from a sample to estimate the variance of data in the population is only one of many possible estimates. We cannot take into account the influence of chance in estimating that variance using the standard normal distribution. We can, however, accomplish this using the **Student's *t* distribution.**[2]

---

[2] The word "Student" in statistical terminology is always capitalized. It is a pseudonym used by W. S. Gossett in many of his publications.

STUDENT'S *t* DISTRIBUTION

The Student's *t* distribution is a member of the Gaussian family of distributions. By that we imply that the Student's *t* distribution is mathematically "related" to the Gaussian distribution. Like the standard normal distribution, the Student's *t* distribution is a standard distribution with a scale to which we can convert observed values. Unlike when we used the standard normal distribution, however, we do not assume that the population's distribution of means from all possible samples of a certain size is shaped like the Student's *t* distribution, differing only in the value of its mean and variance. Rather, we continue to assume that the population's distribution of all possible estimates of the mean is a Gaussian distribution.[3]

In Chapter 3, we converted the sample's mean to the standard normal scale to avoid having to use calculus to calculate probabilities. This is also an advantage of converting to the Student's *t* scale. Conversion to the Student's *t* scale provides an additional advantage that we will examine in a moment. First, let us see how to convert observed values to Student's *t* values.

Recall that the standard normal distribution is a Gaussian distribution with a mean equal to zero and a variance equal to one. The Student's *t* distribution also has a mean equal to zero and a variance equal to one. Therefore, conversion of the sample mean to the Student's *t* scale is accomplished in exactly the same way as is conversion to the standard normal scale. Specifically, we subtract the population's mean from the sample's mean and divide by the standard error (Equation 4.4).

$$t = \frac{\overline{Y} - \mu_{\overline{Y}}}{SE} \tag{4.4}$$

where t = Student's *t* value.

The calculation in Equation 4.4 looks just like the calculation of a standard normal deviate (Equation 4.1). The Student's *t* distribution is not, however, the same as the standard normal distribution: What distinguishes them from each other is that the Student's *t* distribution has three, rather than two, parameters. That is to say, three summary measures are needed to fully characterize the Student's *t* distribution mathematically. In addition to a mean and variance, the Student's *t* distribution has a third parameter called **degrees of freedom.**

As previously stated, we are interested in the Student's *t* distribution because it takes into account the fact that we are estimating the variance of data in the population, as well as the population's mean, from our sample's observations. Degrees of freedom reflect the amount of information that a sample contains for estimating the variance of data in the population. At first, we might imagine that the amount of information in a sample is the same as the number of observations in that sample. This is almost correct. Actually, the amount of information in a sample that can be used to

---

[3]Because of the central limit theorem (Chapter 3), we are comfortable making this assumption for the distribution of estimates of the mean especially if the sample is large.

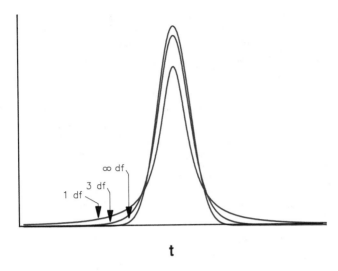

FIGURE 4.1 Student's *t* distribution. The dispersion of the Student's *t* distribution decreases as the degrees of freedom increase. When the degrees of freedom are equal to infinity, the Student's *t* distribution is the same as the standard normal distribution.

estimate the variance of data in the population is equal to the number of observations in the sample minus one.

To see why we subtract one from the sample's size to get the degrees of freedom in a sample, let us take another look at Equation 4.3. Notice that our estimate of the variance of data in the population requires an estimate of the population's mean. One way to interpret degrees of freedom is to say that this parameter tells us the amount of information we have left after we account for the other parameters we have to estimate. Thus, the degrees of freedom (*df*) for a univariable sample of a continuous variable must be equal to the sample's size minus one since we must use an estimate of the population's mean to estimate the variance of data in the population:[4]

$$df = n - 1 \tag{4.5}$$

Figure 4.1 shows the Student's *t* distribution for a few different degrees of freedom values. Notice that the distribution becomes less dispersed or spread out as the number of degrees of freedom increases. That implies that statistical significance can be achieved with a smaller Student's *t* value or that confidence intervals will be narrower when we have more degrees of freedom.

The degrees of freedom reflect how much information we have to estimate the variance of data in the population. By using degrees of freedom, we are taking into account the influence of chance in estimating that variance. The larger our sample size, the more degrees of freedom we have and the less we expect chance to influence our

[4]Another way to interpret degrees of freedom is to say that this parameter is equal to one when we have the smallest possible sample that allows the variance of data in the population to be estimated. We cannot estimate that variance from a single observation (our estimate would always be equal to zero); thus, the smallest number of observations that will allow estimation of the variance of data in the population is two.

estimate of the variance of data in the population since larger samples are expected to approximate the population's parameters more closely. Degrees of freedom in the Student's t distribution cause us to "penalize" ourselves for our uncertainty in estimation of the variance of data in the population. The larger our sample's size, the less the penalty.

For a moment, let us consider an extreme value for degrees of freedom. Suppose we had an infinitely large sample. Then, we would have infinite degrees of freedom. The Student's t distribution with an infinite number of degrees of freedom is exactly the same as the standard normal distribution. When we think about it, that makes good sense. If we have an infinitely large sample, then we have, in fact, observed the entire population. If we observe the entire population, we are certain that our estimate of the variance of data in the population is not an estimate at all, but rather it is exactly equal to that variance. Therefore, we need not penalize ourselves and we can use the standard normal distribution. In practice, this is never the case. With large samples, however, the penalty for uncertainty is very small.[5]

The Student's t distribution is the first of several distributions that we will encounter in *Statistical First Aid* that are related to the standard normal distribution. One characteristic that we will discover about all members of the Gaussian family except the standard normal distribution is that degrees of freedom is one of their parameters. In each case, degrees of freedom will be used to reflect the amount of information in a sample. Thus, understanding degrees of freedom is an important step in understanding many statistical procedures.

INTERVAL ESTIMATION

We can use the Student's t distribution in inference or interval estimation for a mean from a univariable sample of continuous data. Let us first consider interval estimation. We calculate a $(1 - \alpha)\%$, two-tailed confidence interval for the population's mean in the same way that we did using the standard normal distribution (see Equation 3.7). Now, however, we recognize that we should use a Student's t value with $n - 1$ degrees of freedom rather than a standard normal deviate. Equation 4.6 shows how a two-tailed confidence interval is calculated using the Student's t distribution. For a one-tailed confidence interval, we simply add *or* subtract from the sample's mean the product of the standard error and a Student's t value corresponding to an area of α in one tail and $n - 1$ degrees of freedom.

$$\mu = \overline{Y} \pm (t_{\alpha/2,\, df=n-1} \cdot \mathrm{SE}) \qquad (4.6)$$

where $t_{\alpha/2,\, df=n-1}$ = Student's t value corresponding to an area of $\alpha/2$ in each tail of the Student's t distribution with $n - 1$ degrees of freedom (Table B.2).

---

[5]When the degrees of freedom are equal to 60 (corresponding to a sample size of 61 in the current application), the Student's t value for $\alpha = 0.05$ is equal to 2.00, which is quite close to 1.96.

Example 4.1 In Example 3.1, we were interested in estimating the mean diastolic blood pressure in a population of patients diagnosed as hypertensive. In that example, we randomly selected 11 patients for whom we recorded diastolic blood pressure and determined a point and interval (99%, two-tailed) estimate for the population's mean using the standard normal distribution. Now that we realize that the standard normal distribution is inappropriate when we must estimate the variance of data in the population as well as the population's mean from the sample's observations, let us recalculate estimates of the population's mean using an appropriate method.

From Example 3.1, we find the following observations:

Patient	Diastolic Blood Pressure
HR	96
FW	114
RG	125
IH	105
VW	97
HL	96
ZH	131
CW	117
TD	107
ER	111
EM	123

First, we calculate the sample's mean as our point estimate for the population's mean. This calculation is unchanged from that in Example 3.1:

$$\overline{Y} = \frac{\Sigma Y_i}{n} = \frac{96 + 114 + \cdots + 123}{11} = \frac{1{,}222}{11} = 111.1 \text{ mm Hg}$$

Next, we determine the squared deviation of each observation from that sample's mean. Again, our calculations are identical to those in Example 3.1:

Patient	Y_i	$Y_i - \overline{Y}$	$(Y_i - \overline{Y})^2$
HR	96	−15.1	227.74
FW	114	2.9	8.46
RG	125	13.9	193.46
IH	105	−6.1	37.10
VW	97	−14.1	198.55
HL	96	−15.1	227.74
ZH	131	19.9	396.37

Patient	Y_i	$Y_i - \overline{Y}$	$(Y_i - \overline{Y})^2$
CW	117	5.9	34.92
TD	107	−4.1	16.74
ER	111	−0.1	0.01
EM	123	11.9	141.83
Total	1,222	0.0	1,482.91

Then, we calculate our estimate of the variance of data in the population:

$$s^2 = \frac{\Sigma(Y_i - \overline{Y})^2}{n-1} = \frac{1,482.91}{11 - 1} = 148.291 \text{ mm Hg}^2$$

The estimate of the variance of data in the population is then used to calculate the standard deviation of the distribution of means from all possible samples (the standard error):

$$\text{SE} = \sqrt{s^2/n} = \sqrt{148.291/11} = \sqrt{13.481} = 3.67 \text{ mm Hg}$$

Note that the standard error obtained here is exactly the same as the standard error value obtained in Example 3.1. Now, however, we do something a little bit different from what was done in Example 3.1. Instead of consulting Table B.1 to determine the standard normal deviate that corresponds to an area of 0.01 (0.005 in each tail), we look at Table B.2 for a Student's t value corresponding to $\alpha/2 = 0.01$ and $n - 1 = 10$ degrees of freedom. We find that Student's t value to be equal to 3.169. Now, we can use Equation 4.6 to determine a two-tailed, 99% confidence interval for the population's mean:

$$\mu = \overline{Y} \pm (t_{\alpha/2=0.01,10df} \cdot \text{SE}) = 111.1 \pm (3.169 \cdot 3.67) = 99.5, 122.7 \text{ mm Hg}$$

Note that the confidence interval we have calculated here is wider than the confidence interval in Example 3.1, which used the standard normal deviate (101.6, 120.5). The wider confidence interval using the Student's t distribution reflects greater uncertainty about the value of the population's mean because of the fact that we have had to estimate the variance of data in the population using the sample's observations.

INFERENCE

Recall from Chapter 3 that statistical inference involves testing a specific hypothesized condition for a population's parameter (usually a measure of location such as the mean) described in the null hypothesis. For most univariable samples, it is difficult to imagine what value we should hypothesize for the population. For instance, consider Example 4.1, where we examined diastolic blood pressure measurements on 11 patients. Our objective was to estimate the mean diastolic blood pressure in the population from which those patients were selected for observation. That is a logical purpose for collecting those data. It is difficult however, to conceive of what hypothesis might be tested using those observations. To perform statistical inference about the population's mean, we need to state a specific value for the population's mean. Often, with univariable samples, there is no hypothetical value of interest. Thus, interval estimation is used more commonly than inference for univariable samples.

There is, nevertheless, one kind of univariable sample in which inference makes sense. That is when we have a **paired sample** of continuous data. The most common type of paired sample is when we make two measurements of the same characteristic under different conditions for each subject. Example 3.2 includes such a paired sample. There, each patient received, at different times, a placebo and an antihypertensive agent. The variable that is examined using statistical inference in that case is the difference in diastolic blood pressure measurements. Since each observation includes only one difference, this is a univariable sample. The sensible null hypothesis for such a paired sample is that the mean of those differences is equal to zero in the population, indicating that the measurements are the same under the two conditions.

Less commonly, we might see paired samples in which similar, but not identical, individuals are compared one to the other. Again, the variable examined consists of the differences in the measurements of a characteristic between the two members of the pair. It is important to remember, however, that a legitimate paired sample will allow a particular individual to be compared to one and only one other individual. For example, a paired sample might consist of individuals compared to a sibling. It would usually not be appropriate, however, to use univariable methods to compare groups that are balanced or matched according to, say, age or gender.[6] That sort of sample is called a **group matched sample** rather than a paired sample.

To perform statistical inference on the mean from a univariable sample, we convert the sample's mean to a Student's t statistic using the method in Equation 4.7. Recall that this formula is the same as the one we used to convert the sample's mean to a standard normal deviate (Equation 4.1). First, we subtract the value of the population's mean specified in the null hypothesis from the estimated value of the population's mean calculated from our sample's observations. This has the effect of converting the mean of the distribution of all possible estimates of the mean to zero. Then, we divide that difference by the standard error. This converts the variance of the distribution of all possible samples' means to a value of one:

$$t = \frac{\overline{Y} - \mu_0}{SE} \tag{4.7}$$

Since the method of calculating a Student's t value is identical to the method of calculating a standard normal deviate, the difference between the standard normal and the Student's t tests is only the standard distribution to which we compare our

---

[6]In that case, it might be possible to construct several different pairs for the same individual if the sample contains more than one comparison individual of the same age group and gender.

converted sample's mean. The Student's *t* value is compared to a value from Table B.2 corresponding to a specified α and $n - 1$ degrees of freedom. If the calculated value is equal to or larger than the value from Table B.2, we reject the null hypothesis.

Example 4.2   Let us reconsider the clinical study described in Example 3.2. Recall that, in this study, we randomly selected 11 hypertensive patients and randomized each patient to receive either a placebo followed by an antihypertensive agent or the antihypertensive agent followed by a placebo, each for a specified period of time. At the end of each treatment period, we measured diastolic blood pressure. Subtracting each patient's pressure on the antihypertensive agent from the pressure on placebo, we made the following observations:

Patient	Difference
HR	7
FW	14
RG	27
IH	5
VW	2
HL	1
ZH	31
CW	19
TD	9
ER	9
EM	21

In Example 3.2 we tested the null hypothesis that the population from which this sample was derived has a mean of differences in diastolic blood pressure equal to zero by converting the mean of differences calculated from the sample to the standard normal scale. Now, we realize that this was inappropriate since it is necessary to estimate the variance of data in the population from the sample's observations. Now, let us reanalyze these data using the Student's *t* distribution.

In Example 3.2, we determined that our alternative hypothesis should be two-tailed and that we would allow a 5% chance of committing a Type I error. We will maintain those decisions here. From Table B.2, we find that the rejection region corresponding to 0.025 in each tail is equal to $t = \pm 2.228$ and beyond. Note that this is larger than the standard normal deviate used in Example 3.2 (where $z = \pm 1.96$). Thus, we will need to have a larger mean of differences using the Student's *t* distribution to reject the null hypothesis than we did using the standard normal distribution. This is the only distinction between this example and Example 3.2.

From our sample, the estimate of the population's mean is:

$$\overline{Y} = \frac{\Sigma Y_i}{n} = \frac{7 + 14 + \cdots + 21}{11} = \frac{145}{11} = 13.2 \text{ mm Hg}$$

And the estimate of the variance of data in the population is:

$$s^2 = \frac{\Sigma(Y_i - \overline{Y})^2}{n-1} = \frac{-6.2^2 + 0.8^2 + \cdots + 7.8^2}{11 - 1} = \frac{1,017.636}{10} = 101.764 \text{ mm Hg}^2$$

Next, from that variance estimate, we determine the standard error:

$$\text{SE} = \sqrt{\frac{s^2}{n}} = \sqrt{\frac{101.764}{11}} = \sqrt{9.25} = 3.04 \text{ mm Hg}$$

Finally, we convert our sample's estimate of the population's mean (assuming that the population's mean is equal to zero) to the Student's t scale:

$$t = \frac{\overline{Y} - \mu_0}{\text{SE}} = \frac{13.2 - 0}{3.04} = 4.33$$

Now, we compare the converted mean to values in the Student's t distribution. Since 4.33 is more extreme than 2.228, we reject the null hypothesis, accepting, by elimination, the alternative hypothesis which says that the antihypertensive agent changes the diastolic blood pressure.

In this example, using the Student's t rather than the standard normal distribution did not result in a different conclusion. If, however, a value between 1.96 and 2.228 had been observed, the two methods would have had different results. The correct conclusion in that case would have been that the null hypothesis could not be rejected (which would be the conclusion reached using the Student's t distribution).

||| SUMMARY

In this chapter, we have recognized that chance influences our sample's estimate of the variance of data in the population as well as the sample's estimate of the population's mean. When we use the standard normal distribution to make estimates or to test hypotheses about the population's mean, we are assuming that we know the value of the variance of data in the population. In practice, this is not true. Thus, the standard normal distribution is not appropriate to include entirely the role of chance in estimation or inference about the population's mean even when the distribution of all possible means from samples is a Gaussian distribution.

To take into account the fact that we are estimating the variance of data in the population, we use the Student's t distribution instead of the standard normal distribution. The Student's t distribution is similar to the standard normal distribution, with an additional parameter: degrees of freedom. The number of degrees of freedom reflects the amount of information contained in a sample that is available for estimation of the variance of data in the population. In a univariable sample of continuous data, that amount of information is equal to the sample's size minus one:

$$df = n - 1 \tag{4.5}$$

Estimation and inference for the population's mean using the Student's t distribution is the same as those procedures using the standard normal distribution, with the exception of calculation of the number of degrees of freedom and its use in locating a Student's t value in a table of Student's t values. With univariable samples, estimation is usually of more interest than is inference. A two-tailed, $(1 - \alpha)\%$ confidence interval for the population's mean is calculated by adding to and subtracting from the point estimate of the mean the product of a Student's t value from Table B.2 (corresponding to $\alpha/2$ and $n - 1$ degrees of freedom) and the standard error:

$$\mu = \overline{Y} \pm (t_{\alpha/2, df=n-1} \cdot \text{SE}) \tag{4.6}$$

The reason for a greater interest in interval estimation rather than inference in univariable samples is the difficulty we encounter when trying to formulate an appropriate null hypothesis to test. An exception is when we have a paired sample. In that case, the data of interest are the differences between paired observations, and the usual null hypothesis is that the mean of those differences is equal to zero in the population. To test that null hypothesis, we convert the sample's mean of differences to a Student's t value and compare it to a value from Table B.2:

$$t = \frac{\overline{Y} - \mu_0}{\text{SE}} \tag{4.7}$$

||| PRACTICE PROBLEMS

4.1 The mean arterial partial pressure of oxygen (PO_2) in a sample of 18 patients was found to be equal to 87.5 mm Hg. The standard deviation of data in the population of PO_2 measurements estimated from that sample of patients was equal to 25.1 mm Hg. Calculate an interval estimate for the population's mean arterial PO_2 within which we are 95% confident that the true value is included.

4.2 Using the observations in Problem 4.1, test the null hypothesis that the mean arterial PO_2 is actually 60 mm Hg versus the alternative that it is higher than 60 mm Hg. Allow a 1% chance of making a Type I error.

4.3 Suppose that we are interested in the effectiveness of a particular dietary intervention on body mass index (weight/height^2). In what is called a crossover trial, we randomly assign ten obese persons to receive either the experimental intervention first, followed by the standard dietary counseling, or the standard dietary counseling, followed by the experimental intervention. Each of the treatment programs is continued for 4 weeks before determining the body mass index (kg/m^2) and changing the method of treatment. The following results are observed:

Experimental	Standard
23.4	28.2
27.2	29.3
30.3	27.9
22.7	27.6
28.5	24.8
33.3	33.8
29.3	33.1
26.1	30.0
23.0	27.7
31.9	34.4

Assuming that there is no effect of the first treatment carried over to the second period of treatment, test the null hypothesis that the mean of differences in body mass index is actually zero in the population that was sampled versus the alternative that it is not equal to zero. Allow a 5% chance of making a Type I error.

4.4 From the observations in Problem 4.3, calculate a 99%, two-tailed interval estimate for the mean of differences in body mass index.

CHAPTER 5

Ordinal Dependent Variables

Ordinal data differ from continuous data in that they include a limited number of potential values. In addition, ordinal data do not necessarily have equal distances or intervals between potential values. There are some types of information in health research that are naturally measured on an ordinal scale. An example of ordinal data that we discussed in Chapter 2 was stage of disease. Another example is visual acuity. Even though visual acuity is measured on a quantitative scale that could theoretically be thought of as continuous, in practice, we measure only a limited number of values.

Thus, data on an ordinal scale can include measurements that are quantitative only in the sense that they can be ordered (such as stage of disease) or measurements that are truly quantitative but are usually measured using only a limited number of possible values (such as visual acuity). We use the same statistical procedures on both types of ordinal data. These procedures are based on the relative ranks of the measurements.

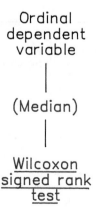

Ordinal dependent variable

|

(Median)

|

Wilcoxon signed rank test

FLOWCHART 3 Univariable analysis of an ordinal dependent variable. Point estimates are indicated in red. Statistical procedures are in red and underlined.

Although some data of interest to health researchers naturally occur on an ordinal scale, it is much more common in health research for ordinal data to be constructed from continuous data (we will see why this is done in a moment). That conversion is accomplished by ranking continuous observations in the same way that we would determine the relative ranks of ordinal observations.

We will often convert data to ranks in health statistics, so let us take a moment to learn how it is done. It does not really matter whether we rank observations from lowest to highest or from highest to lowest, but it is conventional to do the former (in *Statistical First Aid*, we will follow this convention). The only tricky part is ranking observations that have the same value. These are known as **tied observations.** Tied observations should all be assigned the same rank. The rank that we assign to tied observations is the mean of the ranks that they would have received if they were to be given separate ranks. It is easiest to understand how this is done by looking at an example.

Example 5.1   Convert the continuous data in Example 3.2 to an ordinal scale by determining the relative ranks of the observations.

Patient	Difference	Rank
HR	7	4
FW	14	7
RG	27	10
IH	5	3
VW	2	2
HL	1	1
ZH	31	11
CW	19	8
TD	9	5.5
ER	9	5.5
EM	21	9

Here, we have two differences equal to 9 mm Hg. These are tied observations. They are the fifth and sixth largest observations in this data set. To each, we assign the mean of those ranks. Thus, they are each assigned:

$$\frac{5 + 6}{2} = 5.5$$

Note that this method of assigning ranks to tied observations results in the largest rank being equal to the number of observations. We can quickly check the ranks that we have assigned by comparing the largest rank to the sample's size.

In Example 5.1, we converted data that occur naturally on a continuous scale to an ordinal scale. It is important for us to realize that, when we convert continuous data to an ordinal scale, we lose information. Consider the differences in diastolic blood pressure in Example 5.1. Patient ZH had the largest change in blood pressure and, therefore, was assigned the rank of 11. That ordinal information tells us only that this was the largest change. We must look at these data on a continuous scale to see how large that change was. Why, then, should we be interested in converting continuous data to an ordinal scale if we lose information in the process? The reason is that the loss of information is accompanied by a reduction in the number of assumptions that must be made to use statistical procedures designed to analyze continuous data.

When we performed inference or estimation on continuous data in Chapter 4, we made an assumption about the distribution of information in the population. When we were interested in inference or estimation for the population's mean, we assumed that the means from all possible samples had a Gaussian distribution.[1] The central limit theorem (see Chapter 3) tells us that means have a tendency to have a Gaussian distribution even if the data do not. It also tells us that this tendency increases as the sample's size increases. For small samples, on the other hand, we might not be able to assume a Gaussian distribution for all possible samples' means.

Statistical methods for ordinal data make no assumptions about the distribution of estimates of the population's parameters. Thus, we might want to analyze continuous data by converting those continuous data to an ordinal scale. When data are naturally ordinal or converted to an ordinal scale, we do not have to make the assumption that the estimates from all possible samples have a Gaussian distribution. For this reason, methods for ordinal data are called distribution-free or **nonparametric** methods, especially when they are applied to continuous data converted to an ordinal scale. It is important to remember, however, that nonparametric methods are not completely free of assumptions. Regardless of the statistical method we use, we always assume that dependent variable values were obtained by a random sample of the population of interest (as discussed in Chapter 2).

ESTIMATION

Since nonparametric methods do not assume any particular distribution for estimates from all possible samples, they cannot be thought of as directly estimating values of the population's parameters. Thus, estimation is not usually considered to be of interest when we are analyzing ordinal data. We can, however, use the median to describe the location and the interquartile range to describe the dispersion of continuous data converted to an ordinal scale.

---

[1]Remember that the population distribution used for interval estimation or statistical inference is the distribution of sample estimates, not the distribution of data.

Recall that the median is the physical center of a distribution in which half of the data occur above the median and half the data occur below the median. The median is not influenced by how far apart measurements are from one another. Rather, the median reflects the relative order of the data. Thus, the same median is found for a set of observations, regardless of the scale of measurement. With continuous data for which we are concerned about the distribution of estimates from all possible samples, we can use the median as a resistant estimate of the mean. This estimate is resistant to the influence of extreme observations in the sample that might not represent the distribution of data in the population.

Like the median, quartiles are not affected by how far apart observations are from one another. Quartiles simply divide observations into four groups, each containing the same number of observations. These quartiles are the same regardless of whether we consider data on a continuous or an ordinal scale. In Chapter 2, we found that two-thirds of the interquartile range (the distance between the first and third quartiles) can be used as a resistant estimate of the standard deviation of data in the population.

INFERENCE

The first requirement in statistical inference is that we have a null hypothesis to test. So far, we have only encountered null hypotheses that make statements about the population's parameters. Since a nonparametric method of inference is not concerned with parameters, we must have a different sort of null hypothesis. In the case of paired samples, the null hypothesis addressed by nonparametric tests is that a balance exists between positive and negative differences (this is parallel to the hypothesis that the mean of differences is equal to zero).

There are several different nonparametric tests that can be used to analyze paired samples of ordinal data or continuous data converted to an ordinal scale. In *Statistical First Aid,* we will consider only the most popular method: the **Wilcoxon signed-rank test.**

The first step in the Wilcoxon signed-rank test is to rank the differences as we did in Example 5.1. In that example, all the patients showed a positive difference in systolic blood pressures (i.e., blood pressure was consistently lower under treatment). Most paired samples do not result in differences all in the same direction. Rather some differences are positive and some are negative. In the Wilcoxon signed-rank test, we ignore the sign of the differences when assigning a rank. In other words, we rank the absolute value of the difference. After ranks have been assigned, we then apply the sign of the difference to the rank (thus, creating "signed ranks"). Differences of zero are a problem since zero cannot be thought of as being positive or negative. There are various methods that have been suggested to handle differences of zero. Here, we will use the most commonly encountered method which is simply to ignore observations with differences of zero. Let us take a look at how ranking is done when we have differences with various signs such as the data in Example 5.2.

Example 5.2   Suppose we are interested in the effectiveness of a new educational intervention for weight loss. To study this intervention, we enrolled 15 overweight patients and
measured their weight before and six months after the intervention. Further suppose that the
results in the following table were observed for those 15 patients. Determine signed ranks for
each patient.

Weight Before	Weight After	Difference	| Difference |*	Rank	Signed Rank
139	146	−7	7	4	−4
222	183	39	39	14	14
156	146	10	10	6	6
190	190	0	0	—	—
147	149	−2	2	1	−1
199	195	4	4	3	3
196	175	21	21	12	12
224	211	13	13	7	7
138	119	19	19	11	11
150	158	−8	8	5	−5
184	198	−15	15	10	−10
160	184	−14	14	8.5	−8.5
172	141	31	31	13	13
157	143	14	14	8.5	8.5
149	146	3	3	2	2

*Vertical bars indicate an absolute value.

Note that the largest rank is *not* equal to the sample size when we have differences of zero.
Rather, the largest rank is equal to the number of observations with nonzero differences.

Conversion of observations to a test statistic with the Wilcoxon signed-rank test is
very different from the methods we have learned thus far. Here, there are two test
statistics that we calculate from the signed ranks: one is the total of the positive ranks
(T_+) and the other is the total of the negative ranks (T_-).

$$T_+ = \Sigma \, \text{positive ranks} \tag{5.1}$$

$$T_- = \Sigma \, \text{negative ranks} \tag{5.2}$$

If we are interested in a one-tailed test, which of the two statistics is to be
compared to a value in the table (Table B.3) is determined by which of the two
statistics the alternative hypothesis implies will be the smaller. For instance, if we are
interested in a one-tailed alternative hypothesis that states that the positive differences

are larger than the negative differences, the total of the negative ranks is the appropriate test statistic since it is hypothesized to be the smaller of the two statistics. For the data in the previous example, a one-tailed alternative hypothesis might state that weight after the intervention is less than weight before the intervention. Since the differences were found by subtracting the weight after the intervention from the weight before the intervention, this alternative hypothesis suggests that the total of the positive ranks should be greater than the total of the negative ranks. Thus, the sum of the negative ranks should be used to test the null hypothesis with this alternative hypothesis.

If, on the other hand, we are interested in the one-tailed alternative hypothesis that states that the negative differences are larger than the positive differences (e.g., that the weight after the intervention is larger than the weight before the intervention), we would expect the total of the negative ranks to be greater than the total of the positive ranks. In that case, the sum of the positive ranks is the appropriate test statistic. For a two-tailed test, we calculate both the total of the positive ranks and the total of the negative ranks and choose the total that is actually the smaller of the two test statistics.

Let us take a moment to examine the table of Wilcoxon signed-rank statistics (Table B.3). Notice that the values in that table get smaller as we consider smaller α values. This is the opposite of Tables B.1 and B.2. When we learned about the standard normal and Student's t tests, we rejected the null hypothesis if the absolute value of the calculated test statistic was equal to or larger than the value in the table. In the Wilcoxon signed-rank test, we do just the opposite. Here, the null hypothesis will be rejected if the calculated test statistic is *equal to or smaller* than the value in the table corresponding to our chosen α. The Wilcoxon signed-rank test is the only procedure that we will learn in which the statistic gets smaller as the chance of making a Type I error decreases.

Example 5.3 Using the data from the study of the effectiveness of a new educational intervention for weight loss presented in Example 5.2, test the null hypothesis that weight gain equals weight loss versus the alternative that weight gain does not equal weight loss. Allow a 5% chance of making a Type I error.

First, let us calculate the two test statistics for the Wilcoxon signed-rank test from the ranks assigned in Example 5.2.:

$$T_+ = 14 + 6 + 3 + 12 + 7 + 11 + 13 + 8.5 + 2 = 76.5$$

$$T_- = 4 + 1 + 5 + 10 + 8.5 = 28.5$$

Since we have no reason to believe that it would be impossible for the education intervention to be associated with an increase in weight, the alternative hypothesis in this example is two-tailed. Thus, the appropriate test statistic is the smaller of T_+ and $T_- \cdot T_- = 28.5$ is the smaller. Now we consult Table B.3 to find the Wilcoxon signed-rank statistic that is associated with a sample's size of 14 (remember that we are ignoring the observation with a difference of zero and that our sample's size is equal to the number of nonzero differences for the Wilcoxon signed-rank test) and an α equal to 0.05. That statistic is equal to 21. Since our calculated value is greater than the value in the table, we are unable to reject the null hypothesis.   ⊟

It is important to remember that, although tests of statistical inference for ordinal dependent variables require fewer assumptions than corresponding tests for continuous dependent variables, there are some remaining assumptions of which we must be aware. *All* statistical procedures assume that the composition of the sample differs from the composition of the population only by chance.[2] In other words, we are always assuming that we have a random sample.

STATISTICAL POWER OF NONPARAMETRIC TESTS

As discussed earlier in this chapter, continuous data can be converted to an ordinal scale to circumvent some of the assumptions required for analysis of continuous dependent variables. We also learned that information is lost when continuous data are converted to an ordinal scale. We gain flexibility by performing such a conversion, but we must pay a price. The resultant loss of information can mean a loss of statistical power. Remember that we learned in Chapter 3 that statistical power means the ability to avoid a Type II error (incorrectly failing to reject a false null hypothesis).

Loss of power occurs when the assumptions required by a statistical procedure for a continuous dependent variable are satisfied, but instead we choose to convert our continuous data to an ordinal scale for analysis. In other words, it occurs when it would have been appropriate to use a statistical procedure designed for a continuous dependent, but we used a nonparametric procedure instead. It does not occur when the assumptions required by a statistical procedure for a continuous dependent variable are *not* satisfied and we convert to an ordinal scale. Thus, if we find a greater ability to reject a null hypothesis using a nonparametric test than with a test designed for continuous dependent variables, we can surmise that the assumptions of the test designed for continuous data were violated and that the nonparametric test is more appropriate. This is true of all nonparametric tests, not just the Wilcoxon signed-rank test.[3]

---

[2] There are some aspects of composition that might differ between the sample and the population, but special statistical procedures must be used to take those differences into account. The aspect of the composition that is being examined in estimation or inference, however, must reflect differences only due to chance.

[3] Unfortunately, the converse is not true. If the parametric test appears to have greater power, that might be a reflection of greater power of parametric tests or the result of violated assumptions.

The decision regarding whether or not to convert data to another scale is a common one in analysis of health research data. Unfortunately, it is not often an easy decision to make.[4] In *Statistical First Aid*, we will look only at the loss of power that can occur when we make an incorrect decision.

One way to examine power is by considering *P*-values. We learned in Chapter 3 that a *P*-value is the minimum value of α that we could have used in an analysis and still have rejected the null hypothesis. The greater the power of a statistical procedure, the smaller the *P*-value will be. In Example 5.4, we use this principle to examine the power of the Wilcoxon signed-rank test relative to the Student's *t* test in a situation in which it would have been possible to use the Student's *t* test.

Example 5.4   Test the null hypothesis that the mean of differences in weight loss before and after the new educational intervention in Example 5.2 is equal to zero versus the alternative that it is not equal to zero. Allow a 5% chance of making a Type I error. Compare the result of this approach to that obtained in Example 5.3.

Weight Before	Weight After	Difference (Y_i)	$Y_i - \overline{Y}$	$(Y_i - \overline{Y})^2$
139	146	−7	−14.2	201.64
222	183	39	31.8	1,011.24
156	146	10	2.8	7.84
190	190	0	−7.2	51.84
147	149	−2	−9.2	84.64
199	195	4	−3.2	10.24
196	175	21	13.8	190.44
224	211	13	5.8	33.64
138	119	19	11.8	139.24
150	158	−8	−15.2	231.04
184	198	−15	−22.2	492.84
160	184	−14	−21.2	449.44
172	141	31	23.8	566.44
157	143	14	6.8	46.24
149	146	3	−4.2	17.64
Total		108	0	3,534.40

[4]In *Statistical First Aid*, we will not discuss the methods that statisticians use to make this decision.

To test directly a null hypothesis about the mean of differences in the population, we need to use the Student's t procedure discussed in Chapter 4. To apply the Student's t procedure, we first calculate the sample's estimate of the mean of the differences in weight:

$$\overline{T} = \frac{\Sigma \Upsilon_i}{n} = \frac{108}{15} = 7.2$$

Next, we calculate the sample's estimate of the variance of data in the population and the standard error of the distribution of all possible means of differences in weight from samples containing 15 observations:

$$s^2 = \frac{\Sigma (\Upsilon_i - \overline{\Upsilon})^2}{n - 1} = \frac{3,534.40}{15 - 1} = 252.46$$

$$SE = \sqrt{\frac{s^2}{n}} = \sqrt{\frac{252.46}{15}} = 4.10$$

Finally, we convert the mean of differences to a Student's t statistic:

$$t = \frac{\overline{\Upsilon} - \mu_0}{SE} = \frac{7.2 - 0}{4.10} = 1.76$$

To compare this analysis with the Wilcoxon signed-rank test, let us first look at Table B.2 to find the smallest value of α we could have had and still rejected the null hypothesis. In that table, we find $t_{\alpha/2=0.10,\,14df} = 1.761$. Therefore, the P-value for this approach is approximately equal to 0.10. Now, we consult Table B.3 to look for $T = 28.5$. We find that value is between $T_{\alpha/2=0.10,\,n=14} = 25$ and $T_{\alpha/2=0.20,\,n=14} = 31$. In other words, the P-value for the Wilcoxon signed-rank test is $0.10 < P < 0.20$. Thus, the P-value of the Student's t test is slightly smaller than that for the Wilcoxon signed-rank test, suggesting lower power of the Wilcoxon signed-rank test if assumptions of the Student's t test are satisfied.

In Example 5.4, we find that the apparent loss of statistical power when using the Wilcoxon signed-rank test instead of the Student's t test does not affect our conclusion for this particular set of observations. Using either method, we fail to reject the null hypothesis. In most instances, the loss of statistical power due to use of a nonparametric test will be small[5] and will not affect the conclusion we draw in statistical inference. This will be true unless the P-value is close to our chosen value of α (i.e., unless we are close to the borderline of statistical significance).

---

[5]Some nonparametric tests are associated with a substantial loss of power, but they are not commonly used (for the very reason that they have low statistical power). The nonparametric tests that we present in *Statistical First Aid* are among the most powerful tests available.

| ‖   SUMMARY

To perform statistical analysis of ordinal dependent variables, the values of those variables are converted into relative ranks. This is done regardless of whether the variables are from data that naturally occur on an ordinal scale or from continuous data that we wish to convert to an ordinal scale. Such a conversion of continuous data to ranks is done to allow statistical analysis without assuming that the distribution of estimates from all possible samples is a Gaussian distribution.

Conversion of data to ranks can be accomplished by assigning the rank of one to the smallest value, two to the next larger value, and so on. Observations that have the same value, called tied observations, are assigned the mean of the ranks they would have received if they were given separate ranks.

Estimation of parameters of a population's distribution is not often pursued for ordinal dependent variables since no particular distribution is assumed. This lack of assumptions concerning distributions and parameters has led to procedures for ordinal data being referred to as distribution-free or nonparametric procedures. Even so, the median and the interquartile range can be determined from ordinal data and used as resistant estimators of the population's mean and the standard deviation of data in the population.

The most common method for performing statistical inference on a single ordinal variable is the Wilcoxon signed-rank test. The test statistics for that procedure are the sum of the ranks for the negative differences and the sum of the ranks for the positive differences between paired observations. Unlike for other test statistics, we reject the null hypothesis if the calculated Wilcoxon signed-rank test statistic is smaller than the value in the table. For a two-tailed test, we calculate both the sum of the negative ranks and the sum of the positive ranks and choose the smaller of the two. A one-tailed test uses either the sum of the positive ranks or the sum of the negative ranks. Which of the two sums is used depends on the alternative hypothesis. Specifically, the appropriate test statistic is the sum that is assumed, according to the alternative hypothesis, to be the smaller of the two sums.

When continuous data are converted to an ordinal scale for statistical analysis, we gain the ability to ignore certain assumptions about the distribution of estimates derived from all possible samples. We cannot, however, ignore the assumption that dependent variable values are randomly selected from the population. As a result of this conversion to an ordinal scale, however, we have the potential for losing statistical power. That is to say, it can become more difficult to reject a false null hypothesis. This loss of statistical power occurs when the assumptions of the statistical procedure for continuous data were not violated, but we analyzed the data as if it were ordinal. The loss of power is usually small and often has no effect on the conclusions we draw in inference.

| ‖   PRACTICE PROBLEMS

5.1 In Problem 4.3, we were interested in the effectiveness of a particular dietary intervention on body mass index. In a crossover trial, we randomly assigned ten obese persons to receive either the experimental intervention first, followed by the standard dietary counseling, or the standard dietary counseling, followed by the experimental intervention. Each of the treatment programs was continued for 4 weeks before determining the body mass index (kg/m^2) and changing the method of treatment. The following results were observed:

Experimental	Standard
23.4	28.2
27.2	29.3
30.3	27.9
22.7	27.6
28.5	24.8
33.3	33.8
29.3	33.1
26.1	30.0
23.0	27.7
31.9	34.4

Convert these observations to an ordinal scale.

5.2 Assuming that there is no effect of the first treatment carried over to the second period of treatment, test the null hypothesis that persons on the experimental intervention in the crossover trial considered in Problem 5.1 gained body mass to the same degree that they lost body mass versus the alternative that they did not. Allow a 5% chance of making a Type I error.

5.3 Compare your conclusion in Problem 5.2 to the conclusion drawn in Problem 4.3. Which approach to these data was more appropriate?

CHAPTER 6

Nominal Dependent Variables

Much of the data that we encounter in health research is measured on a nominal scale.[1] We learned in Chapter 2 that a nominal variable consists of dichotomous (yes/no) information. For an individual, a nominal variable indicates either the presence or absence of some characteristic (e.g., disease or no disease). When information is combined for several individuals, nominal variables are often summarized as relative frequencies or probabilities by dividing the number of individuals with the characteristic by the total number of individuals.

FLOWCHART 4 Univariable analysis of a nominal dependent variable. Point estimates are indicated in red. Statistical procedures are in red and underlined.

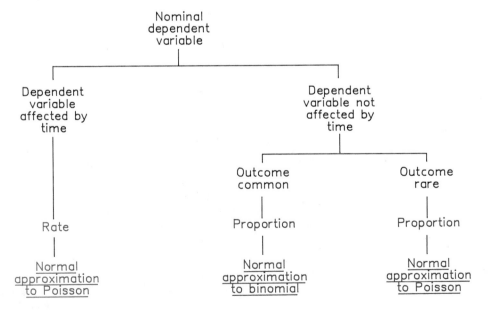

[1]Continuous or ordinal data can also be converted to a nominal scale. If this is done, information is lost.

POINT ESTIMATES

There are two special probabilities that we use in health research when we wish to talk about the probability of disease. These are called **prevalence** and **risk.** In its most common form, prevalence is the probability that someone in a population has a particular disease at a particular point in time.[2] It is calculated from a sample's observations by dividing the number of persons in the sample with the disease by the total number of persons in the sample (Equation 6.1). Risk is the probability that a person will develop a particular disease over a specified period of time. It is calculated from a sample's observations by dividing the number of persons in a sample that develop the disease during the time period by the total number of disease-free persons in the sample at the beginning of the time period (Equation 6.2). The number of disease-free persons in a sample at the beginning of a time period is called the number "at risk."

$$\text{Prevalence} = \frac{\text{Number with disease at time } t}{\text{Total number at time } t} \tag{6.1}$$

$$\text{Risk} = \frac{\text{Number developing disease from time 0 to time } t}{\text{Total number without disease at time 0}} \tag{6.2}$$

Both prevalence and risk are probabilities with properties just like those described for probabilities in Chapter 1. For example, prevalence or risk can have any value between zero and one. They are both most often considered to be conditional probabilities. For instance, we might be interested in the prevalence of neuropathy under the condition of diabetes or the risk of coronary heart disease, given that a patient smokes. The distinction between prevalence and risk is that prevalence addresses the proportion of persons with a characteristic at a point in time, while risk addresses the proportion of persons who develop a characteristic over a specified period of time. This is an important distinction, for prevalence can be estimated from a single examination, while estimation of risk involves an examination to determine which persons do and do not have the characteristic and a second examination after a period of time to discover how many persons, who initially did not have the characteristic, have developed the characteristic during the time interval.

Example 6.1 Suppose that we are interested in the probability of retinopathy among diabetics. We examine 500 persons with diabetes and find 6 persons with diabetic retinopathy. Five years later, we reexamine the 494 persons who did not have retinopathy and find that 68 have developed retinopathy since the first examination. From those observations, we wish to estimate the prevalence and risk of diabetic retinopathy in the population from which these persons were sampled.

[2]More precisely, this is called a point prevalence.

There are two different points in time for which we could estimate prevalence. Our estimate of prevalence at the first examination is:

$$\text{Prevalence}_{\text{1st exam}} = \frac{\text{Number with retinopathy at 1st exam}}{\text{Total number in sample}} = \frac{6}{500} = 0.012$$

The estimate of prevalence at the second exam is:

$$\text{Prevalence}_{\text{2nd exam}} = \frac{\text{Number with retinopathy at 2nd exam}}{\text{Total number in sample}} = \frac{68 + 6}{500} = 0.136$$

Although we can calculate two different estimates of retinopathy prevalence corresponding to the two examinations, we can estimate only one risk from this study. Since risk, in this example, is the probability of developing diabetic retinopathy over a five-year time period, our interest must be only in persons who do not have retinopathy at the beginning of the time period. At the second examination, we find how many of the 494 persons without retinopathy have developed that condition. Thus, our estimate of the five-year risk of diabetic retinopathy is:

$$\text{Risk}_{\text{5-yr}} = \frac{\text{Number developing retinopathy over 5 years}}{\text{Number without retinopathy at 1st exam}} = \frac{68}{494} = 0.138$$

Although the most common form in which a nominal dependent variable is presented is as a probability, we will also find this sort of information presented as a **rate.** A probability has no units of measurement. A rate has 1/time as the unit of measurement. A probability can have any value between zero and one. A rate can have any value between zero and infinity. The measure of rate that we use in health research is called **incidence** (I). We measure incidence by dividing the number of new cases of a disease by the number of persons "at risk" times the length of the time period during which we observe development of the disease (Equation 6.3). This product of the number of persons "at risk" times the length of the time period during which we observe development of the disease that appears in the denominator of incidence is known as the number of person-years of observation.

$$\text{Incidence} = I = \frac{\text{Number developing disease}}{\text{Number at risk} \cdot \text{Time period of observation}}$$

$$= \frac{\text{Number developing disease}}{\text{Number of person-years}} \qquad \textbf{(6.3)}$$

Prevalence, risk, and incidence are measurements of disease frequency. Most of the diseases of interest to health researchers are rare. Therefore, values of prevalence, risk, and incidence are usually small numbers. To avoid dealing with these small numbers, prevalence and risk are often presented as a larger number times 10^{-5} (so many cases per 10^5 persons),[3] and incidence is frequently given as a larger number times 10^{-5} years

---

[3]This is known as scientific notation. 10^{-5} is equal to one over ten to the fifth power or $1/100,000$. 10^5 is equal to ten to the fifth power or $100,000$.

(number of cases per 10^5 person-years). For more common diseases, prevalence and risk are usually expressed as a percentage (cases per 100 persons). Since incidence has the units 1/time, it cannot be expressed as a percentage.

Example 6.2 Let us consider further the study of diabetic retinopathy described in Example 6.1. We are told that 494 persons were free of retinopathy at the beginning of a five-year period of observation. During that period, 68 persons developed retinopathy. Now, let us assume that, on the average, the 68 persons developed retinopathy after 2.5 years. What, then, is our estimate of the incidence of diabetic retinopathy in the population sampled?

The numerator of incidence is the same as the numerator of risk calculated in Example 6.1. We have observed 68 new cases of retinopathy. What differs in estimation of incidence is calculation of the denominator. When we calculated risk, the denominator consisted only of the 494 persons at risk. For incidence, we need to consider how long each of those 494 were at risk to develop retinopathy.

The general principle here is that a person is no longer at risk once they have the disease. For those persons who did not develop retinopathy, they were at risk for the entire five-year period of observation. Since there were $494 - 68 = 426$ persons who did not have retinopathy at the end of five years, one component of the denominator of incidence is $426 \cdot 5 = 2,130$ person-years. For those 68 persons who developed retinopathy, we are told that they spent an average of 2.5 years at risk (i.e., on the average, they took 2.5 years to develop the disease). Therefore, those 68 persons contribute $68 \cdot 2.5 = 170$ person-years to the denominator. Thus, our estimate of incidence is:

$$\text{Incidence} = I = \frac{\text{Number developing disease}}{\text{Number at risk} \cdot \text{Time until disease develops}}$$

$$= \frac{68}{2130 + 170} = 0.02957 \text{ per year or } 2957 \text{ per } 10^5 \text{ year}$$

INTERVAL ESTIMATES

Thus far, we have discussed interval estimation for means of continuous data using the distribution of means from all possible samples of a given size assumed to be a Gaussian distribution. Distributions of probabilities representing nominal data are not Gaussian distributions since a Gaussian distribution assumes that there are an infinite number of evenly spaced values. Rather, probabilities have a **binomial distribution** or a **Poisson distribution.** Whether a binomial or a Poisson distribution is appropriate for a distribution of probability estimates depends on the magnitude of the population's probability. A general rule of thumb is that probabilities between 0.05 and 0.95 should be assumed to have a binomial distribution of estimates. If a probability is not within that range and, in addition, a large number of observations (≥ 100) have been made in the sample, the probability estimates can be assumed to have a

Poisson distribution.[4] Incidence estimates are always assumed to have a Poisson distribution.[5]

With nominal data, we can take either of two approaches. For small samples (when the number of people with the condition or the number of people without the condition are less than 5), we should use **exact methods.** With those methods, we must calculate probabilities from the mathematical formulas for the binomial or Poisson distributions to perform estimation or inference.[6] However, when the number of people with the condition and the number of people without the condition are both equal to or greater than 5, we can use **normal approximations** instead of exact methods. These methods rely on the fact that probabilities and rates estimated from samples of nominal data have population distributions that very closely resemble Gaussian distributions when large samples are taken.[7] Normal approximations are computationally much easier to perform than are exact methods. In *Statistical First Aid,* we will consider only normal approximations.

Normal approximations to the binomial distribution or the Poisson distribution convert the sample's statistics to standard normal deviates in the same way that a mean from a sample of a Gaussian distribution was converted in Chapter 3 (see Equation 3.5). The sample's statistic in the binomial distribution is the observed probability[8] (p) that estimates the population's probability expressed by the parameter theta (θ). The sample's estimate p and the population's parameter θ can stand for a prevalence, risk, or any other probability. We can convert p (the observed probability) to a standard normal deviate by subtracting the population's value and dividing by the standard error (Equation 6.4):

$$z = \frac{p - \theta}{SE_p} \tag{6.4}$$

Notice that Equation 6.4 is the same as Equation 3.5 (for conversion of a sample's mean to the standard normal scale) except that here we use p and θ as the sample's statistic and the population's parameter instead of $\overline{Y}$ and μ. Another difference is not obvious from Equation 6.4. The method for calculating the standard error of p (Equation 6.5) is quite different (and much easier) from the method for calculating the standard error of the mean:

$$SE_p = \sqrt{\frac{p \cdot (1 - p)}{n}} \tag{6.5}$$

[4]Actually, the Poisson distribution is a simplification of the binomial distribution. It is also correct, but less convenient, to assume a binomial distribution for probabilities outside the range of 0.05 to 0.95.

[5]One way to think of the reason for this is to realize that the denominator of an incidence can be infinitely large if we express the incidence in an infinitely small period of time. For instance, one person-year is equal to 365.25 person-days (or 31,557,600 person-seconds).

[6]Most sets of nominal data in health research have large enough samples that exact methods are not necessary. Therefore, we will not discuss those exact methods in *Statistical First Aid.*

[7]The parameters of the binomial and Poisson distributions are similar to means, therefore the central limit theorem can be applied to these distributions.

[8]Notice that we use a lowercase p to represent any probability (as we did in Chapter 1). To represent the special probability that results from a test of statistical inference (i.e., the P-value), we use an uppercase P.

Let us take a moment to look more closely at the standard error for p (Equation 6.5). Notice that, for a given sample's size and value of p, only one value for the standard error is possible. This is distinct from the standard error of $\overline{Y}$ (Equation 3.4), which can have any of an infinite number of values for a given sample's size and value of $\overline{Y}$. Which value of the standard error of the mean is the correct one depends on the value of the variance of data in the population, and that variance usually must be estimated from the sample's observations. This is why we used the Student's t distribution rather than the standard normal distribution for interval estimation and inference of the population's mean (see Chapter 4). For p, however, we do not need to estimate anything in addition to the parameter θ, and there is no need to penalize ourselves for estimation of the variance of data in the population.[9] Thus, the standard normal distribution, rather than the Student's t distribution, is appropriate for interval estimation of a probability using the normal approximation to the binomial.

Now let us see how we calculate an interval estimate for a probability assumed to come from a binomial population distribution. To do that, we algebraically rearrange Equation 6.4 to solve for θ. Thus, a one-tailed, $(1 - \alpha)\%$ confidence interval is calculated as shown in Equation 6.6.

$$\theta = p + (z_\alpha \cdot SE_p) \qquad (6.6)$$

where z_α = standard normal deviate representing an area of α in one tail.

A two-tailed, $(1 - \alpha)\%$ confidence interval is calculated as shown in Equation 6.7.

$$\theta = p \pm (z_{\alpha/2} \cdot SE_p) \qquad (6.7)$$

where $z_{\alpha/2}$ = standard normal deviate representing an area of $\alpha/2$ in each tail.

Example 6.3 Calculate a two-tailed, 95% confidence interval for the five-year risk of developing diabetic retinopathy based on the information given in Example 6.1.

Recall that the five-year risk of retinopathy in Example 6.1 was estimated as follows:

$$Risk_{5\text{-yr}} = \frac{\text{Number developing retinopathy over 5 years}}{\text{Number without retinopathy at 1st exam}} = \frac{68}{494} = 0.138$$

The standard error of that estimate is:

$$SE_p = \sqrt{\frac{p \cdot (1 - p)}{n}} = \sqrt{\frac{0.138 \cdot (1 - 0.138)}{494}} = 0.0155$$

---

[9]Conversion of the sample's estimate of the population's probability to a standard normal deviate allows us to take the role of chance in estimation of that probability into account. The role of chance in estimation of the variance of data in the population to allow calculation of the standard error is the same as the role of chance in estimation of the probability in the normal approximation to the binomial. Thus, we do not need to consider two separate effects of chance for nominal data as we did for continuous data.

Therefore, the 95% two-tailed confidence interval is:

$$\theta = p \pm (z_{\alpha/2} \cdot \text{SE}) = 0.138 \pm (1.96 \cdot 0.0155) = 0.108, 0.168$$

When we are interested in calculating an interval estimate of an incidence or a small probability (such as the prevalence or risk of a rare disease) from a large sample, we can use the normal approximation to the Poisson rather than the normal approximation to the binomial. Conversion of the sample's estimate from the Poisson distribution to the standard normal scale follows the same general procedure that we have used to convert probabilities from a binomial population distribution to the standard normal scale (Equation 6.4). There are three important distinctions between the normal approximation to the binomial and the normal approximation to the Poisson, however.

The first difference is in the population's parameter for which we calculate an interval estimate. In the normal approximation to the binomial distribution, the estimate converted to a standard normal deviate is a probability. The estimate converted to a standard normal deviate in the normal approximation to the Poisson, however, is *not* an incidence nor is it a probability. Rather, the parameter of the Poisson distribution that is converted to a standard normal deviate is the number of persons with the characteristic of interest (i.e., the numerator of the probability or incidence). The symbol for this parameter is lambda (λ). The sample's estimate of λ is symbolized by the letter a. Thus, the parameter for which we can directly calculate an interval estimate from the incidence of retinopathy in Example 6.2 is the number of persons developing retinopathy over the period of observation, not the number of persons developing that condition per person-year.

The second difference is that we do not directly convert the sample's estimate of the number of persons with the characteristic of interest (i.e., a) to the standard normal scale when we use the normal approximation to the Poisson. Rather, we convert the *square root* of a to a standard normal deviate. The reason we must do this is that $\sqrt{a}$, rather than a, tends to come from a distribution that can be approximated by the Gaussian distribution when the sample's size is large.

The third difference is that the standard error used in the normal approximation to the Poisson is not dependent on the number of persons with the characteristic in the sample nor is it dependent on the number of observations in the sample. Instead, the standard error of $\sqrt{a}$ is equal to the same value regardless of the magnitude of a. Specifically, the standard error is equal to $\frac{1}{2}$ for all values of a. Thus, conversion of the square root of the number of persons with the condition is accomplished as shown in Equation 6.8.

$$z = \frac{\sqrt{a} - \sqrt{\lambda}}{\frac{1}{2}} \tag{6.8}$$

Now, we can rearrange Equation 6.8 algebraically to calculate an interval estimate for $\sqrt{a}$, the square root of the numerator of a probability or incidence. This, however, is not quite what we want. We would like to have an interval estimate of the population's incidence or probability rather than an interval estimate for the number of persons with the characteristic in the population (λ). To obtain an interval estimate for a probability or a rate, we square the limits of the confidence interval for $\sqrt{\lambda}$ (i.e., $[\sqrt{a} + (z_{\alpha} \cdot \frac{1}{2})]^2$) and divide those limits by the number of persons (for a probability) or by the number of person-years (for an incidence) in the sample. Thus, $(1 - \alpha)\%$ one-tailed confidence intervals are calculated as follows:

$$\theta = \frac{[\sqrt{a} + (z_{\alpha} \cdot \frac{1}{2})]^2}{n} \tag{6.9}$$

$$I = \frac{[\sqrt{a} + (z_{\alpha} \cdot \frac{1}{2})]^2}{\text{person-years}} \tag{6.10}$$

Two-tailed $(1 - \alpha)\%$ confidence intervals can be determined from the following:

$$\theta = \frac{[\sqrt{a} \pm (z_{\alpha/2} \cdot \frac{1}{2})]^2}{n} \tag{6.11}$$

$$I = \frac{[\sqrt{a} \pm (z_{\alpha/2} \cdot \frac{1}{2})]^2}{\text{person-years}} \tag{6.12}$$

Example 6.4 In Example 6.2, we estimated the incidence of diabetic retinopathy to be 0.02957 per year. Calculate an estimate of that incidence within which we are 95% confident that the population's value lies.

Since we have no reason to believe that the incidence of diabetic retinopathy in the population deviates in a particular direction from our point estimate, we should calculate a two-tailed confidence interval. For an interval estimate of an incidence, the normal approximation to the Poisson is used. Thus, we use Equation 6.12:

$$I = \frac{[\sqrt{a} \pm (z_{\alpha/2} \cdot \frac{1}{2})]^2}{\text{person-years}} = \frac{[\sqrt{68} \pm (1.96 \cdot \frac{1}{2})]^2}{2,300} = 0.02296, 0.03701 \text{ per year}$$

Therefore, we are 95% confident that the incidence of diabetic retinopathy in the population of diabetics sampled is within the interval from 0.02296 to 0.03701 per year.

Note. Unlike other interval estimates that we have calculated, the point estimate of incidence from Example 6.2 (0.02957 per year) does not lie in the middle of the confidence interval. That is because distributions of samples' estimates of incidence are not symmetric around a population's incidence. The same is true of probabilities of rare characteristics if the normal approximation to the Poisson is used.

INFERENCE

Inference for a single nominal variable can involve normal approximations to the binomial (Equation 6.4) or the Poisson (Equation 6.8) distributions. As with other univariable data sets, however, the occasions when we are interested in testing a hypothesis about a single nominal variable are quite limited. Remember that, to conduct statistical inference, we must be able to state a null hypothesis describing a specific parameter's value or a specific condition. In Chapter 4, we found one such hypothesis when we had a single continuous variable that was the difference between two measurements on each individual or pairs of individuals. In Chapter 5, we looked at a parallel procedure for ordinal data or continuous data converted to an ordinal scale by ranking. Now let us examine a similar procedure for nominal data.

Suppose that we are interested in comparing two treatments for which we can only evaluate an outcome measured using nominal data. An example might be two analgesics for which we ask each subject to choose which gave the greater pain relief. If the two treatments do not differ in their ability to relieve pain, we would expect half of the persons indicating a preference to favor the first treatment (and half to favor the second treatment). Thus, we can state a specific null hypothesis that the probability that a person showing a preference will favor the first treatment is equal to 0.50 in the population being sampled. Then, we can use the normal approximation to the binomial (since the probability stated in the null hypothesis is between 0.05 and 0.95). This procedure is demonstrated in Example 6.5.

Example 6.5   Suppose that we are interested in comparing aspirin with a new analgesic for treatment of arthritis. To make this comparison, we gave 50 arthritis patients a supply of both medications, labeling the new analgesic as drug A and aspirin as drug B. After a two-week period of time, we asked these patients which of the medications seemed to give greater relief from pain. Twelve of the 50 patients reported no preference for either of the medications. Of the 38 patients who reported a preference, 27 thought that drug A (the new analgesic) was more effective in relieving pain. Allowing a 5% chance of making a Type I error, test the null hypothesis that the medications are the same in their abilities to relieve pain in the population being sampled.

We have no prior reason to believe, if the null hypothesis is false, that it would be impossible for patients to prefer aspirin over the new medication. Therefore, we should consider the two-tailed alternative hypothesis that there is a preference for one of the two medications.

We start by calculating a point estimate for the probability that a patient in the population sampled will have a preference for the new medication. (Note that the results of inference would be exactly the same if we chose the probability that a patient would prefer aspirin instead of the probability that a patient would prefer the new medication.)

$$p\,(\text{Prefer new med}) = \frac{\text{Number preferring new med}}{\text{Number having a preference}} = \frac{27}{38} = 0.71$$

Next, we calculate the standard error of that point estimate. Here we use θ rather than p in Equation 6.5 since inference is performed assuming that the null hypothesis is true. According to the null hypothesis, $\theta = 0.50$.

$$SE_p = \sqrt{\frac{\theta \cdot (1 - p)}{n}} = \sqrt{\frac{0.50 \cdot (1 - 0.50)}{38}} = 0.0811$$

Finally, we convert the observed probability to a standard normal deviate using Equation 6.4.

$$z = \frac{p - \theta}{\text{SE}_p} = \frac{0.71 - 0.50}{0.0811} = 2.59$$

From Table B.1, we find that a standard normal deviate of 2.59 is associated with an area of 0.0048 in each tail. Therefore, the two-tailed P-value for this test of inference is 0.0096. Since 0.0096 is less than 0.05, we reject the null hypothesis.

The normal approximation to the binomial distribution can also be used for statistical inference performed on continuous (or ordinal[10]) data converted to a nominal scale. This type of conversion might be used for the same reason that continuous data are sometimes converted to an ordinal scale. That is to say, the assumptions of statistical procedures designed for continuous data can be circumvented by converting those continuous data to a nominal scale.

The conversion of continuous data to a nominal scale is accomplished by indicating whether the continuous data values are above or below a specified value. For example, we could convert changes in body weight (measured as continuous data) to a nominal scale by indicating whether or not each individual lost weight. When this approach is used for statistical inference on continuous data to avoid assumptions of the Student's *t* test, it is called the **sign test.** That name reflects the fact that the data are reduced to yes/no (plus/minus) indications of the state of a nominal variable. Then a normal approximation to the binomial is used to test the null hypothesis that the probability of differences with a particular "sign" (positive = yes and negative = no) is equal to some hypothesized value (usually 0.50).

Although you might encounter the sign test in health research literature, we do not recommend its use if the Wilcoxon signed-rank test could be used instead. When we convert continuous data to a nominal scale, we lose even more information than when we convert continuous data to an ordinal scale. In the latter case, we lose information about how far apart measurements are from one another, but we retain information about the relative order of the observations. When we convert to a nominal scale, however, we lose all quantitative information about the sample's observations except the direction in which they deviate from some specified value. This loss of information means a loss of statistical power and, thus, an increased chance of making a Type II error in inference.

---

[10]The procedures described here could be used on ordinal as well as continuous data. Since statistical procedures for ordinal data do not require assumptions about the distribution of estimates from all possible samples, however, there is little motivation for converting ordinal data to a nominal scale.

SUMMARY

Nominal data can be summarized by probabilities or by rates. Two special types of probabilities that we encounter in health research are prevalence and risk. Prevalence of a disease is the probability that an individual chosen at random from a population will have that particular disease.

$$\text{Prevalence} = \frac{\text{Number with disease at time } t}{\text{Total number at time } t} \tag{6.1}$$

Risk is the probability that a disease-free individual in the population will develop the disease during a specified period of time.

$$\text{Risk} = \frac{\text{Number developing disease from time 0 to time } t}{\text{Total number without disease at time 0}} \tag{6.2}$$

Rates are different from probabilities in that rates contain a measure of time in their denominator. The most commonly used rate in health research is the incidence of disease. Incidence is the number of cases of disease that develop per unit of person-time (or per person-year).

$$\text{Incidence} = I = \frac{\text{Number developing disease}}{\text{Number at risk} \cdot \text{Time period of observation}}$$

$$= \frac{\text{Number developing disease}}{\text{Number of person-years}} \tag{6.3}$$

Estimates of probabilities and rates do not come from Gaussian distributions. Instead, they are assumed to come from either binomial or Poisson distributions. Interval estimation and inference for probabilities and rates are usually accomplished using a normal approximation. The justification for using a Gaussian distribution for interval estimation and inference on probabilities and rates is that, like means of continuous data, estimates of probabilities and rates from all possible samples tend to come from distribution similar to a Gaussian distribution, especially when the samples' sizes are large (this is an application of the central limit theorem).

Standard errors for probabilities and rates are different from standard errors for continuous data. For probabilities within the range of 0.05 to 0.95, the standard error is a function of the probability itself.

$$\text{SE}_p = \sqrt{\frac{p \cdot (1 - p)}{n}} \tag{6.5}$$

For probabilities outside that interval that are estimated from large samples and for rates, the standard error used in interval estimation and inference is equal to a constant ($\frac{1}{2}$). Since we do not have to make a separate estimate of the variance of data in the population (as we do for continuous data), we do not have to use the Student's t distribution to take into account errors in estimating that variance. Rather, normal approximations to the binomial and Poisson distributions use the standard normal distribution.

In calculating interval estimates or performing tests of statistical inference on probabilities that are assumed to have binomial population distributions, we use the probability observed in the sample (p) as the point estimate of the probability in population (θ).

For inference:

$$z = \frac{p - \theta}{SE_p} \tag{6.4}$$

For one-tailed interval estimates:

$$\theta = p + (z_\alpha \cdot SE_p) \tag{6.6}$$

For two-tailed interval estimates:

$$\theta = p \pm (z_{\alpha/2} \cdot SE_p) \tag{6.7}$$

In interval estimation and inference on probabilities or rates that are assumed to come from a Poisson population distribution, however, we use only the square root of the numerator of the point estimate of the probability or rate (i.e., the number of times the event occurs) in our calculations. For inference using the normal approximation to the Poisson, we convert the square root of the numerator to a standard normal deviate.

$$z = \frac{\sqrt{a} - \sqrt{\lambda}}{\frac{1}{2}} \tag{6.8}$$

In the case of interval estimation, we first calculate a confidence interval for the square root of the numerator of the probability or rate. Then, the limits of that confidence interval are converted to limits of a confidence interval for the probability or rate by squaring and dividing by the number of persons or number of person-years in the sample.

For one-tailed interval estimates:

$$\theta = \frac{[\sqrt{a} + (z_\alpha \cdot \frac{1}{2})]^2}{n} \tag{6.9}$$

$$I = \frac{[\sqrt{a} + (z_\alpha \cdot \frac{1}{2})]^2}{\text{person-years}} \tag{6.10}$$

For two-tailed interval estimates:

$$\theta = \frac{[\sqrt{a} \pm (z_{\alpha/2} \cdot \frac{1}{2})]^2}{n} \tag{6.11}$$

$$I = \frac{[\sqrt{a} \pm (z_{\alpha/2} \cdot \frac{1}{2})]^2}{\text{person-years}} \tag{6.12}$$

As with other univariable analyses, statistical inference on a single nominal dependent variable is less often of interest than is estimation. The reason for this preference for estimation is the difficulty in formulating an appropriate null hypothesis. When such a null hypothesis can be constructed, however, we can use the normal approximation to the binomial or Poisson distributions to test it. A special case of inference is the sign test, which can be applied to continuous or ordinal data converted to a nominal scale. We do not recommend this conversion since it involves a substantial loss of information and it is seldom necessary to avoid assumptions of tests designed for continuous or ordinal data.

||| PRACTICE PROBLEMS

6.1 At the beginning of a three-year study of peripheral neuropathy among diabetic patients, we identified 300 insulin-dependent persons with juvenile-onset diabetes for at least ten years, none of whom had peripheral neuropathy. At the end of the period of observation, 18 of those persons had developed peripheral neuropathy. What is the point estimate for the three-year risk of peripheral neuropathy in the population from which this sample was drawn? What is the 95%, two-tailed interval estimate for that risk?

6.2 Assuming that the 18 persons who developed peripheral neuropathy became ill, on the average, in the middle of the three-year period of observation, what is the point estimate for the incidence of peripheral neuropathy in the population from which this sample was drawn? What is the 95%, two-tailed interval estimate for that incidence?

6.3 In a particular geriatrics practice, 1,200 of 2,000 patients were found to have senile cataracts. Calculate point and interval (95%, two-tailed) estimates of the population's prevalence of senile cataracts.

6.4 The national prevalence of senile cataracts among persons in the same age interval as the patients in Problem 6.3 is 0.45. Test the null hypothesis that the patients in that geriatrics practice are from a population with a prevalence of senile cataracts that is the same as the national prevalence. As an alternative, consider the possibility that the population's prevalence is different from the national prevalence. Allow a 5% chance of making a Type I error.

PART THREE

Understanding Bivariable Analysis

When a sample contains two variables, we use statistical procedures that are called bivariable methods. In bivariable analysis, the variable of primary interest (i.e., the one for which we would like to make estimates or test hypotheses) is called the dependent variable. The variable that describes conditions under which we would like to make those estimates or test hypotheses is called the independent variable. For example, suppose that we were interested in the relationship between the dose of an antihypertensive medication and the diastolic blood pressure of hypertensive patients. Here, we are measuring two variables[1] on each individual: dose and diastolic blood pressure. Diastolic blood pressure is the variable of primary interest. If we wish to make estimates, we are interested in estimating diastolic blood pressure. If our interest is in inference, we will test a null hypothesis that makes some statement about diastolic blood pressure. Dose, on the other hand, sets the conditions for either estimation or inference. In estimation, our interest will be in making estimates of the diastolic blood pressure that would be expected for patients receiving a specific dose. In inference, our null hypothesis would be that diastolic blood pressure is the same, regardless of dose. Thus, diastolic blood pressure is the dependent variable and dose is the independent variable.

The ability to distinguish between the dependent and independent variables is an important part of learning to select an appropriate statistical procedure. This usually can be accomplished by asking ourselves which variable in a set of variables is of primary interest. That variable is then the dependent variable. Sometimes, however, a set of variables might contain more than one variable that is of primary interest in addressing different research questions. For example, suppose that we were studying methods for prevention of coronary heart disease. In such a study, we might measure two different variables. One of these might measure morbidity and the other might measure mortality. For each of those variables, we would like to make estimates or test hypotheses. This would reflect our interest in two different research questions. The first question concerns

---

[1]Note that we are thinking about a pair of *variables* here in which *one value* for each of *two variables* is measured for each individual. This is different from a pair of *observations* of the same variable that we discussed in Chapter 4, in which *two values* of *one variable* are measured for each individual.

the effect of methods of prevention on coronary heart disease morbidity. The second question concerns the effect of those methods on coronary heart disease mortality. Thus, both of those variables are dependent variables. Most often in health research, we would conduct separate analyses to examine each of those dependent variables. It is even possible for the dependent variable in one analysis to function as an independent variable in another analysis. For example, when analyzing coronary heart disease mortality as the dependent variable, we might include coronary heart disease morbidity as an independent variable to permit us to take into account (i.e., control for) levels of coronary heart disease morbidity when examining mortality.

In the introduction to Part Two, Understanding Univariable Analysis, we learned that selecting a method of statistical analysis involves determination of the type of data represented by the dependent variable. Now, we have not only a dependent variable, but also an independent variable. The next step in choosing an analytic approach is to identify the type of data represented by the independent variable. In the flowcharts at the beginning of each of the remaining chapters, you will notice that determining the type of data represented by the independent variable is the first decision we are asked to make as part of the process of selecting a statistical procedure. The types of data that we consider for independent variables are the same as those used for dependent variables: continuous, ordinal, and nominal. Thus, for two variables, methods of analysis (called bivariable methods) are selected, in part, by answering the following three questions:

1. Which is the dependent and which is the independent variable?
2. What type of data is represented by the dependent variable?
3. What type of data is represented by the independent variable?

As were chapters in Part Two (Understanding Univariable Analysis), chapters in Part Three (Understanding Bivariable Analysis) are labeled according to the answer to the second question (i.e., according to the type of data represented by the dependent variable). Within each chapter, there are sections that address methods of analysis that are appropriate for independent variables representing continuous, ordinal, and nominal data.

CHAPTER 7

Continuous Dependent Variables

To understand how we analyze bivariable samples containing a continuous dependent variable, there are a few new concepts that we will need to discuss: covariance, partitioning sums of squares, variance of linear combinations, weighted averages, and purposive and naturalistic sampling. These might sound like difficult concepts, but you will see that they are merely extensions of concepts we already understand.

CONTINUOUS INDEPENDENT VARIABLE

As shown in Flowchart 5, when we have a continuous dependent variable and a continuous independent variable, we may have a choice of two types of analysis. One of these is commonly called **correlation analysis.** Correlation analysis is used to examine how two continuous variables vary together. That is to say, it is concerned with how much change in one variable is associated with a change in another variable. For example, if we consider diastolic blood pressure and dose of an antihypertensive medication, correlation analysis could tell us if diastolic blood pressure decreases or increases as dose increases and how strong the relationship is between those two variables. The other type of analysis is commonly called **regression analysis.** Regression analysis is used to estimate[1] values of the dependent variable for specific values of the independent variable. For example, regression analysis would allow us to estimate the diastolic blood pressure we could expect for a patient who receives a given dose of antihypertensive medication.

---

[1]Statisticians refer to estimation of values of the dependent variable in regression as **prediction.** We will avoid use of that term in this context for two reasons. First, we want to emphasize that estimation in regression is the same basic process as estimation elsewhere in statistics. Second, we do not want to imply that regression analysis can make estimates beyond the range of values in the sampled population (such as prediction of future events). We are concerned that the use of prediction here might give that impression.

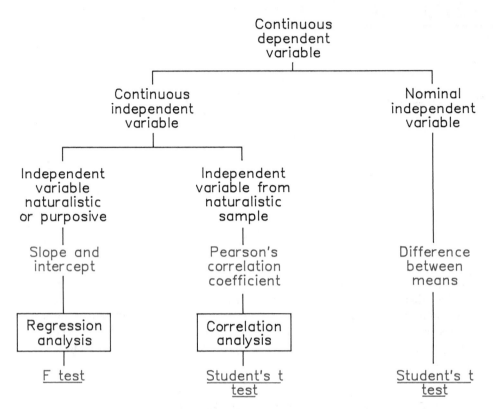

FLOWCHART 5 Bivariable analysis of a continuous dependent variable. Point estimates are indicated in red. Statistical procedures are in red and underlined. Common names for a general class of statistical procedures appear in boxes.

We have said that we may have a choice between correlation analysis and regression analysis. However, to use correlation analysis properly, a particular condition must be fulfilled. This condition places a restriction on the sampling method that was used to obtain values for the independent variable (see Flowchart 5).

To help you understand this restriction for correlation analysis, let us take a moment to review what we already know about sampling. Recall from Chapter 2 that we always assume that the sample we are examining with statistical methods is a random one. That is to say, we expect the distribution of values in the sample to differ from the distribution of values in the population from which the sample was drawn only by chance. The universality of this assumption, however, applies only to values of the dependent variable. When we have an independent variable, we assume that values of the dependent variable in the sample are a random sample of the dependent variable's values in the population *associated with each value of the independent variable*. In the example of diastolic blood pressure and dose of an antihypertensive agent, we assume that the sample's values of diastolic blood pressure for a specific dose are a random subset of the population's values of diastolic blood pressure associated with that dose.

The distribution of the sample's values of the independent variable may be a random sample of the distribution of those values in the population, or their distribution in the sample may be determined by the researcher. For example, if we were studying dose of a particular medication, we would probably plan our experiment so that a certain number of persons would receive each dose of interest. If we had a sample of 50 persons, we might assign 10 persons each to receive 5, 10, 15, 20, and 25 mg of the medication. Hence, no attempt would be made to produce a distribution of doses in the sample that were a random sample of any population to which we wish to apply the results of our study. Rather, that sample's distribution would be selected to allow us to have uniform statistical power in estimation of dose-specific responses. When a study is constructed in such a way that the researcher determines the sample's distribution of the independent variable, we say that a **purposive sample** was taken.

Purposive sampling is the usual way in which doses of a medication are assigned to persons in a study. When we think of naturally occurring independent variables such as dietary salt intake or serum cortisol levels, however, we can imagine collecting a sample in which the distribution of the independent variable is influenced only by its distribution in the population and by chance. For example, suppose we are interested in studying the relationship between diastolic blood pressure and dietary salt intake. One way to collect a sample of 50 persons would be to find 10 persons for each of 5 groups in which each group is identified by a specific level of salt intake. This would give us a purposive sample. Alternatively, we could collect a sample of 50 persons, regardless of their salt intake. Then, the sample's distribution of levels of dietary salt intake would be a random sample of the population's distribution. A sample in which values of the independent variable are randomly chosen from the population's values is called a **naturalistic sample.** In naturalistic sampling, we assume that the sample's distributions of both the dependent and independent variables are randomly drawn from their distributions in the population.

Regression analysis can be used regardless of how the independent variable has been sampled. Correlation analysis, on the other hand, assumes that the sample's distribution of the independent variable is representative of its distribution in the population (i.e., that a naturalistic sample has been taken). Violation of this assumption can lead to errors in estimating the strength of the association between the independent and dependent variables in the population. Misuse of correlation analysis is a common mistake in health research. As we read the health research literature, we must make sure that a naturalistic sample has been taken if correlation analysis has been used to analyze data.

CORRELATION ANALYSIS

ESTIMATION   Correlation analysis is concerned with the direction and strength of the association between two continuous variables. In other words, it examines how two variables vary together, or their **covariance.** Covariance is closely related to variance of data except that covariance measures how much two variables vary or change *together,* while variance measures how much one variable itself varies or changes. Because of the close relationship between these two measurements of variation, we might expect the method of calculating covariance to be similar to the method for calculating variance. To examine this similarity, let us first recall (from Equation 3.2) how variance of data is estimated in a sample.

$$s^2 = \frac{\Sigma(Y_i - \overline{Y})^2}{n - 1} = \frac{\Sigma(Y_i - \overline{Y})(Y_i - \overline{Y})}{n - 1} \tag{7.1}$$

In Equation 7.1, we see that variance is estimated by adding up deviations of each observation from the sample's mean and then multiplying this result by itself, and dividing by the sample's size minus one. This same general procedure is used to estimate covariance, but we now need to consider *both* the dependent and independent variables. The first thing we need to do is to assign different letters to represent the independent and dependent variables. The convention is to use X for the independent variable and Y for the dependent variable. Then, we calculate the sample's estimate of the population's covariance,[2] as shown in Equation 7.2. The numerator of covariance is called the **sum of cross products.**

$$COV = \frac{\Sigma(Y_i - \overline{Y})(X_i - \overline{X})}{n - 1} \tag{7.2}$$

Recall that variance has a range from 0 to $+\infty$. In other words, variance can never have a negative value. Covariance, on the other hand, can have a positive or negative value.[3] A positive covariance value indicates that the two variables have a **direct** relationship. That is to say, as values of the independent variable increase, so do values of the dependent variable. A negative value of covariance indicates that the two variables have an **inverse** relationship. This implies that values of the dependent variable decrease as values of the independent variable increase.

To see how the covariance reflects the direction and the strength of the association between the independent and dependent variables, let us take a look at Figure 7.1. The graphs in Figure 7.1 are **scatterplots.** In a scatterplot, values of the dependent variable appear on the ordinate or Y-axis, and values of the independent variable appear on the abscissa or X-axis. Individual observations (called **data points**) are plotted according to their values of the dependent and independent variables.

If we draw lines in a scatterplot representing the means of the two variables (as we have done in Figure 7.1), we divide the scatterplot into quadrants. Data points in each of those quadrants have a particular effect on the value of the covariance. Observations that occur in the upper right-hand quadrant have values of the independent and dependent variables that are both greater than their respective means. For observations

---

[2]For a single continuous variable, we have assumed that the population has a Gaussian distribution. When we have two continuous variables together in the same analysis, we assume that the population consists of two Gaussian distributions combined into one distribution. This combined distribution is called a "bivariate normal distribution." The parameters of the bivariate normal distribution are the means and variances of the two continuous variables and their covariance.

[3]The range of covariance is from $-\sqrt{s_Y^2 s_X^2}$ to $+\sqrt{s_Y^2 s_X^2}$.

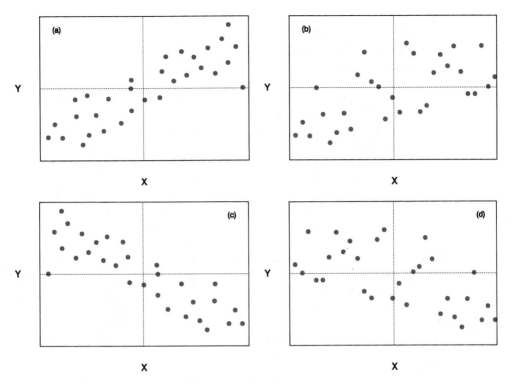

FIGURE 7.1 Scatterplots showing various relationships between dependent and independent variables: (a) strong direct association, (b) weak direct association, (c) strong inverse association, and (d) weak inverse association.

in this quadrant, both deviations in the numerator of the covariance will be positive. Those observations will increase the magnitude of the covariance's estimate in a positive direction. Observations that occur in the lower left-hand quadrant have independent and dependent variable values that are both less than their respective means. For observations in this quadrant, both deviations in the numerator of the covariance will be negative. Since the product of two negative values is equal to a positive value, those observations will also increase the magnitude of the covariance's estimate in a positive direction. Notice that, for direct associations between the independent and dependent variables, the majority of the data points are in these two quadrants. That arrangement of data points will result in a positive value of the covariance. The stronger the direct association between the variables, the greater the proportion of observations that are confined to these two quadrants (the upper right-hand and the lower left-hand).

Now, let us examine inverse associations between the independent and dependent variables. With inverse associations, the majority of data points occur in the upper left-hand and the lower right-hand quadrants. In those quadrants, one of the variable's values is greater than the mean of that variable, and the other variable's value is less than its mean. Thus, one of the deviations in the numerator of the covariance will be positive and the other will be negative. Since the product of a positive number and a negative number is equal to a negative number, observations in these two quadrants will result in negative covariance. The stronger the inverse association between the independent and dependent variables, the greater the proportion of observations that are confined to these two quadrants.

Thus, covariance appears to reflect accurately the type and strength of the association between a continuous dependent variable and a continuous independent variable. Covariance has one drawback as a measure of the strength of the association between two continuous variables, however: the value of the covariance changes as the variance of the two variables changes. This is not a desirable property since we would like to think of the strength of the association between two variables as independent of how dispersed they are. For example, suppose that we measure serum cholesterol before and after some sort of intervention and we wish to measure the strength of the association between those two measurements. Most often, we would record serum cholesterol as so many mg/dl. If, however, we recorded serum cholesterol as mg/l, the variances of our measurements would be 1/100th those recorded as mg/dl. Similarly, the covariance of those two serum cholesterol measurements recorded as mg/l would be 1/100th those recorded as mg/dl, yet it is not logical to believe that the strength of the association should be different simply because we have used a different scale.

Example 7.1   Let us reconsider the clinical study described in Problem 3.4. In that study, eight patients known to be hypercholesterolemic had serum cholesterol levels (mg/dl) measured before and after a 30-day regimen on a drug designed to lower serum cholesterol levels. The following results were observed:

Patient	Before	After
1	281	269
2	259	245
3	272	271
4	264	248
5	253	229
6	297	276
7	312	289
8	275	260

Estimate the covariance between these two cholesterol measurements.

Before we calculate the covariance, let us take a moment to recall our previous interest in these data and to compare that to our current interest. In Practice Problem 3.4, we were interested in the mean of the differences in cholesterol levels before and after a 30-day drug regimen. When making point and interval estimates of the population's mean of differences from these data, we used the differences between paired values as our dependent variable and we had no independent variable. Thus, in Problem 3.4, these data represented a univariable data set. Now, however, we are interested in the association between the initial cholesterol level and the cholesterol level after treatment. In the present case, the cholesterol level after treatment is the dependent variable, and the cholesterol level before treatment is the independent variable.[4] Thus, these same data that represented a univariable data set in Problem 3.4 now represent a bivariable data set! It is important to understand that recognition of which variable is the dependent variable and how many variables a set of data contains both depend to some degree on the question being asked.

To solve the current problem (i.e., to estimate the covariance), we first need to calculate the sum of cross products (the numerator of covariance) for the two variables. To do that, we must calculate estimates of the means for the two variables. Using the sums at the bottom of the following table:

$$\overline{X} = \frac{\Sigma X_i}{n} = \frac{2,213}{8} = 276.625 \text{ mg/dl}$$

$$\overline{Y} = \frac{\Sigma Y_i}{n} = \frac{2,087}{8} = 260.875 \text{ mg/dl}$$

Then the deviations of each of those variables from their means and the cross products can be calculated as shown below:

Before (X_i)	After (Y_i)	$(X_i - \overline{X})$	$(Y_i - \overline{Y})$	$(Y_i - \overline{Y})(X_i - \overline{X})$
281	269	4.375	8.125	35.547
259	245	−17.625	−15.875	279.797
272	271	−4.625	10.125	−46.828
264	248	−12.625	−12.875	162.547
253	229	−23.625	−31.875	753.047
297	276	20.375	15.125	308.172
312	289	35.375	28.125	994.922
275	260	−1.625	−0.875	1.422
2,213	2,087	0	0	2,488.625

Using Equation 7.2, we estimate the covariance as follows:

$$COV = \frac{\Sigma(Y_i - \overline{Y})(X_i - \overline{X})}{n - 1} = \frac{2,488.625}{7} = 355.518 \ (\text{mg/dl})^2$$

[4]In calculation of covariance (or in any other aspect of correlation analysis), the distinction between which variable is the dependent variable and which is the independent variable is less important than it is for other types of analyses. The reason for this is that the same assumptions (e.g., that the observations result from a random sample of the population's values) are made for both variables. Identical results will be obtained regardless of which variable is considered to be the dependent variable.

Now, let us examine the effect of the scale of measurement that we use on the covariance's estimate. Rather than using mg/dl, suppose we measured serum cholesterol as mg/l. Then the previous table would be as follows:

Before (X_i)	After (Y_i)	($X_i - \overline{X}$)	($Y_i - \overline{Y}$)	($Y_i - \overline{Y}$) ($X_i - \overline{X}$)
28.1	26.9	0.4375	0.8125	0.35547
25.9	24.5	−1.7625	−1.5875	2.79797
27.2	27.1	−0.4625	1.0125	−0.46828
26.4	24.8	−1.2625	−1.2875	1.62547
25.3	22.9	−2.3625	−3.1875	7.53047
29.7	27.6	2.0375	1.5125	3.08172
31.2	28.9	3.5375	2.8125	9.94922
27.5	26.0	−0.1625	−0.0875	0.01422
221.3	208.7	0	0	24.88625

And the covariance's estimate would be:

$$COV = \frac{\Sigma(Y_i - \overline{Y})(X_i - \overline{X})}{n - 1} = \frac{24.88625}{7} = 3.55518 \ (mg/l)^2$$

which is 1/100th of the estimate for serum cholesterol measured in mg/dl.

This effect of the scale of measurement makes covariance, by itself, not very useful as an indicator of the strength of association between the dependent and independent variables. Instead, we would like to be able to calculate a number that is the same regardless of the scale of measurement. In other words, we would like to correct for artificial differences in the variances of the data represented by the two variables, such as occurs when the scale of measurement changes. This can be done by simply dividing the covariance by the square root of the product of the two variances (Equation 7.3). This corrected covariance measurement is known as the **correlation coefficient.**[5] We use the symbol ρ (Greek letter rho) to indicate the population's value of the correlation coefficient and r to indicate the sample's estimate of ρ.

$$r = \frac{\dfrac{\Sigma(Y_i - \overline{Y})(X_i - \overline{X})}{n - 1}}{\sqrt{\dfrac{\Sigma(Y_i - \overline{Y})^2}{n - 1} \cdot \dfrac{\Sigma(X_i - \overline{X})^2}{n - 1}}} = \frac{\Sigma(Y_i - \overline{Y})(X_i - \overline{X})}{\sqrt{\Sigma(Y_i - \overline{Y})^2 \cdot \Sigma(X_i - \overline{X})^2}} \tag{7.3}$$

---

[5] The correlation coefficient described here is also known as Pearson's correlation coefficient. It is, by far, the most commonly used correlation coefficient for two continuous variables.

Example 7.2   Calculate the correlation coefficient for the serum cholesterol measurements in Example 7.1.

In Example 7.1, we found that the sum of the cross products for the two cholesterol measurements was equal to 2,488.625. To estimate the correlation coefficient, we must also calculate the sums of squares for the two variables.

Before (X_i)	After (Y_i)	$(X_i - \overline{X})$	$(X_i - \overline{X})^2$	$(Y_i - \overline{Y})$	$(Y_i - \overline{Y})^2$
281	269	4.375	19.141	8.125	66.016
259	245	−17.625	310.641	−15.875	252.016
272	271	−4.625	21.391	10.125	102.516
264	248	−12.625	159.391	−12.875	165.766
253	229	−23.625	558.141	−31.875	1,016.016
297	276	20.375	415.141	15.125	228.766
312	289	35.375	1,251.391	28.125	791.016
275	260	−1.625	2.641	−0.875	0.766
2,213	2,087	0	2,737.875	0	2,622.875

Then, using Equation 7.3, we find the following correlation coefficient:

$$r = \frac{\Sigma(Y_i - \overline{Y})(X_i - \overline{X})}{\sqrt{\Sigma(Y_i - \overline{Y})^2 \cdot \Sigma(X_i - \overline{X})^2}} = \frac{2,488.625}{\sqrt{2,622.875 \cdot 2,737.875}} = 0.9287$$

The correlation coefficient is a good measure of the direction and strength of the association between two continuous variables. It is not altered by changes that influence estimates of the variance of the data, such as a change in the scale of measurement. The correlation coefficient has a range from −1 to +1. A correlation coefficient equal to +1 indicates a perfect direct relationship between the dependent and the independent variables. In a perfect direct relationship, the value of the dependent variable *increases* by the same amount for each unit increase in the value of the independent variable. A correlation coefficient of −1 indicates a perfect inverse relationship. In a perfect inverse relationship, the value of the dependent variable *decreases* by the same amount for each unit increase in the value of the independent variable. A correlation coefficient of 0 indicates no relationship between the dependent and the independent variables. What we imply by no relationship between those variables is that there is not a consistent (i.e., in one direction only) change in the value of the dependent variable for each unit change in the value of the independent variable.

Other than for values of −1, 0, and +1, correlation coefficients, by themselves, are not easy to interpret. Take, for instance, a correlation coefficient of 0.50. We know that two variables with a correlation coefficient of 0.50 have a direct relationship that is not perfect. It would be a mistake, however, to think that an association with a correlation coefficient of 0.50 is half as strong as an association with a correlation coefficient of 1.00. To make this sort of interpretation, we need to examine the **coefficient of determination (R^2)**. The coefficient of determination is easily calculated by squaring the correlation coefficient (Equation 7.4).

$$R^2 = r^2 \tag{7.4}$$

The coefficient of determination helps us to interpret the value of a particular correlation coefficient by telling us the proportion of variation in the dependent variable that is associated with variation or changes in the independent variable. For a correlation coefficient of 0.50, the coefficient of determination is $0.50^2 = 0.25$. In other words, 0.25 (or 25%[6]) of the observed variability in serum cholesterol measurements among persons after the dietary intervention is associated with serum cholesterol measurements before the intervention. Therefore, a correlation coefficient of 0.50 describes an association that is one-quarter as strong as does a correlation coefficient of 1.00.

Example 7.3 In Example 7.2, we found a correlation coefficient of 0.9287 when examining the relationship between serum cholesterol measurements before and after an intervention. Convert that correlation coefficient to a coefficient of determination.

Using Equation 7.4, we find that a correlation coefficient of 0.9287 is equal to a coefficient of determination of 0.8625.

$$R^2 = r^2 = 0.9287^2 = 0.8625$$

Thus, we estimate that 0.8625 or 86.25% of the variation in serum cholesterol levels after treatment is due to (or at least associated with) the serum cholesterol levels prior to treatment.

So far, we have looked at the correlation coefficient as a measure of the strength of the association between two continuous variables and how that correlation coefficient can be interpreted by calculating the coefficient of determination. We have only discussed point estimates of those two coefficients. It is also possible to calculate an interval estimate for either the correlation coefficient or for the coefficient of determination. Calculation of these interval estimates, however, is somewhat complicated[7] and not often encountered in the health research literature. Therefore, we will not describe those interval estimates in *Statistical First Aid*.

INFERENCE   Inference, as you will recall from Chapter 3, is a process of assuming a specific value for a population's parameter and comparing the actual point estimate

---

[6] Often, coefficients of determination are reported as percentages. For example, a coefficient of determination of 0.25 could be said to indicate that 25% of the variation in the dependent variable is associated with or explained by the independent variable.

[7] Interval estimates for the correlation coefficient and the coefficient of determination involve conversion of those coefficients to Fisher transformed values.

from our sample to that hypothesized value. For a correlation coefficient, we most often assume that the population's value is equal to zero (meaning that there is no association between the two variables in the population). The assumption in the null hypothesis that the population's correlation coefficient is equal to zero is an important one. Correlation coefficients estimated from a sample's observations have a Gaussian distribution only when the population's correlation coefficient is equal to zero. The methods for statistical inference about correlation coefficients that we will consider in *Statistical First Aid* depend on a Gaussian distribution. Thus, the methods described in *Statistical First Aid* are applicable only when we are testing the null hypothesis that the population's correlation coefficient is equal to zero.

The first thing we need to test the null hypothesis that the population's correlation coefficient is equal to zero is a standard error for the correlation coefficient. Equation 7.5 shows that the standard error for the correlation coefficient includes the point estimate of the correlation coefficient.

$$SE_r = \sqrt{\frac{1 - r^2}{n - 2}} \qquad (7.5)$$

Recall from Chapter 6 that we used the standard normal distribution when testing hypotheses about a probability from a binomial distribution. The explanation for the use of the standard normal distribution was that the standard error of a probability from the binomial distribution was a function of the sample's size and the estimate of the population's probability. Since we do not need to take uncertainty in estimation of the population's probability into account twice, there was no need to penalize ourselves for any uncertainty in estimation of the standard error. At first, it might seem that we have a parallel situation with the correlation coefficient. The correlation coefficient, however, is much more complicated than is a probability.

As we learned in Chapter 6, a probability is simply the number of persons with a characteristic divided by the total number of persons. Only the numerator of a sample's estimate of a probability is in doubt (i.e., the sample's size is known precisely). Therefore, a probability estimated from a sample contains only one number that must be estimated. A correlation coefficient, on the other hand, contains the estimate of the covariance divided by the square root of the product of the variances of the two variables (Equation 7.3). To make these calculations, we must estimate two other population's parameters: the mean of the dependent variable and the mean of the independent variable. We are uncertain about the population's values of those means. Since they are included in the estimate of the standard error, we must penalize ourselves for this uncertainty as we did in estimation and inference for the mean (Chapter 4). Thus, when testing the null hypothesis that the population's correlation coefficient is equal to zero, we use the Student's t distribution with $n - 2$ degrees of freedom (we lose two degrees of freedom since we are estimating two population's means).

$$t = \frac{r - \rho_0}{SE_r} = \frac{r - 0}{SE_r} \qquad (7.6)$$

Example 7.4 Test the null hypothesis that the correlation coefficient obtained in Example 7.2 is equal to zero versus the alternative that it is not equal to zero. Allow a 5% chance of making a Type I error.

In Example 7.2, we estimated the population's correlation coefficient to be equal to 0.9287 from a sample of eight hypercholesterolemic patients. To test the null hypothesis that the population's correlation coefficient is actually equal to zero, we must first calculate the standard error of this correlation coefficient. We do that by using Equation 7.5.

$$SE_r = \sqrt{\frac{1 - r^2}{n - 2}} = \sqrt{\frac{1 - 0.9287^2}{8 - 2}} = 0.1514$$

Then, using Equation 7.6, we convert our sample's estimate of the population's correlation coefficient to a Student's t value.

$$t = \frac{r - \rho_0}{SE_r} = \frac{0.9287 - 0}{0.1514} = 6.134$$

That Student's t value is associated with $8 - 2 = 6$ degrees of freedom. From Table B.2, we find that a Student's t value for 6 degrees of freedom and an α of 0.05 split between the two tails of its distribution is equal to 2.447. Since our calculated Student's t value (6.134) is greater than the value in the table (2.447), we reject the null hypothesis that the population's correlation coefficient is actually equal to zero and accept, by elimination, that it is not equal to zero.   ▭

REGRESSION ANALYSIS

ESTIMATION   In correlation analysis, we were concerned with estimating the strength of the association between two continuous variables. In regression analysis, we are concerned with estimating the components of a mathematical model that reflects the relationship between the dependent and independent variables in the population. To do this, we first make the assumption that the relationship is a straight line.[8]

Two population's parameters are needed to describe a straight line (Equation 7.7). They are the intercept (called α) and the slope (called β).[9]

$$Y = \alpha + \beta X \tag{7.7}$$

Figure 7.2 shows a straight line and its relationship to the intercept and slope. We can think of the intercept as the elevation of the line above the X-axis. Mathematically, it is the value of the dependent variable when the independent variable is equal to zero. The slope can be thought of as an indicator of how fast the line leaves or approaches the X-axis. Mathematically, the slope is the number of units that the dependent variable changes for each unit change in the independent variable.

---

[8] It is because of this assumption that regression analysis is sometimes referred to as **linear regression** or **simple linear regression**. A straight-line relationship is also assumed in correlation analysis.

[9] It is unfortunate that α and β are used to symbolize the slope and intercept in regression analysis as well as the probabilities of making a Type I and a Type II error in statistical inference. We should be careful to note that, in spite of the similarity of symbols, describing a straight line and statistical inference are separate procedures.

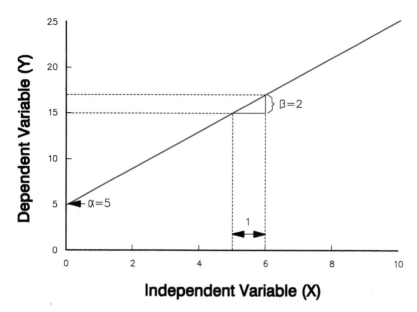

FIGURE 7.2 A straight line and its relationship to the intercept (α) and the slope (β). The intercept is the value of the dependent variable (here, equal to 5) when the independent variable is equal to zero. The slope is the amount that values of the dependent variable change (here, equal to 2) as values of the independent variable change one unit.

Equation 7.7 implies that, in the population, there is one and only one value of the dependent variable corresponding to each value of the independent variable. This is not really how we think of the relationship between the dependent and independent variables in statistics. Rather, we assume that there is a large number of values of the dependent variable in the population corresponding to each value of the independent variable. The distribution of those values of the dependent variable in the population is assumed to be a Gaussian distribution (Figure 7.3).

The specific value of the dependent variable that lies on the straight line in Figure 7.3 is the mean of the distribution of dependent variable values corresponding to a particular value of the independent variable. Thus, a more accurate mathematical description of the straight-line relationship between the dependent and independent variables includes the mean of the dependent variable. Equation 7.8 illustrates this relationship:

$$\mu_{Y_X} = \alpha + \beta X \tag{7.8}$$

where μ_{Y_X} = the population's mean of the dependent variable corresponding to a specific value of the independent variable.

Our first task in regression analysis is to estimate values for the population's slope and intercept from the sample's observations. The sample's estimates of the intercept

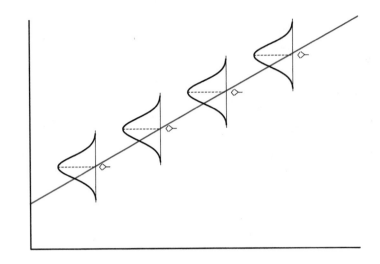

Independent Variable (X)

FIGURE 7.3 An illustration of the way in which we think of the relationship between the dependent and independent variables in statistics. For each value of the independent variable, we assume that there is a large number of values of the dependent variable that have a Gaussian distribution.

and slope are symbolized by a and b. To distinguish it from the sample's estimate of the overall mean of the dependent variable $(\overline{Y})$, we symbolize the estimate of the mean of the dependent variable corresponding to a specific value of the independent variable (μ_{Y_x}) as $\hat{Y}$ (called "Y hat"). Thus, the sample's estimate of the straight-line relationship between the dependent and independent variables is as follows:

$$\hat{Y} = a + bX \tag{7.9}$$

Our job now is to choose values of a and b that describe a straight line that best fits the observations in the sample. To understand how we do this, let us take a look at the relationship between those observations and the best-fitting straight line (Figure 7.4).

For each value of the dependent variable observed in the sample (Y_i), there is a corresponding value estimated by the straight line $(\hat{Y}_i)$. If we take each difference between an observed value of the dependent variable and its value estimated from the regression equation, square that difference, and add up all the squared differences $[\Sigma(Y_i - \hat{Y}_i)^2]$, we would find that different lines give us different sums. We want to choose the particular straight line that best fits our observations. That is tantamount to wanting the particular straight line that gives us the smallest sum of the squared differences between the observed and estimated values of the dependent variable. The

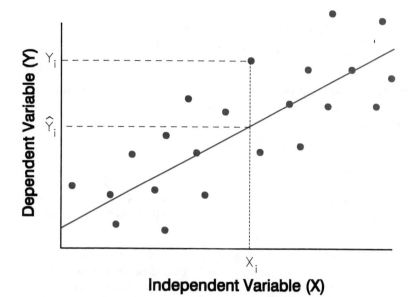

Independent Variable (X)

FIGURE 7.4 The relationship between observations obtained in a sample (points) and the best-fitting straight line. Least squares regression analysis finds the straight line that minimizes the differences between the observed values of the dependent variable (Y_i) and the values estimated by the straight line ($\hat{Y}_i$).

procedure that we use to find this straight line is, thus, called the method of **least squares.**

The first parameter[10] of the least squares regression line that we estimate is the slope. We can find the slope of the line that minimizes the square of the sum of the differences between the observed and estimated values of the dependent variable if we use the following calculation:

$$b = \frac{\Sigma(Y_i - \overline{Y})(X_i - \overline{X})}{\Sigma(X_i - \overline{X})^2} \qquad (7.10)$$

To estimate the intercept of the line, we use our estimate of the slope and the knowledge that the best-fit line will always pass through the point corresponding to

---

[10] Previously, we have used the term "parameter" to refer to the population's mean, variance, or probability that tells us about the shape of the population's distribution. Actually, a parameter is any single number that describes the population's data. Thus, the slope and the intercept of the straight line estimating values of the dependent variable corresponding to values of the independent variable in the population are also parameters.

the means of both the dependent and independent variables.[11] Thus, the overall mean of the dependent variable can be found by the following calculation:

$$\overline{Y} = a + b\overline{X} \tag{7.11}$$

We know the means of the dependent and independent variables in the sample and the sample's estimate of the slope. Therefore, we can estimate the intercept by algebraically rearranging Equation 7.11.

$$a = \overline{Y} - b\overline{X} \tag{7.12}$$

Example 7.5   Estimate a regression line describing serum cholesterol levels after treatment as a function of serum cholesterol levels before treatment, based on the observations in Example 7.1.

To estimate a regression line, we need to calculate four things from the sample's observations: the sum of the cross products, the sums of squares for the independent variable, and the means for both variables. All of these have been calculated in previous examples. In Example 7.1, we found that the sample's mean for the dependent variable (serum cholesterol after treatment) is equal to 260.875 mg/dl; the sample's mean for the independent variable (serum cholesterol before treatment) is equal to 276.625 mg/dl; and the sum of the cross products is equal to 2,488.625 (mg/dl)^2. In Example 7.2, we found that the sum of squares for the independent variable is equal to 2,737.875 (mg/dl)^2. Those results are summarized in mathematical notation below:

$$\Sigma(Y_i - \overline{Y})(X_i - \overline{X}) = 2{,}488.625 \ (mg/dl)^2$$
$$\Sigma(X_i - \overline{X})^2 = 2{,}737.875 \ (mg/dl)^2$$
$$\overline{Y} = 260.875 \ mg/dl \qquad \overline{X} = 276.625 \ mg/dl$$

The first part of the equation for the regression line that we estimate is the slope. The slope of the sample's observations is calculated using Equation 7.10.

$$b = \frac{\Sigma(Y_i - \overline{Y})(X_i - \overline{X})}{\Sigma(X_i - \overline{X})^2} = \frac{2{,}488.625}{2{,}737.875} = 0.909$$

Next, we estimate the intercept. The intercept of the sample's observations is calculated using Equation 7.12.

$$a = \overline{Y} - b\overline{X} = 260.875 - (0.909 \cdot 276.625) = 9.423 \ mg/dl$$

Thus, the estimated regression equation is:

$$\hat{Y} = 9.423 + 0.909X$$

[11]It can be shown mathematically to always be true that the sum of the squared deviations between observed and expected values of the dependent variable will be at a minimum when and only when the regression line passes through the means of both the dependent and independent variables. Remember that the mean is the most frequent value of a variable from a Gaussian distribution. Thus, it is the single value we are best able to estimate.

We have seen how we can calculate point estimates for the slope and the intercept of the straight line that allow estimation of values of the dependent variable for each value of the independent variable. These point estimates are our single best guess at their corresponding values in the population. Like point estimates of the mean, however, the point estimates of the slope and intercept have a very low probability of being exactly equal to the population's slope and intercept. The solution to this problem in regression analysis is the same as the solution in estimation of the mean. Specifically, we could calculate confidence intervals for the slope and intercept.[12] This is done less often for the slope and intercept than for the mean in health research. For this reason and because of the close relationship between interval estimation and inference, we will not discuss the mechanics of interval estimation as part of regression analysis in *Statistical First Aid*.

INFERENCE   As we have learned in previous chapters, an important component in statistical hypothesis testing is the variation of values of the dependent variable. Up to now, we have considered only one type of variation of data which is expressed by the variance (or its square root, the standard deviation). In Chapter 3, we found that the variance of data is estimated in the sample by dividing the sum of squares by the sample's size minus one (Equation 7.13).

$$s^2 = \frac{\Sigma(Y_i - \overline{Y})^2}{n - 1}$$

(7.13)

In regression analysis, we can think of more than one source of variation of data represented by the dependent variable. In fact, there are three ways to think about variation of values of a continuous dependent variable when we have a continuous independent variable. To understand inference in regression analysis, it is helpful to examine these sources of variation.

One of the sources of variation of data in regression analysis is the same as the variation with which we are already familiar. In regression analysis, it convenient to think of the variance of data represented by the dependent variable as calculated in Equation 7.13 as a measure of the **total variation** of values of the dependent variable. The numerator in Equation 7.13 is called the **total sum of squares,** and the denominator is called the **total degrees of freedom.** In regression analysis, the total sum of squares divided by the total degrees of freedom is called the **total mean square.** Only the name is new, however. The total mean square is exactly the same as the variance of data represented by the dependent variable.

$$s^2 = \frac{\Sigma(Y_i - \overline{Y})^2}{n - 1} = \frac{\text{Total sum of squares}}{\text{Total degrees of freedom}} = \text{Total mean square}$$

(7.14)

The numerator and the denominator of the total mean square (i.e., the variance of data represented by the dependent variable) each consist of two components of special

---

[12] We also can calculate interval estimates for estimated values of the dependent variable.

interest in regression analysis. Dividing a sum of squares into its component parts is a useful process that we will encounter in several statistical procedures. This process is called **partitioning the sum of squares.**

We touched on one of the components of the total sum of squares in our discussion of the least squares method for determining the regression line. This is a measure of the variation of data resulting from differences between the sample's observations and the estimated straight line. It is referred to as the **residual sum of squares.** The residual sum of squares is the sum of the squared differences between the observations and the corresponding estimates from the straight line $[\Sigma(Y_i - \hat{Y}_i)^2]$.

The degrees of freedom of the residual sum of squares is equal to the total number of observations minus the number of parameters that must be estimated to calculate the residual sum of squares. To calculate the residual sum of squares, we must first estimate the parameters of the straight line so that we can calculate $\hat{Y}_i$. Thus, the two parameters that we have to estimate to calculate the residual sum of squares are the population intercept and slope. Therefore, the value of the **residual degrees of freedom** is found by subtracting two from the sample's size. The residual sum of squares divided by the residual degrees of freedom is called the **residual mean square** $(s_{Y|X}^2$ or the variance of Y given $X)$.

$$s_{Y|X}^2 = \frac{\Sigma(Y_i - \hat{Y}_i)^2}{n - 2} = \frac{\text{Residual sum of squares}}{\text{Residual degrees of freedom}} = \text{Residual mean square} \quad (7.15)$$

Thus, we can calculate part of the total variation in data represented by the dependent variable. This is the residual or *unexplained* variation in values of the dependent variable after we utilize the information about those values provided by the regression line. The rest of the variation of data, therefore, must be that which is *explained* by the regression line. We called the variation in data represented by the dependent variable that is explained by the regression line the **regression sum of squares.** One way to calculate the regression sum of squares is by summing the squared differences between the overall mean of the dependent variable and the estimated values $[\Sigma(\hat{Y}_i - \overline{Y})^2]$. It is easier, however, to recognize that the residual sum of squares and the regression sum of squares added together equal the total sum of squares. Thus, the regression sum of squares can be found by subtracting the residual sum of squares from the total sum of squares.[13]

$$\text{Regression sum of squares} = \text{Total sum of squares} - \text{Residual sum of squares}$$
$$= \Sigma(Y_i - \overline{Y})^2 - \Sigma(Y_i - \hat{Y}_i)^2 \quad (7.16)$$

The **regression degrees of freedom** can also be found by subtracting the residual degrees of freedom from the total degrees of freedom. In bivariable regression analysis,

---

[13] Note that we can add the residual and regression sums of squares to obtain the total sum of squares. We also can add the residual and regression degrees of freedom and obtain the total degrees of freedom. We *cannot*, however, add the residual and regression mean squares and obtain the total mean square (this must be found by dividing the total sum of squares by the total degrees of freedom). Remembering this distinction will help you to avoid a mistake commonly made by students of statistics.

the value of the regression degrees of freedom is always equal to one $[(n - 1) - (n - 2) = 1]$.

Regression degrees of freedom

$$= \text{Total degrees of freedom} - \text{Residual degrees of freedom} \quad \text{(7.17)}$$

$$= (n - 1) - (n - 2) = 1$$

The regression sum of squares divided by the regression degrees of freedom is equal to the **regression mean square** (S^2_{reg}).

$$s^2_{\text{reg}} = \frac{\Sigma(\acute{Y}_i - \overline{Y})^2}{1} = \frac{\text{Regression sum of squares}}{\text{Regression degrees of freedom}} \quad \text{(7.18)}$$

$$= \text{Regression mean square}$$

Let us take a moment to think about the regression mean square and what it tells us about regression analysis. A regression line gives us a value for the dependent variable that is our best guess at the population's value that corresponds to a specific value of the independent variable. If we did not know the relationship between the dependent and independent variables, our best guess for a value of the dependent variable would be the mean of the dependent variable (see Chapter 2). The way that we calculate the regression sum of squares reflects this fact. To calculate the regression sum of squares, we sum the squared differences between our best guess knowing the regression line $(\acute{Y})$ and our best guess not knowing the regression line $(\overline{Y})$. Thus, the degree to which our ability to guess the population's mean is improved by knowing the relationship between the dependent and independent variables is reflected in the magnitude of the regression sum of squares.

Example 7.6   Estimate the three sources of variation for data represented by the dependent variable (serum cholesterol after treatment) in the population from which the observations in Example 7.1 were drawn.

First, let us estimate the total variation of data represented by the dependent variable. In Example 7.2, we calculated the sum of the squared deviations between the sample's values of the dependent variable and the mean of that variable. This total sum of squares was equal to 2,622.875 $(\text{mg/dl})^2$. The value of the total degrees of freedom is equal to the sample's size minus one or $8 - 1 = 7$. Remember that the total mean square is just another name for the variance of the dependent variable, and it is calculated by dividing the total sum of squares by the total degrees of freedom (Equation 7.14):

$$s^2 = \text{Total mean square} = \frac{\text{Total sum of squares}}{\text{Total degrees of freedom}}$$

$$= \frac{\Sigma(Y_i - \overline{Y})^2}{n - 1} = \frac{2,622.875}{7} = 374.696 \ (\text{mg/dl})^2$$

Next, we estimate the variation in data represented by the dependent variable that is left unexplained by the regression equation. This residual mean square is calculated by dividing the residual sum of squares by the residual degrees of freedom. To calculate the residual sum of squares, we must use the regression equation to estimate values of the dependent variable for each observed value of the independent variable. That regression equation was estimated in

Example 7.5:

$$\hat{Y} = 9.423 + 0.909X$$

To calculate estimated values for the dependent variable, we substitute an observed value of the independent variable for X in the regression equation. For example, the estimated value of the dependent variable for the first value of the independent variable (281 mg/dl) is found as follows:

$$\hat{Y} = 9.423 + 0.909X = 9.423 + (0.909 \cdot 281) = 264.852 \text{ mg/dl}$$

Those estimated values of the dependent variable are then subtracted from each observed value of the dependent variable, and that difference is squared. This procedure is illustrated in the following table.

Before (X)	After (Y)	$\hat{Y}_i$	$(Y_i - \hat{Y}_i)$	$(Y_i - \hat{Y}_i)^2$
281	269	264.9	4.148	17.206
259	245	244.9	0.146	0.021
272	271	256.7	14.329	205.320
264	248	249.4	−1.399	1.957
253	229	239.4	−10.400	108.160
297	276	279.4	−3.396	11.533
312	289	293.0	−4.031	16.249
275	260	259.4	0.602	0.362
2,213	2,087		0	360.808

Then, the residual mean square is calculated by dividing the residual sum of squares by the residual degrees of freedom (Equation 7.15).

$$s_{Y|X}^2 = \text{Residual mean square} = \frac{\Sigma(Y_i - \hat{Y}_i)^2}{n - 2} = \frac{\text{Residual sum of squares}}{\text{Residual degrees of freedom}}$$

$$= \frac{360.808}{6} = 60.135 \text{ (mg/dl)}^2$$

Finally, we calculate the sample's estimate of the regression sum of squares by subtracting the residual sum of squares from the total sum of squares (Equation 7.16).

Regression sum of squares = Total sum of squares − Residual sum of squares

$$= \Sigma(Y_i - \overline{Y})^2 - \Sigma(Y_i - \hat{Y}_i)^2 = 2,622.875 - 360.808 = 2,262.067 \text{ (mg/dl)}^2$$

The regression mean square is found by dividing the regression sum of squares by the regression degrees of freedom (Equation 7.18).

$$s_{reg}^2 = \text{Regression mean square} = \frac{\Sigma(\hat{Y}_i - \overline{Y})^2}{1} = \frac{\text{Regression sum of squares}}{\text{Regression degrees of freedom}}$$

$$= \frac{2,262.067}{1} = 2,262.067 \text{ (mg/dl)}^2$$

So, there are three sources of variation of data represented by the dependent variable which we can measure in regression analysis. The total variation is the same as the variance of data represented by the dependent variable. In regression analysis, we can think of two components of the numerator and denominator of that total variation. One component is used to calculate the variation of data for which we are unable to account by knowing the regression line. The residual mean square calculated from the sample's observations estimates this variation. The other component is used to calculate the variation in data represented by the dependent variable for which we are able to account by the regression line. This source of variation is estimated by the regression mean square calculated from the sample's observations. These sources of variation are summarized in Table 7.1.

Recall that our purpose in examining the three sources of variation in regression analysis was to prepare us to perform statistical inference. When we tested inferences about means or probabilities in previous chapters, we began by calculating standard errors for those estimates. In regression analysis, we might wish to test hypotheses about the population's slope or the population's intercept. Thus, we need to calculate standard errors for estimates of the slope and intercept. Now that we understand sources of variation in regression analysis, we are ready to examine how those standard errors are calculated.

The standard errors for all estimates in regression analysis include the residual mean square ($s^2_{Y|X}$). Those standard errors are larger for larger residual mean squares. Thus, we can make more precise estimates when there is little unexplained variation in data represented by the dependent variable (i.e., when the residual mean square is

TABLE 7.1   The three sources of variation of data represented by the dependent variable in regression analysis with one independent variable. Note that the residual plus regression degrees of freedom equals the total degrees of freedom. Likewise, the residual plus the regression sums of squares equals the total sum of squares. The mean squares are found by dividing the sum of squares by the degrees of freedom.

Source	Degrees of Freedom	Sum of Squares	Mean Square
Total	$n - 1$	$\Sigma(Y_i - \overline{Y})^2$	$s^2_Y = \dfrac{\Sigma(Y_i - \overline{Y})^2}{n - 1}$
Residual	$n - 2$	$\Sigma(Y_i - \hat{Y}_i)^2$	$s^2_{Y|X} = \dfrac{\Sigma(Y_i - \hat{Y}_i)^2}{n - 2}$
Regression	1	$\Sigma(\hat{Y}_i - \overline{Y})^2$	$s^2_{reg} = \dfrac{\Sigma(\hat{Y}_i - \overline{Y})^2}{1}$

small). This is a relationship that we might have expected, for the same relationship exists between the variance of data and the standard error of the mean.

In regression analysis, however, there is an additional wrinkle. All standard errors in regression analysis also include the sum of squares of the *independent* variable $[\Sigma(X_i - \overline{X})^2]$. The sum of squares of the independent variable has an inverse relationship with the standard error of the distribution of estimates of values of the dependent variable. That is to say, as the sum of squares of the independent variable increases, the standard error of values of the dependent variable decreases. From this, we can conclude that the greater the variation in the independent variable, the more precise are our estimates of regression parameters.

At first, it might seem nonsensical that greater variation in the independent variable should lead to greater precision in estimation of values of the dependent variable. To understand why this relationship exists, imagine drawing a straight line through two points. If you had the choice of selecting two points that are close together or two points that are far apart, you would probably choose the points that are far apart to draw that line. You would feel more confident that you were drawing the line correctly the further the two points were from one another. For that same reason, regression analysis can estimate parameters of a straight line with greater precision when the observations are at extreme values of the independent variable.

Before we look at the specifics of how we test hypotheses about the slope and intercept, let us examine one more characteristic that these procedures share. Both procedures use the Student's t distribution rather than the standard normal distribution. The reasons for that choice are that both standard errors contain the residual mean square and that the residual mean square from the sample is only an estimate of that value in the population. Recall that the number of degrees of freedom of the residual mean square is equal to the sample's size minus two. That value is the number of degrees of freedom used to locate a Student's t value in Table B.2.[14]

First, let us examine how hypotheses about the slope can be tested. The standard error of the slope is the square root of the residual mean square divided by the sum of squares of the independent variable (Equation 7.19).

$$SE_b = \sqrt{\frac{s_{Y|X}^2}{\Sigma(X_i - \overline{X})^2}} \tag{7.19}$$

To test the null hypothesis that the slope of the line in the population is equal to some specific value (usually zero, but not always, as shown in Example 7.7). We convert the sample's estimate of the slope to a Student's t value (Equation 7.20).

$$t = \frac{b - \beta_0}{SE_b} \tag{7.20}$$

---

[14]We need not pay a penalty for insecurity about estimates of values of the independent variable, for the independent variable is assumed to be measured without error.

Example 7.7   First test the null hypothesis that the slope of the regression line estimated in Example 7.5 is actually equal to zero in the population versus the alternative that it is not equal to zero. Then test the null hypothesis that the slope of that regression line is actually equal to one in the population versus the alternative that it is not equal to one. In both tests, allow a 5% chance of making a Type I error.

First, let us consider why we might be interested in testing these specific null hypotheses. If the population's slope is equal to zero, then the value of the independent variable does not affect the estimated value of the dependent variable. We can see that this is true by looking at the regression equation. If the slope is equal to zero, then it does not matter what value of the independent variable is considered: the estimated value of the dependent variable will always be equal to the intercept.

$$\hat{Y} = \alpha + (0 \cdot X) = \alpha$$

In this example, that would imply that the level of serum cholesterol after treatment does not depend on the level before treatment. Rather, a population's slope of zero would suggest that the level of serum cholesterol after treatment is equal to a constant value (i.e., the intercept).

If the population's slope is equal to a value other than zero, then values of the dependent variable can be estimated, in part, from values of the independent variable. The simplest form of that relationship is when values of the dependent variable differ from values of the independent variable by a constant amount (i.e., the value of the intercept). That relationship occurs when the population's slope is equal to one.

$$\hat{Y} = \alpha + (1 \cdot X) = \alpha + X$$

In this example, that would imply that the level of serum cholesterol after treatment differs from the level before treatment by the same amount, regardless of the level before treatment. In this example, the amount that serum cholesterol changes would be equal to 9.423 mg/dl (the intercept).

Now, let us test those hypotheses. Both hypotheses are tested using Equation 7.20, and both involve comparing the calculated Student's t value to the value from Table B.2 corresponding to an α of 0.05 and $8 - 2 = 6$ degrees of freedom ($t = 2.447$). Both Student's t values also are calculated using the same standard error. To calculate the standard error, we need to recall that the residual mean square was found to be equal to 60.135 mg/dl^2 in Example 7.6 and that the sum of squares for the independent variable is equal to 2,737.875 mg/dl^2 (from Example 7.2). Then, the standard error for the estimate of the slope is calculated using Equation 7.19:

$$SE_b = \sqrt{\frac{s_{Y|X}^2}{\Sigma(X_i - \overline{X})^2}} = \sqrt{\frac{60.135}{2,737.875}} = 0.148$$

In testing the null hypothesis that the population's slope is equal to zero, we calculate (using Equation 7.20) the following Student's t value:

$$t = \frac{b - \beta_0}{SE_b} = \frac{0.909 - 0}{0.148} = 6.142$$

Since 6.142 is greater than 2.447 (from Table B.2), we reject the null hypothesis that the population's slope is equal to zero and accept, by elimination, the alternative hypothesis that the population's slope is not equal to zero.

Next, we calculate the Student's t value associated with the null hypothesis that the population's slope is equal to one.

$$t = \frac{b - \beta_0}{SE_b} = \frac{0.909 - 1}{0.148} = -0.615$$

Since the absolute value of -0.615 is less than 2.447, we cannot reject the null hypothesis that the population's slope is equal to one.   ▭

Next, let us consider testing hypotheses about the intercept. Like inference about the slope, inference about the intercept involves conversion of the point estimate to a Student's t value by subtracting the value of the intercept specified in the null hypothesis and dividing by the standard error for the sample's estimate of the intercept. That calculation is shown in Equation 7.21.

$$t = \frac{a - \alpha_0}{SE_a} \tag{7.21}$$

The intercept is the value of the dependent variable when the independent variable is equal to zero. The general procedure that we use for testing hypotheses about the intercept is not limited, however, to the situation in which the independent variable is equal to zero. Rather, it can be used to test the null hypothesis that the population's value of the dependent variable corresponding to any specific value of the independent variable is equal to any particular quantity. Even so, testing hypotheses about the value of the intercept in the population is not often of interest in health research.[15] We will not, therefore, examine the method that is used to calculate the standard error for the estimate of the intercept in *Statistical First Aid*.

The purpose of regression analysis is to estimate a straight line that describes the relationship between the dependent and independent variables. So far, we have looked at point estimation and inference for components of the straight-line equation. In addition to (or instead of) examining those components, it is often of interest to ask whether or not a straight-line relationship exists at all in the population from which our sample was obtained. The null hypothesis that addresses this question states that knowledge of values of the independent variable does nothing to improve estimation of values of the dependent variable. This is known as the **omnibus null hypothesis.**

To understand how we might address the omnibus null hypothesis, let us recall the three variance estimates that result from partitioning the total sum of squares. If the null hypothesis is true, each of those three (total mean square, residual mean square, and regression mean square) is estimating the same quantity, namely the variance of data represented by the dependent variable.[16] Thus, we can test the

---

[15]One circumstance in which this might be of interest is when we wish to determine if a dose equal to zero (i.e., no exposure to a drug) is associated with a particular level of the dependent variable.

[16]One way to think about the reason we expect all of these mean squares to be equal is to view the regression mean square and the residual mean square as "conditional" estimates of the population's variance that differ from the "unconditional" variance estimate (the total mean square) only if a certain condition is met. That condition is met when the regression line reduces some of the variation in estimation of values of the dependent variable. Under that condition, the regression mean square will be larger than expected and the residual mean square will be smaller than expected. Otherwise, on the average, they will be equal.

omnibus null hypothesis by determining whether these three variance estimates are equal.

We need only compare two of the three variance estimates to refute the contention that all three are equal. By convention, the estimates we compare are the regression mean square and the residual mean square. These variance estimates are compared as a ratio. This ratio is calculated by dividing the explained variation (regression mean square) by the unexplained information (the residual mean square). The ratio is called an **F ratio** (Equation 7.22). The F ratio does not have a Gaussian distribution; rather, a ratio of two variances has an **F distribution**.[17] We will see in a little while, however, that the F distribution is a member of the Gaussian family of distributions.

$$F = \frac{s^2_{\text{reg}}}{s^2_{Y|X}} = \frac{\text{Regression mean square}}{\text{Residual mean square}} \qquad (7.22)$$

When the regression line does nothing to reduce the variation in estimation of dependent variable values, the regression mean square is equal to the residual mean square. Under that circumstance, the F ratio will be equal to one. Thus, the omnibus null hypothesis is reflected in the F ratio by a value of one.

Table B.4 gives us various values of the F distribution. Notice that Table B.4 indicates only one-tailed α values. The reason for this is that alternative hypotheses concerning the F ratio are one-tailed only. If the omnibus null hypothesis is true (meaning that the regression mean square is equal to the residual mean square), then the population's F ratio will be equal to one. If the omnibus null hypothesis is not true, then the regression line must account for some of the variation in the dependent variable. Under this condition, the regression mean square must be larger than the residual mean square, and the population's F ratio must be greater than one. We consider it to be impossible that knowing the regression line would provide less information about values of the dependent variable in the population than not knowing the regression line. Thus, alternative hypotheses concerning the F ratio are always one-tailed in regression analysis.

When we use the Student's t distribution, the number of degrees of freedom is employed to take into account our insecurity in estimating the population's variance of data. By the same token, the F ratio contains two estimates of the variance of data in the population, each with its own degrees of freedom. Therefore, degrees of freedom in both the denominator and in the numerator must be taken into account when we use the F distribution. Notice that Table B.4 provides us with F values corresponding to different numerator and denominator degrees of freedom.

Example 7.8 Test the omnibus hypothesis for the regression line estimated in Example 7.5. Allow a 5% chance of making a Type I error.

To calculate the F ratio as shown in Equation 7.22, we need to know the regression mean square and the residual mean square. These were estimated in Example 7.6, where the regression

---

[17]The F distribution is named after Sir Ronald A. Fisher, a British geneticist and statistician who laid the groundwork for much of modern statistics.

mean square was 2,262.067 $(mg/dl)^2$ and the residual mean square was 60.135 $(mg/dl)^2$.

$$F = \frac{s^2_{reg}}{s^2_{Y|X}} = \frac{\text{Regression mean square}}{\text{Residual mean square}} = \frac{2,262.067}{60.135} = 37.62$$

We then compare this F ratio to the F value from Table B.4 corresponding to one degree of freedom in the numerator, $8 - 2 = 6$ degrees of freedom in the denominator, and an α equal to 0.05. That F value is equal to 5.99. Since 37.62 is greater than 5.99, we reject the omnibus null hypothesis.

When we discuss regression analysis with more than one independent variable in Chapter 10, we will find that testing the omnibus null hypothesis is quite interesting. It is helpful to learn about that test in the simpler situation in which we have only one independent variable, but it is not very useful here. The reason for a lack of enthusiasm about the omnibus null hypothesis in bivariable regression analysis is that, contrary to initial appearances, it tests nothing new. We tested the omnibus null hypothesis early in our discussion of bivariable regression analysis when we tested the null hypothesis that the slope of the regression line in the population is equal to zero.

To see why this is true, let us take another look at what is being tested in the omnibus null hypothesis. Recall that this hypothesis states that knowledge of values of the independent variable does nothing to improve estimation of values of the dependent variable (over knowledge of the mean of the dependent variable). There is only one situation in which this could be true. That would be when the regression line is flat or, in other words, the slope is equal to zero.[18] In that circumstance, the intercept would be equal to the population's mean and our estimates of values of the dependent variable would not be affected by different values of the independent variable.

$$\hat{Y} = \alpha + 0 \cdot \beta = \alpha = \overline{Y} \tag{7.23}$$

If both the Student's t test of the null hypothesis that the population's slope is equal to zero and the F test of the omnibus null hypothesis are testing the same thing, we might suspect that the Student's t distribution and the F distribution are related. In fact, they are. If you take the square root of the F value obtained in Example 7.8, you will find that it is equal to the Student's t value obtained in Example 7.7. In general, an F value with one degree of freedom in the numerator and $n - 2$ degrees of freedom in the denominator is equal to the square of a Student's t statistic with $n - 2$ degrees of freedom. Therefore, the F distribution is a member of the Gaussian family of distributions[19] by virtue of its relationship to the Student's t distribution.

---

[18] The slope is such an important parameter in regression analysis that it is often called the **regression coefficient** rather than the slope.

[19] Recall that a family of distributions includes those that are related in some mathematical manner (see Chapter 2). This does not imply, however, that the distributions in a family appear similar when examined graphically. In fact, the standard normal and Student's t distributions are symmetrical around the mean of the distribution. The F distribution is skewed (i.e., it has a long tail in one direction).

RELATIONSHIP BETWEEN CORRELATION AND REGRESSION ANALYSIS

In regression analysis, we estimate the parameters of a straight line that can be used in turn to estimate values of the dependent variable corresponding to specific values of the independent variable. A natural question to ask about this estimated straight line is: "For how much of the variability of the dependent variable does it account?" If we recall the sources of variation in regression, we can see a logical way to answer this question. The component of the total variation in data represented by the dependent variable that is explained by the straight line is reflected by the regression sum of squares. The total variation in data represented by the dependent variable is reflected by the total sum of squares. Therefore, the proportion of variation of data represented by the dependent variable for which the straight line accounts can be found by dividing the regression sum of squares by the total sum of squares. This is called the coefficient of determination (R^2).

$$R^2 = \frac{\Sigma(\hat{Y}_i - \overline{Y})^2}{\Sigma(Y_i - \overline{Y})^2} = \frac{\text{Regression sum of squares}}{\text{Total sum of squares}} \qquad (7.24)$$

Recall from our discussion of correlation analysis that the square of the correlation coefficient tells us the proportion of the variation of data represented by the dependent variable that is associated with the independent variable. This was also called the coefficient of determination (R^2). The use of identical terms in regression and correlation analyses to label this concept is not coincidental. In fact, these two coefficients are algebraically identical. The link is even stronger between regression and correlation analysis when we find that the square of the Student's t value used to test the null hypothesis that the population's correlation coefficient is equal to zero is exactly equal to the F value obtained when testing the omnibus null hypothesis for the regression line.

This close association between correlation and regression analyses might cause us to forget an important distinction between these two approaches to a continuous dependent variable and a continuous independent variable. That distinction is that correlation analysis is appropriate when and only when we have a naturalistic sample of values of the independent variable (see Flowchart 5). It is imperative that we do not forget this distinction, for we can create a correlation coefficient of almost any magnitude, depending on how the independent variable is sampled. If our method of sampling has no relevance to the distribution of the independent variable in the population for which we would like to estimate the correlation coefficient, then the sample's estimate of the correlation coefficient has no relevance to that population.

Since the coefficient of determination is simply the square of the correlation coefficient, it also is interpretable if and only if the independent variable has been sampled naturalistically. This is a common source of confusion since the coefficient of determination is often provided by computer programs when a regression analysis has been requested. We must keep in mind, however, that the coefficient of determination has meaning only when the distribution of values of the independent variable in the sample is representative of the distribution of those in the population (i.e., we have a naturalistic or random sample of the independent variable). Computer regression programs do not know when the coefficient of determination is an appropriate summary of the relationship between the dependent and independent variables. We must be prepared to ignore it unless the independent variable is from a naturalistic sample.

ORDINAL INDEPENDENT VARIABLE

When a sample contains a continuous dependent variable, we can choose among a variety of statistical procedures for continuous or nominal independent variables. There are not, however, any well-accepted procedures used in health research for a sample consisting of a continuous dependent variable and an ordinal independent variable. Such a sample is analyzed either by converting the continuous data represented by the dependent variable to an ordinal scale and using techniques discussed in Chapter 8 or by creating a collection of nominal variables from the ordinal data represented by the independent variable and using procedures described in Chapter 10.

NOMINAL INDEPENDENT VARIABLE

Recall that the purpose of an independent variable is to define conditions under which we make estimates or draw inferences about the dependent variable. When the independent variable is nominal, that variable identifies two groups[20] between which we compare values of the dependent variable. For example, suppose we are interested in comparing systolic blood pressure between two groups of individuals: one receiving drug X and the other receiving a placebo. The dependent variable in that case is systolic blood pressure, and the independent variable is a nominal variable that is an indicator of group membership (drug or placebo).

ESTIMATION

The most common method of comparing values of the dependent variable between two groups is by comparing the means of the two groups. Those means are compared by examining their difference. In the example of comparison of systolic blood pressure between persons receiving a drug versus those receiving a placebo, we would examine the difference between the means of systolic blood pressure measurements in the two groups. The reason for examining differences between means is that a linear combination (such as a sum or a difference) of means has a Gaussian distribution if the means have a Gaussian distribution.[21]

---

[20]Remember that, to a statistician, a nominal variable can contain only two values. Therefore, a single nominal independent variable divides a sample into two and only two groups. If the sample contains more than two groups, it must contain more than one nominal independent variable.

[21]Let us not forget the central limit theorem that tells us that means have a tendency to have a Gaussian distribution even if the data from which they are calculated do not.

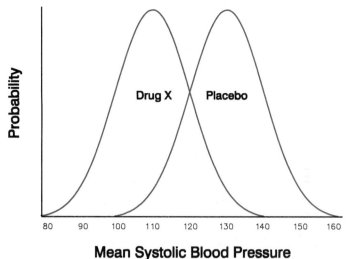

FIGURE 7.5 Distributions of means of systolic blood pressure measurements in two groups of individuals for all possible samples of a given size. For simplicity, we have assumed that the distributions differ only in location and that their standard errors are the same.

INFERENCE

The point estimate that we use when we have a continuous dependent variable and a nominal independent variable is the sample's difference between the means of the dependent variable values divided into groups according to the two values of the nominal independent variable. To test hypotheses (or calculate interval estimates) for that difference, we need to estimate the standard error of the difference. To see how that standard error can be calculated, let us examine a distribution of the differences between means for our example of systolic blood pressure measured in two treatment groups. Let us suppose that the distributions of the mean systolic blood pressures for a particular sample's size in each of the two groups are as shown in Figure 7.5.

Next, let us imagine the distribution of differences between mean systolic blood pressures that we could calculate in samples with means from the distributions illustrated in Figure 7.5. The range of means of blood pressure measurements in the treated group plotted in Figure 7.5 is from 80 to 140 mm Hg for the persons receiving drug X and is from 100 to 160 mm Hg for the persons receiving the placebo.[22] Therefore, the extreme values for differences between the means of blood pressure measurements among persons receiving drug X and those receiving the placebo is from −80 mm Hg (80 minus 160 mm Hg) to 40 mm Hg (140 minus 100 mm Hg). The distribution of those differences between means is illustrated in Figure 7.6.

[22]Actually, a Gaussian distribution is assumed to extend from −∞ to ∞. To think about a finite range of values, however, we are assuming that means that have a very low probability of being observed do not exist. We have used the same low probability to truncate distributions in Figures 7.5 and 7.6.

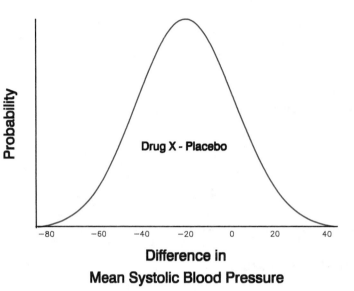

Probability

Drug X - Placebo

−80   −60   −40   −20   0   20   40

Difference in

Mean Systolic Blood Pressure

FIGURE 7.6 Distribution of differences between means of systolic blood pressure measurements in two groups. The standard error of this distribution is greater than the standard error of each distribution in Figure 7.5.

Notice that the spread of the distribution in Figure 7.6 is greater than the spread of the individual distributions in Figure 7.5. In fact, the range of the distribution of differences between means (−80 to 40 mm Hg = 120 mm Hg) is twice the range of each of the individual distributions of means (80 to 140 mm Hg = 60 mm Hg and 100 to 160 mm Hg = 60 mm Hg). If we were to calculate the variances of the means (i.e., the square of their standard errors) of the two distributions in Figure 7.5 and the distribution in Figure 7.6, we would find that the variance of the distribution of differences between means (Figure 7.6) is twice the variance of each of the distributions of means (Figure 7.5). In general, the standard error of a difference between means[23] is equal to the square root of the sum of their standard errors squared (Equation 7.25).

$$SE_{\overline{Y}_1 - \overline{Y}_2} = \sqrt{SE_1^2 + SE_2^2} \tag{7.25}$$

where

$SE_{\overline{Y}_1 - \overline{Y}_2}$ = standard error of the differences between the mean of group 1
and the mean of group 2

SE_1, SE_2 = standard errors for the means of groups 1 and 2

In Figure 7.5, we made the standard errors of the two distributions of means equal to the same value. We did this for simplicity, but it is most often the case that those standard errors are not equal to the same value. There are two reasons that they might differ. One reason might be that the variances of data in the two groups differ. The other reason might be that the number of observations in the two groups are not the

---

[23] This is also the standard error for a sum of two means.

same. To understand the influence of the variance of data and the number of observations in each group on standard error estimates, let us recall the calculation of the standard error for the distribution of means from Equation 3.4. The standard error of the mean is equal to the square root of the variance of data divided by the sample's size. Thus, we can rewrite Equation 7.25 as follows:

$$\mathrm{SE}_{\overline{Y}_1 - \overline{Y}_2} = \sqrt{\mathrm{SE}_1^2 + \mathrm{SE}_2^2} = \sqrt{\frac{s_1^2}{n_1} + \frac{s_2^2}{n_2}} \tag{7.26}$$

where

s_1^2, s_2^2 = variances for the distributions of data for groups 1 and 2
n_1, n_2 = number of observations in groups 1 and 2

Equation 7.26 can be used if the population's variances of data for the two groups (identified by values of the nominal independent variable) of values of the dependent variable are different or if they are the same. Most often, we assume that the population's variances of data represented by the dependent variable in the two groups are the same. That is to say, we assume that, if the population's distributions of data for the two groups differ, they differ only in their means and that the variances of data in the two groups are equal to the same value. There are two advantages to making such an assumption. First, calculation of degrees of freedom is much simpler if we assume that the population's variances of data are the same. Second, this assumption allows us to use all the observations in a sample (i.e., dependent variable values associated with both groups) to estimate a single variance of data rather than having to estimate separate variances for each of the two groups. Thus, we can have greater confidence in that estimate and greater power (ability to avoid a Type II error) in statistical inference.

When we assume that the population's variance of data represented by the dependent variable is the same in the two groups, we use information from both groups to estimate that population's variance. It is important to keep in mind that assuming that the population's variances of data represented by the dependent variable are equal does not require the sample's estimates of the variance observed in each of the two groups to have the same value. Rather, we expect that the sample's observations in each of those groups will give us somewhat different variance estimates by chance alone even if they are estimating exactly the same population's variance. To understand how we derive a single estimate of the population's variance of data from the sample's two estimates, we need to learn an important statistical concept: a **weighted average.**

In everyday language, the terms "average" and "mean" are considered to be synonyms. In statistics, we draw a distinction between these two. An average or weighted average is the sum of the products of each observation or estimate times a particular number (called a weight), divided by the sum of the weights. This is easier to see if we look at Equation 7.27:

$$\mathrm{Weighted\ average} = \frac{\Sigma(w_i \cdot Y_i)}{\Sigma w_i} \tag{7.27}$$

where w_i = weight for the ith observation or estimate.

The purpose of a weighted average is to provide greater weight to observations or estimates in which we have greater confidence and less weight to those in which we have less confidence that they truly reflect values in the population. A mean is a special type of weighted average in which each observation is given a weight equal to one. This implies that we are unable to say that one observation is closer to the population's mean than is any other observation.

$$\overline{X} = \frac{\Sigma(1 \cdot Y_i)}{\Sigma 1} = \frac{\Sigma Y_i}{n} \tag{7.28}$$

Now, let us apply this principle of weighted averages to estimation of the population's variance of data when we have estimates of that variance from two groups of dependent variable values. We know from Chapter 4 that the number of degrees of freedom is used in the Student's t distribution to reflect the degree of precision with which we can estimate the population's variance of data. The greater the number of degrees of freedom, the less the penalty we have to pay for estimating the population's variance from the sample's observations. Since degrees of freedom can be used in that context to reflect how precisely we can estimate the population's variance of data, it makes sense for us to use degrees of freedom as the weights for the variance estimates for each of the two groups in our sample. The weighted average of those two variance estimates using degrees of freedom as the weights is called a **pooled estimate** of the variance of data or the **pooled variance (s_p^2)**.

$$s_p^2 = \frac{\Sigma(df_i \cdot s_i^2)}{\Sigma df_i} = \frac{[(n_1 - 1) \cdot s_1^2] + [(n_2 - 1) \cdot s_2^2]}{(n_1 - 1) + (n_2 - 1)} \tag{7.29}$$

That pooled estimate of the variance of data is used in estimating the standard error of the difference between the means, as shown in Equation 7.30.

$$SE_{\overline{Y}_1 - \overline{Y}_2} = \sqrt{\frac{s_p^2}{n_1} + \frac{s_p^2}{n_2}} \tag{7.30}$$

Now that we understand how to calculate the standard error for the difference between two means, we are ready to see how we can test hypotheses about that difference. The most commonly addressed null hypothesis for a difference between means is that the difference in the population is equal to zero. This is tantamount to hypothesizing that the means for the two groups are equal to each other.

Hypothesis testing about the population's difference between two means involves converting the observed difference to a Student's t statistic with $(n_1 - 1) + (n_2 - 1) = n_1 + n_2 - 2$ degrees of freedom. That calculation is presented in Equation 7.31.

$$t = \frac{(\overline{Y}_1 - \overline{Y}_2) - (\mu_1 - \mu_2)}{SE_{\overline{Y}_1 - \overline{Y}_2}} \tag{7.31}$$

Example 7.9 Suppose we conduct a clinical trial of a drug that is designed to lower systolic blood pressure. We randomly assign 20 persons to receive either the drug (12 persons) or a placebo (8 persons) and observe the following results.

Patient	Treatment (X_i)	Systolic Blood Pressure (Y_i)
LM	Drug	120
ER	Placebo	127
TN	Drug	104
WS	Drug	111
OB	Placebo	120
CD	Placebo	133
AM	Drug	117
PH	Drug	105
FB	Drug	114
VG	Placebo	136
HJ	Drug	103
LK	Placebo	124
CH	Drug	100
SA	Placebo	140
WG	Placebo	132
MA	Drug	116
IG	Drug	106
ND	Drug	115
SH	Placebo	128
KJ	Drug	109

Test the null hypothesis that the means of systolic blood pressure in the population from which this sample was drawn are the same for persons taking the drug as they are for persons taking a placebo. As an alternative, consider the possibility that those means are not the same. Allow a 5% chance of making a Type I error.

Before we can test a hypothesis about the difference between the means of systolic blood pressure in the population, we need to calculate a point estimate for that difference. We do this by calculating the mean of each of the two groups in our sample and then calculating the difference between those means:

$$\overline{Y}_{\text{Drug}} = \frac{\Sigma Y_{i\,\text{Drug}}}{n_{\text{Drug}}} = \frac{120 + 104 + \ldots + 109}{12} = 110 \text{ mm Hg}$$

$$\overline{Y}_{\text{Placebo}} = \frac{\Sigma Y_{i\,\text{Placebo}}}{n_{\text{Placebo}}} = \frac{127 + 120 + \ldots + 128}{8} = 130 \text{ mm Hg}$$

$$\overline{Y}_{\text{Drug}} - \overline{Y}_{\text{Placebo}} = 110 - 130 = -20 \text{ mm Hg}$$

Next, we need to estimate the standard error for that difference. The first step in calculating the standard error is to estimate the population's variance of data represented by the dependent variable from each of the groups as if they were separate samples.

For persons receiving the drug:

Υ_i	$(\Upsilon_i - \overline{\Upsilon})$	$(\Upsilon_i - \overline{\Upsilon})^2$
120	10	100
104	−6	36
111	1	1
117	7	49
105	−5	25
114	4	16
103	−7	49
100	−10	100
116	6	36
106	−4	16
115	5	25
109	−1	1
1,320	0	454

$$s^2_{\text{Drug}} = \frac{\Sigma(\Upsilon_{i\,\text{Drug}} - \overline{\Upsilon}_{\text{Drug}})^2}{n_{\text{Drug}} - 1} = \frac{454}{12 - 1} = 41.273 \ (\text{mm Hg})^2$$

For persons receiving the placebo:

Υ_i	$(\Upsilon_i - \overline{\Upsilon})$	$(\Upsilon_i - \overline{\Upsilon})^2$
127	−3	9
120	−10	100
133	3	9
136	6	36
124	−6	36
140	10	100
132	2	4
128	−2	4
1,040	0	298

$$s^2_{\text{Placebo}} = \frac{\Sigma(\Upsilon_{i\,\text{Placebo}} - \overline{\Upsilon}_{\text{Placebo}})^2}{n_{\text{Placebo}} - 1} = \frac{298}{8 - 1} = 42.571 \ (\text{mm Hg})^2$$

Then, we calculate a pooled estimate of the variance of data by using Equation 7.29 to determine a weighted average of these two estimates of the population's variance of data.

$$s_p^2 = \frac{[(n_{Drug} - 1) \cdot s_{Drug}^2] + [(n_{Placebo} - 1) \cdot s_{Placebo}^2]}{(n_{Drug} - 1) + (n_{Placebo} - 1)}$$

$$= \frac{[(12 - 1) \cdot 41.273] + [(8 - 1) \cdot 42.571]}{(12 - 1) + (8 - 1)} = 41.778 \ (mm \ Hg)^2$$

Next, we use that pooled estimate of the variance in calculating the standard error for the difference between the means (Equation 7.30).

$$SE_{\overline{Y}_{Drug} - \overline{Y}_{Placebo}} = \sqrt{\frac{s_p^2}{n_{Drug}} + \frac{s_p^2}{n_{Placebo}}} = \sqrt{\frac{41.778}{12} + \frac{41.778}{8}} = 2.950 \ mm \ Hg$$

Now, we are ready to test whether the two means are equal by testing the null hypothesis that the difference between the means is equal to zero in the population. We do this by using Equation 7.31:

$$t = \frac{(\overline{Y}_{Drug} - \overline{Y}_{Placebo}) - (\mu_{Drug} - \mu_{Placebo})}{SE_{\overline{Y}_{Drug} - \overline{Y}_{Placebo}}} = \frac{110 - 130 - 0}{2.950} = -6.780$$

We compare this calculated Student's t value to the value from Table B.2 that corresponds to $12 + 8 - 2 = 18$ degrees of freedom and a two-tailed α equal to 0.05. Since the absolute value of the Student's t we have calculated (6.780) is greater than the value from the table (2.101), we reject the null hypothesis and accept, by elimination, the alternative that the means in the population are not the same in the drug and placebo groups (i.e., that the difference between the means in the population is not equal to zero).

In Chapter 3, we discussed the relationship between estimation and inference. One of the things we learned in that discussion was that we can perform a test of inference by examining an interval estimate. To do that, we simply observe whether or not the null value is included within the confidence interval. We can do that in univariable, bivariable, or multivariable analysis. There is one common error, however, that we should avoid.

Let us say that we encounter a health research report that compares serum cholesterol levels between two groups of persons. Let us further suppose that the report provides confidence intervals, but we are interested in testing the null hypothesis that there is no difference in means of cholesterol between the two groups (i.e., the population's difference between the groups' means is equal to zero). If the report provided a 95% two-tailed confidence interval for the population's difference between means, it would be entirely proper for us to observe whether or not that confidence interval included zero. If it did not include zero, we could reject the null hypothesis in favor of a two-tailed alternative hypothesis with a 5% chance of making a Type I error. If the confidence interval did include zero, then we should fail to reject that null hypothesis.

Now, suppose that the report contained univariable confidence intervals (i.e., separate confidence intervals for the mean serum cholesterol level in each group) instead of a bivariable confidence interval (i.e., for the difference between means). It might be tempting to observe whether or not those univariable confidence intervals overlapped and conclude that an overlap of univariable confidence intervals is tantamount to failing to reject the null hypothesis that the difference between the means in the population is equal to zero. If we give in to that temptation, we run the risk of making a mistake in our conclusion about the relationship between the means in the population. Univariable confidence intervals are calculated assuming that each mean is from a separate population with a distinct variance, whereas bivariable inference assumes that the two groups are part of the same population with a given variance. Univariable confidence intervals can overlap even when it would be appropriate to reject the bivariable null hypothesis that the difference between the means in the population is equal to zero.

Thus, we need to be very careful in using univariable confidence intervals to test bivariable hypotheses. However, if univariable $(1 - \alpha)\%$ confidence intervals do not overlap, then a test of the null hypothesis that the difference between the means is equal to zero would lead to rejection of that hypothesis, with a chance of making a Type I error equal to or less than α.[24] Also, if univariable confidence intervals overlap both *point estimates,* we can assume that bivariable inference would lead to failure to reject the null hypothesis. The limits of many univariable confidence intervals, however, overlap without including both point estimates. In this situation, we cannot know what to conclude as far as a bivariable null hypothesis is concerned.

||| SUMMARY

In this chapter, we encountered bivariable data sets that contain a continuous dependent variable and an independent variable. In previous chapters, we discussed univariable data sets containing only a dependent variable. In those univariable data sets, our interest was in the dependent variable under all conditions. The independent variable in bivariable data sets, in contrast, specifies special conditions that focus our interest on values of the dependent variable. Continuous independent variables allow us to examine how values of the dependent variable are related to each value of the independent variable along a continuum. Nominal independent variables define two groups of values of the dependent variable between which we can compare estimates of parameters.

The first type of independent variable that we examined in this chapter was a continuous independent variable. When we have a continuous dependent variable and a continuous independent variable, we are interested in the way in which values of the dependent variable vary relative to variation in values of the independent variable. A measure of how two continuous variables vary together is the covariance. The covariance is the sum of the products of the differences between each value of a variable and its mean for both variables. Covariance has the desirable property of having a positive value when there is a direct relationship between the variables (as values of the independent variable increase, so do values of the dependent variable) and a negative value when there is an inverse relationship between the variables (as values of the

---

[24] The actual value of α cannot be determined from this comparison.

independent variable increase, the values of dependent variables decrease). The magnitude of the covariance reflects the strength of the association between the independent and dependent variables.

The covariance, on the other hand, has a distinct disadvantage in that its magnitude is not only a reflection of the strength of the association between the independent and dependent variables, but it is also affected by the scale of measurement. This disadvantage can be overcome by dividing the covariance by the square root of the product of the variances of the data represented by the two variables. The resulting value has a range from -1 to $+1$, with -1 indicating a perfect inverse relationship, $+1$ indicating a perfect direct relationship, and 0 indicating no relationship between the independent and dependent variables. This value is called the correlation coefficient. We symbolize the population's correlation coefficient with ρ and the sample's correlation coefficient with r.

$$r = \frac{\dfrac{\Sigma(Y_i - \overline{Y})(X_i - \overline{X})}{n - 1}}{\sqrt{\dfrac{\Sigma(Y_i - \overline{Y})^2}{n - 1} \cdot \dfrac{\Sigma(X_i - \overline{X})^2}{n - 1}}} = \frac{\Sigma(Y_i - \overline{Y})(X_i - \overline{X})}{\sqrt{\Sigma(Y_i - \overline{Y})^2 \cdot \Sigma(X_i - \overline{X})^2}} \tag{7.3}$$

To evaluate the strength of the association between the independent and dependent variables, we square the correlation coefficient. The square of the correlation coefficient (symbolized by R^2) is known as the coefficient of determination. The coefficient of determination (or that coefficient times 100%) indicates the proportion (or percentage) of variation in the dependent variable that is associated with the independent variable.

Interval estimation of the correlation coefficient is not very commonly used in health statistics. More often, we encounter tests of the null hypothesis that the population's correlation coefficient is equal to zero (indicating no association between the variables). The standard error of the correlation used in testing that null hypothesis is estimated as follows:

$$SE_r = \sqrt{\frac{1 - r^2}{n - 2}} \tag{7.5}$$

Since estimation of the standard error of the correlation coefficient requires estimation of the variances of the data represented by the independent and dependent variables, inference involves conversion of the sample's observations to the Student's t scale to take into account the influence of chance on those estimates. The number of degrees of freedom for that conversion is equal to the sample's size minus two. Two is subtracted from the sample's size because two variances of data in the population are estimated from the sample's observations:

$$t = \frac{r - \rho_0}{SE_r} \tag{7.6}$$

For the correlation coefficient to have relevance, values of both the dependent and independent variables must be randomly sampled from the population of interest. The assumption that the dependent variable is randomly sampled from the population is universal to all statistical procedures. Few procedures assume that the independent variable is also randomly sampled (this is referred to as a naturalistic sample). The value of the correlation coefficient, however, can change dramatically as the distribution of the independent variable in the sample changes (such as can occur when a purposive sample is taken in which the distribution of values of the independent variable in the sample is under the control of the investigator).

Regardless of how the independent variable is sampled, regression analysis can be used to estimate parameters of a straight line that mathematically describes how values of the dependent variable change for various values of the independent variable. The equation for that straight line includes the intercept (the value of the dependent variable when the independent variable is equal to zero) and the slope (the amount that the dependent variable changes for each unit change in the independent variable). The population's intercept is symbolized by α and its estimate from the sample by a. The population's slope is symbolized by β and the sample's estimate by b.

$$\hat{Y} = a + bX \tag{7.9}$$

The sample's estimates of the intercept and slope are derived through the method of least squares. In that method, estimates are chosen to minimize the squared difference between estimated and observed values of the dependent variable. Using the method of least squares, the slope and intercept are estimated using the following calculations:

$$b = \frac{\Sigma(Y_i - \overline{Y})(X_i - \overline{X})}{\Sigma(X_i - \overline{X})^2} \tag{7.10}$$

$$a = \overline{Y} - b\overline{X} \tag{7.12}$$

To understand inference in regression analysis, it is helpful to understand sources of variation of data represented by the dependent variable. There are three sources of variation, each referred to as a sum of squares or, when divided by its degrees of freedom, as a mean square. The total mean square is the same as the variance of data represented by the dependent variable.

$$s^2 = \frac{\Sigma(Y_i - \overline{Y})^2}{n - 1} = \frac{\text{Total sum of squares}}{\text{Total degrees of freedom}} = \text{Total mean square} \tag{7.14}$$

The total variation has two components. One component is the variation in values of the dependent variable that is unexplained by the regression line. When this sum of squares is divided by its degrees of freedom, it is called the residual mean square.

$$s^2_{Y|X} = \frac{\Sigma(Y_i - \hat{Y}_i)^2}{n - 2} = \frac{\text{Residual sum of squares}}{\text{Residual degrees of freedom}} = \text{Residual mean square} \tag{7.15}$$

The other component is the variation in values the dependent variable that is explained by the regression line. This source of variation is called the regression sum of squares or, when divided by its degrees of freedom (always equal to one for bivariable data sets), it is known as the regression mean square.

$$s^2_{\text{reg}} = \frac{\Sigma(\hat{Y}_i - \overline{Y})^2}{1} = \frac{\text{Regression sum of squares}}{\text{Regression degrees of freedom}} = \text{Regression mean square} \tag{7.18}$$

The residual mean square is used in estimation of the standard errors used in regression analysis. For inference about the population's slope, the standard error is calculated from the residual mean square and the sum of squares of the independent variable.

$$SE_b = \sqrt{\frac{s^2_{Y|X}}{\Sigma(X_i - \overline{X})^2}} \tag{7.19}$$

All standard errors in regression analysis include not only the residual mean square but also the sum of squares of data represented by the independent variable. Those standard errors are larger when the unexplained variation in values of the dependent variable (i.e., the residual mean square) is larger, but they are smaller when the variation in values of the independent variable is larger. Point estimates of the slope and intercept, on the other hand, are the same regardless of the variation in the independent variable. Thus, purposive sampling of the independent variable can be used in regression analysis. Tests of inference will have more statistical power (and confidence intervals will be narrower) when the independent variable is sampled with greater variation regardless of whether the sample is naturalistic or purposive.

The intercept is the value of the dependent variable when the independent variable is equal to zero. Other values of the dependent variable are often estimated that correspond to values of the independent variable other than zero. All estimated values of the dependent variable associated with a specific value of the independent variable use the same statistical procedure for inference (or interval estimation).

Inference for the slope or intercept uses the Student's t distribution. The number of degrees of freedom for that distribution is the number of degrees of freedom used in calculation of the residual mean square $(n - 2)$.

In addition to testing specific hypotheses about the slope and intercept in regression analysis, we can test the omnibus hypothesis. The omnibus hypothesis is a statement that knowing values of the independent variable does nothing to improve estimation of values of the dependent variable. It is tested by examining the ratio of the regression mean square and the residual mean square. This ratio is known as the F ratio.

$$F = \frac{s_{reg}^2}{s_{Y|X}^2} = \frac{\text{Regression mean square}}{\text{Residual mean square}} \tag{7.22}$$

The F ratio has a special distribution known as the F distribution. This distribution is similar to the Student's t distribution, but it has two, instead of one, values for degrees of freedom. One value for degrees of freedom is associated with the numerator of the F ratio (always equal to one when we have one independent variable), and the other is associated with the denominator of that ratio (equal to $n - 2$ when we have one independent variable). Table B.4 provides values from the F distribution.

When the null hypothesis that knowing values of the independent variable does nothing to improve estimation of values of the dependent variable is true, we expect the F ratio to be equal to one. When that null hypothesis is false, the explained variation in values of the dependent variable (i.e., the regression mean square) will be greater than the unexplained variation (i.e., the residual mean square) in those values. Then, the F ratio will be greater than one. The F ratio cannot be less than one, since knowing values of the independent variable cannot reduce our ability to estimate values of the dependent variable. Thus, tests of hypotheses using the F ratio are all one-tailed.

When we have only one independent variable, the F ratio also tests the null hypothesis that the slope of the population's regression line is equal to zero. In fact, the square root of the F ratio, in this case, is equal to the Student's t value that we would obtain if we tested the null hypothesis that the population's slope is equal to zero.

Regression analysis can be used regardless of whether values of the independent variable in the sample have a distribution representative of their distribution in the population (the result of naturalistic sampling) or not (the result of purposive sampling). Correlation analysis can only be used if values of the independent variable have been sampled naturalistically. These are distinctions that affect interpretation of results, not ability to calculate those results. Computer programs often provide coefficients of determination as part of regression analysis. We must be mindful of the fact that those coefficients of determination have relevance to the population only when values of the independent variable are from a naturalistic sample.

When the dependent variable is continuous and the independent variable is ordinal, values of the dependent variable are most often converted to an ordinal scale. Procedures for an ordinal dependent variable are discussed in Chapter 8.

A nominal independent variable divides values of the dependent variable into two groups. Comparison of values of the dependent variable between those two groups is accomplished by examining the difference between the means in the groups. The standard error for the difference between means is equal to the square root of the sum of the squares of the standard errors of the means in the groups.

$$SE_{\bar{Y}_1 - \bar{Y}_2} = \sqrt{SE_1^2 + SE_2^2} = \sqrt{\frac{s_1^2}{n_1} + \frac{s_2^2}{n_2}} \qquad (7.26)$$

In calculating the standard error for the difference between two means, we often assume that the variance of the data in the two groups is the same. This allows us to use all of the observations in our sample to estimate a single variance. That estimate of the variance of data is a weighted average of the separate estimates in each group with the degrees of freedom as the weights. The resulting single estimate of the variance of data represented by the dependent variable is known as the pooled variance.

$$s_p^2 = \frac{\Sigma(df_i \cdot s_i^2)}{\Sigma df_i} = \frac{[(n_1 - 1) \cdot s_1^2] + [(n_2 - 1) \cdot s_2^2]}{(n_1 - 1) + (n_2 - 1)} \qquad (7.29)$$

Under the assumption that the variances of data are equal in the two groups, the pooled estimate of the variance is used in place of individual variances when calculating the standard error for the difference between means.

Inference for the difference between means uses the Student's t distribution. The number of degrees of freedom is equal to the sum of the degrees of freedom in the each of two groups $(n_1 - 1 + n_2 - 1)$.

||| PRACTICE PROBLEMS

7.1 Systolic and diastolic blood pressure were measured on 10 healthy persons, and the following results were observed.

Diastolic Blood Pressure	Systolic Blood Pressure
70	116
73	122
65	119
77	133
81	128
68	115
74	120
71	124
82	130
76	125

Estimate the correlation coefficient and the coefficient of determination for the association between diastolic and systolic blood pressure among persons in the population from which the sample was drawn. Test the null hypothesis that the population's correlation coefficient is equal to zero versus the alternative that it not equal to zero. Allow a 5% chance of making a Type I error.

7.2 It is hypothesized that assertiveness training can improve the grade point average of students in medical school. To examine this supposition, a total of 15 students were randomly assigned to either receive such training or not during their first school year. At the end of their medical training, the overall grade point averages were compared between these two groups. The following results were observed.

Training	No Training
98	81
85	86
79	99
86	85
93	78
94	84
88	89
	91

Test the null hypothesis that grade point averages are the same between these two groups (those receiving and those not receiving assertiveness training) in the population from which the sample was drawn versus the alternative that they are not the same in that population. Allow a 5% chance of making a Type I error.

7.3 Suppose that we conducted a clinical trial of a drug to raise the fetal hemoglobin in sickle cell anemia patients. In that trial, we randomly assigned 20 sickle cell patients to receive one of four different doses (mg) of the drug. After a certain period of treatment, we reexamined the percentage of fetal hemoglobin for each sickle cell patient, and the following results were observed.

Patient	Dose	Change in % Fetal Hemoglobin	Patient	Dose	Change in % Fetal Hemoglobin
RT	0	3	KO	10	8
EF	0	−4	DS	10	4
YH	0	0	PW	10	11
CG	0	1	IH	10	16
BE	0	−1	CD	10	9
MA	5	2	KL	15	12
SK	5	0	AE	15	17
LJ	5	7	FM	15	15
AT	5	−1	GO	15	9
ND	5	5	BH	15	18

Estimate the population's regression line for the relationship between dose of this drug and percentage of fetal hemoglobin. Test the omnibus null hypothesis for the population's regression line, allowing a 5% chance of making a Type I error.

7.4 Calculate a correlation coefficient for the association between dose and percentage of fetal hemoglobin from the observations in Problem 7.3. In general, how would you interpret this correlation coefficient? How does that interpretation apply to this particular set of observations?

CHAPTER 8

Ordinal Dependent Variables

As in univariable analysis, ordinal dependent variables in bivariable analysis are most often created from continuous dependent variables to allow analysis without the assumptions required by procedures designed for continuous variables. Recall from Chapter 5 that this conversion is accomplished by ranking the values of the continuous variable.

As can be seen in Flowchart 6, the procedures that we will present here for bivariable analyses are parallel to those presented for continuous dependent variables.

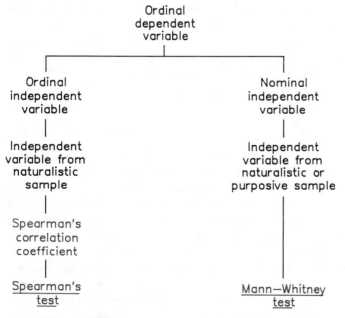

FLOWCHART 6 Bivariable analysis of an ordinal dependent variable. Point estimates are indicated in red. Statistical procedures are in red and underlined.

It should be made clear, however, that these methods also can be applied to dependent variables that naturally occur in an ordinal scale.

CONTINUOUS INDEPENDENT VARIABLE

There are no commonly used procedures in health research statistics to analyze an ordinal dependent variable and a continuous independent variable. When we encounter such a data set, the continuous independent variable is converted to an ordinal scale using the same ranking procedure that we studied in Chapter 5 for continuous dependent variables.

ORDINAL INDEPENDENT VARIABLE

The methods we will discuss here are parallel to those discussed in Chapter 7 for a continuous dependent variable and a continuous independent variable. In that chapter, we encountered two different approaches to this sort of data. First, we looked at correlation analysis. One thing we discovered about correlation analysis was that it is proper only when the independent variable has been sampled in such a way as to make the sample's distribution representative of the distribution of the independent variable in the population (called naturalistic sampling). Now, we will examine a correlation procedure for an ordinal dependent variable and an ordinal independent variable. This procedure allows us to perform a correlation analysis without assuming that either the dependent or the independent variables has a Gaussian distribution. It is important to note, however, that correlation analysis for ordinal variables does not avoid the assumption that the distribution of values of the independent variable (as well as values of the dependent variable) in the sample is representative of its distribution in the population (i.e., the result of a random sample). Any correlation analysis is appropriate only when the independent variable is from a naturalistic sample.

CORRELATION ANALYSIS

ESTIMATION   There are several types of correlation analyses that can be used with an ordinal dependent variable and an ordinal independent variable. By far, the type most commonly used in health research is **Spearman's correlation.** Spearman's correlation coefficient can be used as an estimate of the correlation coefficient that we calculated in Chapter 7 for two continuous variables (Pearson's correlation coefficient) or as a measure of association in its own right. Spearman's correlation coefficient has the same basic interpretation as Pearson's correlation coefficient. For example, it has a range from -1 to $+1$, with -1 indicating a perfect inverse relationship and $+1$ indicating a perfect direct relationship. The square of Spearman's correlation coefficient can also be interpreted in the same way that the coefficient of determination was interpreted in Chapter 7. That is to say, the square of Spearman's correlation coefficient can be considered to indicate the proportion of the variation in the ordinal dependent variable that is shared with the ordinal independent variable.

Spearman's correlation can be calculated for ordinal variables or for continuous variables converted to an ordinal scale. To convert to an ordinal scale, values of both the dependent and the independent variable are ranked in the same way that values of a continuous dependent variable is converted to an ordinal scale in univariable analysis (Chapter 5). That is to say, ranks are assigned to values of the dependent variable, and a separate set of ranks are assigned to values of the independent variable.

We could use the same equation that we used in Chapter 7 to calculate Pearson's correlation coefficient (Equation 7.3) to estimate Spearman's correlation coefficient from those ranks, but there is an easier way. After assigning ranks to values of both the dependent and independent variables, the differences between the ranks for each pair of variables (e.g., rank of a value of the independent variable minus the rank of the corresponding value of the dependent variable for an individual) are calculated. To combine the information from all the pairs of variables, we add the differences in the ranks for the two variables. To keep that sum from always being equal to zero, we square the differences before adding them. The point estimate of Spearman's correlation coefficient is then calculated from the sum of the squared differences between ranks and the sample size (Equation 8.1).

$$r_s = 1 - \frac{6 \cdot \Sigma d_i^2}{n^3 - n} \tag{8.1}$$

where

   r_s = sample's estimate of Spearman's correlation coefficient
   d_i = difference between the ranks of values of the independent and dependent variable for individual i

Example 8.1 Estimate the population's Spearman's correlation coefficient for serum cholesterol levels before and after treatment in the clinical study described in Example 7.1.

The first step in calculating a sample's estimate of Spearman's correlation coefficient is to rank the observations for each of the variables separately. Using the observations from Example 7.1, we get the following ranks.

Patient	Before (X)	Rank of X	After (Y)	Rank of Y
1	281	6	269	5
2	259	2	245	2
3	272	4	271	6
4	264	3	248	3
5	253	1	229	1
6	297	7	276	7
7	312	8	289	8
8	275	5	260	4

Next, we need to find the differences between the rank for the independent variable and the rank for the dependent variable for each individual and square that difference.

Before (X)	Rank X	After (Y)	Rank Y	d	d²
281	6	269	5	1	1
259	2	245	2	0	0
272	4	271	6	−2	4
264	3	248	3	0	0
253	1	229	1	0	0
297	7	276	7	0	0
312	8	289	8	0	0
275	5	260	4	1	1
				0	6

Finally, we use Equation 8.1 to estimate the population's Spearman's correlation coefficient.

$$r_s = 1 - \frac{6 \cdot \Sigma d_i^2}{n^3 - n} = 1 - \frac{6 \cdot 6}{8^3 - 8} = 0.9286$$

Let us take a moment to see how Equation 8.1 works. First, imagine a perfect positive association. In that situation, corresponding values of both the dependent and the independent variables will have the same rank. Thus, the sum of the squared differences between ranks will be zero, and Spearman's correlation coefficient will be equal to +1. Now, imagine a perfect negative association. In that case, values of the independent variable with the lowest ranks will be paired with values of the dependent variable with the highest ranks (and vice versa). If we examined the algebra, we would find that, in this condition, the sum of squared differences between ranks would be equal to $(n^3 - n)/3$ and, thus, Spearman's correlation would be equal to −1.

One of the assumptions of Pearson's correlation coefficient that is circumvented by converting both variables to an ordinal scale concerns the mathematical characteristics of the distributions of the variables. Another assumption that is changed concerns the type of association between the variables. To obtain Pearson's correlation coefficient of +1 (or −1), there must be a linear (straight-line) relationship between the variables. This is not true of Spearman's correlation coefficient. Spearman's correlation coefficient is equal to +1 as long as the order of values of the dependent variable correspond to the order of values of the independent variable. The relationship need not be a straight line in its natural scale. Thus, when there is a question about the existence of a straight-line relationship,[1] Spearman's correlation coefficient might be used instead of Pearson's correlation coefficient. This is illustrated in Example 8.2.

Example 8.2   Suppose that we measured the cardiac index on a sample of 14 persons from a particular population and found the following results when comparing cardiac index with age.

Age (years)	Cardiac Index (liters)
44	2.87
67	2.46
52	2.65
28	3.80
40	3.10
81	2.42
59	2.51
21	3.84
36	3.40
72	2.44
33	3.67
47	2.78
77	2.43
65	2.48

Estimate Pearson's and Spearman's correlation coefficients for the population from which this sample was derived.

First, we will estimate Pearson's correlation coefficient. To begin, we calculate the sums of squares for values of the dependent (cardiac index) and independent (age) variables and their sum of cross products (SCP). Those sums are calculated in the following table.

Age (X)	Cardiac Index (Y)	$X - \overline{X}$	$Y - \overline{Y}$	$(X - \overline{X})^2$	$(Y - \overline{Y})^2$	SCP
44	2.87	−7.6	−0.05	57.3	0.002	0.38
67	2.46	15.4	−0.46	238.0	0.210	−7.08
52	2.65	0.4	−0.27	0.2	0.072	−0.11
28	3.80	−23.6	0.88	555.6	0.778	−20.77
40	3.10	−11.6	0.18	133.9	0.033	−2.09

---

[1]There are a number of techniques that can be used to evaluate the assumption of a straight-line relationship. One of these is to examine a scatterplot, as demonstrated in Example 8.2. We will not discuss alternative methods in *Statistical First Aid*.

Age (X)	Cardiac Index (Y)	$X - \overline{X}$	$Y - \overline{Y}$	$(X - \overline{X})^2$	$(Y - \overline{Y})^2$	SCP
81	2.42	29.4	−0.50	866.0	0.248	−14.70
59	2.51	7.4	−0.41	55.2	0.166	−3.03
21	3.84	−30.6	0.92	934.6	0.850	−28.15
36	3.40	−15.6	0.48	242.5	0.232	−7.49
72	2.44	20.4	−0.48	417.3	0.228	−9.79
33	3.67	−18.6	0.75	344.9	0.566	−13.95
47	2.78	−4.6	−0.14	20.9	0.019	0.64
77	2.43	25.4	−0.49	646.6	0.238	−12.45
65	2.48	13.4	−0.44	180.3	0.192	−5.90
722	40.85	0	0	4,693.3	3.834	−124.48

Then we use Equation 7.3 to calculate the sample's estimate of the population's Pearson's correlation coefficient.

$$r = \frac{\Sigma\,(X_i - \overline{X})(Y_i - \overline{Y})}{\sqrt{\Sigma\,(X_i - \overline{X})^2 \cdot \Sigma(Y_i - \overline{Y})^2}} = \frac{-124.8}{\sqrt{4{,}693.3 \cdot 3.834}} = -0.930$$

Thus, Pearson's correlation coefficient indicates a strong inverse association between age and cardiac index, with 86.5% ($R^2 \cdot 100\%$) of the variation in cardiac index explained by knowing a person's age.

Now, let us calculate Spearman's correlation coefficient. To begin, we rank the observations and find the sum of the squared differences between the ranks for the two variables.

Age (X)	Cardiac Index (Y)	Rank of X	Rank of Y	d	d^2
44	2.87	6	9	−3	9
67	2.46	11	4	7	49
52	2.65	8	7	1	1
28	3.80	2	13	−11	121
40	3.10	5	10	−5	25
81	2.42	14	1	13	169
59	2.51	9	6	3	9
21	3.84	1	14	−13	169
36	3.40	4	11	−7	49
72	2.44	12	3	9	81
33	3.67	3	12	−9	81
47	2.78	7	8	−1	1

Age (X)	Cardiac Index (Y)	Rank of X	Rank of Y	d	d²
77	2.43	13	2	11	121
65	2.48	10	5	5	25
722	40.85				910

The sample's estimate of Spearman's correlation coefficient is calculated using Equation 8.1.

$$r_s = 1 - \frac{6 \cdot \Sigma d_i^2}{n^3 - n} = 1 - \frac{6 \cdot 910}{14^3 - 14} = -1.000$$

Pearson's correlation coefficient suggests that the association between age and cardiac index is strong, but Spearman's correlation coefficient suggests that the association is perfect. To see why this is the case, let us take a look at a scatterplot of age and cardiac index.

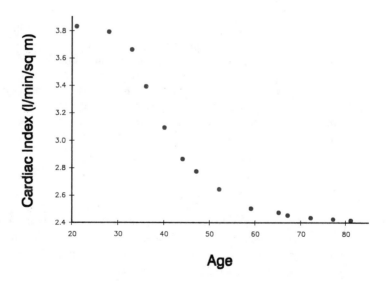

From that scatterplot, we can see that cardiac index decreases as age increases, but the association between age and cardiac index is not a straight-line relationship. The failure of Pearson's correlation coefficient to be equal to one indicates that, for age and cardiac index measured on a continuous scale, there are deviations from a straight line. The perfect relationship between those variables suggested by Spearman's correlation coefficient tells us that a straight line describes cardiac index as a function of age when both are measured on an ordinal scale. We can see that relationship graphically in a scatterplot if we use ordinal scales for both variables.

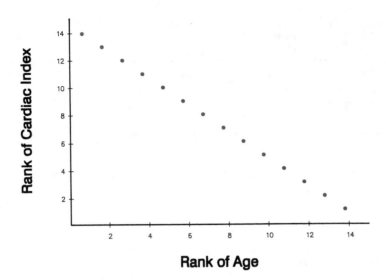

Now we might ask ourselves which correlation coefficient is more appropriate to use in this situation where the relationship is not a straight line. Our first reaction might be to use Spearman's correlation coefficient since it does not assume a straight-line relationship for the actual values of the data. This is the better choice if we are interested in how strongly the two variables are associated in general. It is permissible, however, to calculate Pearson's correlation coefficient for data such as these as long as we remember that Pearson's correlation coefficient tells us about an association that is restricted to a straight line. Thus, the magnitude of Pearson's correlation coefficient is affected not only by the strength of the association but also by how close that relationship is to a straight line.

Equation 8.1 can be used to calculate Spearman's correlation coefficient when each of the observations of a variable value has a distinct rank. That is to say, it is appropriate when none of the ranks are tied. If there are tied ranks, then our estimate of Spearman's correlation coefficient is somewhat incorrect. We can account for those tied ranks by using Equation 8.2 to estimate the coefficient, utilizing correction factors.

$$r_s = \frac{\dfrac{n^3 - n}{6} - \Sigma d_i^2 - \Sigma T_X - \Sigma T_Y}{\sqrt{\left[\dfrac{n^3 - n}{6} - (2 \cdot \Sigma T_X)\right] \cdot \left[\dfrac{n^3 - n}{6} - (2 \cdot \Sigma T_Y)\right]}} \qquad (8.2)$$

where

$\Sigma T_X = \Sigma(t_X^3 - t_X)/12$ (correction factor for the independent variable)
$\Sigma T_Y = \Sigma(t_Y^3 - t_Y)/12$ (correction factor for the dependent variable)
  t_X = the number of tied ranks in each group of tied ranks among ranks of
      values of the independent variable
  t_Y = the number of tied ranks in each group of tied ranks among ranks of
      values of the dependent variable

Example 8.3 Suppose that we are interested in the association between level of pain before and after treatment in patients with arthritis. To evaluate this relationship, we ask ten patients to rate their level of pain on a five-point scale (1 = mild, 5 = severe). Then we treat those patients and ask them to reassess their level of pain. The following results are observed:

Patient	Before (X)	After (Y)
RT	4	2
EJ	4	1
HS	5	2
TJ	3	2
WA	4	2
PG	5	3
LS	5	4
AB	4	3
CH	5	3
DM	3	1

Estimate the degree of association between pain levels before and after treatment in the population from which this sample was taken using Spearman's correlation coefficient.

These data occur naturally on an ordinal scale. Even so, we need to express these ordinal values as ranks to calculate Spearman's correlation coefficient. Thus, to prepare for calculation of Spearman's correlation coefficient, we rank these observations and determine the squares of the differences between ranks.

Patient	Before (X)	After (Y)	Rank of X	Rank of Y	d	d^2
RT	4	2	4.5	4.5	0	0.00
EJ	4	1	4.5	1.5	3	9.00
HS	5	2	8.5	4.5	4	16.00
TJ	3	2	1.5	4.5	−3	9.00

Patient	Before (X)	After (Y)	Rank of X	Rank of Y	d	d²
WA	4	2	4.5	4.5	0	0.00
PG	5	3	8.5	8	0.5	0.25
LS	5	4	8.5	10	−1.5	2.25
AB	4	3	4.5	8	−3.5	12.25
CH	5	3	8.5	8	0.5	0.25
DM	3	1	1.5	1.5	0	0.00
						49.00

Next, we calculate the correction factors (from Equation 8.2) that we will use to estimate Spearman's correlation coefficient. For the independent variable (pain level before treatment), there are three sets of tied ranks. Specifically, there are two ranks equal to 1.5, four ranks equal to 4.5, and four ranks equal to 8.5. Thus, the correction factor for ranks of values of the independent variable is equal to the following:

$$\Sigma T_X = \frac{\Sigma(t_X^3 - t_X)}{12} = \frac{(2^3 - 2) + (4^3 - 4) + (4^3 - 4)}{12} = 10.5$$

For the dependent variable (pain level after treatment), there also are three sets of tied ranks. There are two ranks equal to 1.5, four ranks equal to 4.5, and three ranks equal to 8. The correction factor for ranks of values of the dependent variable is equal to the following:

$$\Sigma T_Y = \frac{\Sigma(t_Y^3 - t_Y)}{12} = \frac{(2^3 - 2) + (4^3 - 4) + (3^3 - 3)}{12} = 7.5$$

Then we use Equation 8.2 to calculate the sample's estimate of Spearman's correlation coefficient.

$$r_s = \frac{\dfrac{n^3 - n}{6} - \Sigma d_i^2 - \Sigma T_X - \Sigma T_Y}{\sqrt{\left[\dfrac{n^3 - n}{6} - (2 \cdot \Sigma T_X)\right] \cdot \left[\dfrac{n^3 - n}{6} - (2 \cdot \Sigma T_Y)\right]}}$$

$$= \frac{\dfrac{10^3 - 10}{6} - 49 - 10.5 - 7.5}{\sqrt{\left[\dfrac{10^3 - 10}{6} - (2 \cdot 10.5)\right] \cdot \left[\dfrac{10^3 - 10}{6} - (2 \cdot 7.5)\right]}} = 0.667$$

If there are not many tied ranks, there is little effect on the value of Spearman's correlation coefficient. Here, however, most of the ranks are tied. To see how much Spearman's correlation coefficient can be affected by many tied ranks, let us calculate that correlation coefficient without correcting for tied ranks. If we had used Equation 8.1 instead of Equation 8.2, we would have gotten the following result:

$$r_s = 1 - \frac{6 \cdot \Sigma d_i^2}{n^3 - n} = 1 - \frac{6 \cdot 49}{10^3 - 10} = 0.703$$

We can see a moderate difference between the corrected Spearman's correlation coefficient (0.667) and the uncorrected Spearman's correlation coefficient (0.703). Thus, a large number of tied ranks has only a moderate effect on the value of Spearman's correlation coefficient, but we should correct for those ties to estimate the coefficient accurately. ▱

INFERENCE Testing the null hypothesis that Spearman's correlation coefficient is equal to zero is usually done using a computer program or a table. Table B.5 can be used for this purpose.[2]

Example 8.4 Test the null hypothesis that the population's Spearman's correlation coefficient, corrected for tied ranks, estimated in Example 8.3 is equal to zero versus the alternative that it is not equal to zero. Allow a 5% chance of making a Type I error.

In Example 8.3, we estimated the population's Spearman's correlation coefficient to be 0.667 from a sample of 10 persons. In Table B.5, we find that Spearman's correlation coefficient associated with a sample's size of 10 and a two-tailed α of 0.05 is equal to 0.648. Since our calculated Spearman's correlation coefficient is larger than the value from the table, we reject the null hypothesis and accept, by elimination, the alternative hypothesis. ▱

REGRESSION ANALYSIS

There are no well-accepted procedures specifically designed to perform a regression analysis on ordinal dependent variables or continuous variables converted to an ordinal scale. Actually, it is not necessary to develop special procedures to perform regression analysis on ordinal dependent variables. To understand why this is so, we need to review what we learned about regression analysis in Chapter 7.

Recall that the purpose of regression analysis is to estimate a straight line that describes values of the dependent variable as a mathematical function of values of the independent variable. To make point estimates of the parameters of the regression line, we do not have to assume that means of values of the dependent variable have a Gaussian distribution. The most important assumption we make in calculating point estimates of the parameters of the regression line is that the relationship between the variables in the population is a straight line.[3] Since we are not concerned about the

---

[2] Table B.5 can be used only if the null hypothesis is that the population's value of Spearman's correlation coefficient is equal to zero. This is the most commonly encountered null hypothesis. Testing of other null hypotheses is more complex and will not be discussed in *Statistical First Aid*.

[3] We also assume the same dispersion of dependent variable values in the population from which the sample was drawn for each value of the independent variable. This is known as the assumption of **homogeneity of variances** or **homoscedasticity**.

distribution of the dependent variable, point estimation of the slope and intercept can be performed on ordinal dependent variables using the same procedures that we described in Chapter 7 for continuous dependent variables.

Inference (or interval estimation) in regression analysis is another matter. In this case, we do assume that the population's distribution of means of values of the dependent variable corresponding to each value of the independent variable is a Gaussian distribution. If we are concerned about this assumption, we should not use the procedures described in Chapter 7 for inference. Thus, we can make point estimates of the slope and intercept when we have an ordinal dependent variable, but we should not perform statistical inference (or calculate interval estimates).[4]

NOMINAL INDEPENDENT VARIABLE

As discussed in Chapter 7, a nominal independent variable has the effect of dividing the dependent variable into two groups. When the dependent variable is continuous, we usually test the null hypothesis that the means of the two groups are equal (i.e., that the difference between means is zero) in the population from which the sample was drawn. For an ordinal dependent variable, we do not assume any particular population's distribution. Thus, we cannot test null hypotheses about parameters that mathematically describe the population's distribution. Rather, we usually test a null hypothesis that is a more general statement about the relationship between the groups, such as the hypothesis that the population's overall distribution of values of the dependent variable are the same in the two groups (instead of a hypothesis about the means of the groups). Without assuming that we have a particular population's distribution of the dependent variable, we cannot make point or interval estimates.[5] Thus, statistical procedures for an ordinal dependent variable and a nominal independent variable are confined to the process of statistical inference. In *Statistical First Aid*, we will discuss only the most commonly used method of inference for an ordinal dependent variable and a nominal independent variable: the **Mann-Whitney test.**

The Mann-Whitney test is used most often as a nonparametric substitute for the Student's *t* test described in Chapter 7. In preparation for this test, we must convert data represented by the continuous dependent variable to an ordinal scale. In that conversion, we use ranking procedures, such as those described in Chapter 5. All of the values of the dependent variable in the sample are ranked without regard to which

---

[4] There is, however, one way that we can test something similar to the omnibus null hypothesis tested in regression analysis for continuous dependent variables. Recall from Chapter 7 that testing the omnibus null hypothesis is tantamount to testing the null hypothesis that Pearson's correlation coefficient is equal to zero. When we have an ordinal dependent variable and an ordinal independent variable, we can test a parallel null hypothesis by performing statistical inference on Spearman's correlation coefficient. Therefore, we can use a test of the null hypothesis that the population's value of Spearman's correlation is equal to zero to substitute for a test of the omnibus null hypothesis in regression analysis when we doubt that the dependent variable has a Gaussian distribution.

[5] There are statistical procedures in which the median is used as a substitute for the mean and a confidence interval is calculated using ordinal data for the difference between medians. These procedures are laborious and very rarely used; therefore, we will not discuss them in *Statistical First Aid*.

group they belong. Then the observations are divided into the groups according to values of the independent variable, and the sum of the ranks for each group is calculated.

The Mann-Whitney test statistic is calculated from the sum of the ranks in one of the groups (chosen arbitrarily), as shown in Equation 8.3.

$$U = (n_1 \cdot n_2) + \frac{n_1 \cdot (n_1 + 1)}{2} - R_1 \qquad (8.3)$$

where

U = the Mann-Whitney test statistic
n_1 = the number of observations in group 1
n_2 = the number of observations in group 2
R_1 = the sum of the ranks in group 1

The choice of which group of dependent variable values is defined as group 1 is arbitrary, and the value of the Mann-Whitney test statistic will be different, depending on that choice. To solve this problem, we calculate the Mann-Whitney U by choosing either group as group 1 and then determining what the Mann-Whitney U value would have been if our choice had been different (we call this alternative value U'). We could use Equation 8.3 to make that calculation; a simpler method, however, is based on the fact that the sum of the two possible Mann-Whitney U values (U and U') is equal to the product of the number of observations in each of the two groups. Then we can use Equation 8.4 as a shortcut method to determine what the Mann-Whitney U value would have been if we had selected the group to be called group 1 differently:

$$U' = (n_1 \cdot n_2) - U \qquad (8.4)$$

where U' = the value of the Mann-Whitney test statistic if the other group had been chosen as group 1.

For a two-tailed alternative hypothesis, the appropriate test statistic to use in the Mann-Whitney test is the larger of U and U'. That test statistic is then compared to values in a table such as Table B.6.

Example 8.5   For the observations presented in Example 7.9, test the null hypothesis that systolic blood pressure is the same in the drug group as it is in the placebo group versus the alternative that blood pressure is not the same in those two groups. Allow a 5% chance of making a Type I error.

The first step in testing this null hypothesis is to rank the values of the dependent variable. In assigning ranks, we do not distinguish to which group the observation belongs.

Drug Group	Rank of Drug	Placebo Group	Rank of Placebo
120	12.5	127	15
104	3	120	12.5

Drug Group	Rank of Drug	Placebo Group	Rank of Placebo
111	7	133	18
117	11	136	19
105	4	124	14
114	8	140	20
103	2	132	17
100	1	128	16
116	10		
106	5		
115	9		
109	6		
	78.5		131.5

Next, we use Equation 8.3 to calculate the Mann-Whitney U statistic. We will arbitrarily pick the drug group as group 1.

$$U = (n_1 \cdot n_2) + \frac{n_1 \cdot (n_1 + 1)}{2} - R_1 = (12 \cdot 8) - \frac{12 \cdot (12 + 1)}{2} - 78.5 = 95.5$$

Then we use Equation 8.4 to determine what the value of the Mann-Whitney U statistic would have been if we had picked the placebo group as group 1.

$$U' = (n_1 \cdot n_2) - U = (12 \cdot 8) - 95.5 = 0.5$$

Since 95.5 is larger than 0.5, we choose 95.5 as our value for the Mann-Whitney U statistic. From Table B.6, we find that a Mann-Whitney U associated with a two-tailed α of 0.05 and 8 and 12 observations in the two groups is equal to 74. Since 95.5 is larger than 74, we reject the null hypothesis that systolic blood pressure in the population is the same for the two groups and accept, by elimination, the alternative hypothesis that systolic blood in the population is not the same for those groups. ⊟

For a one-tailed alternative hypothesis, the appropriate test statistic to use in the Mann-Whitney test is the one that is calculated declaring group 1 as the group hypothesized (by the alternative hypothesis) to have smaller values. For example, if we have two groups called group A and group B, and the alternative hypothesis states that the values in group B are less than in group A, then the number of observations and the sum of the ranks for group B should be used as n_1 and R_1 in Equation 8.3. Thus, for a one-tailed alternative hypothesis, we do not calculate U' (as in Equation 8.4). This is illustrated in the next example.

Example 8.6   For the observations presented in Example 7.9, test the null hypothesis that systolic blood pressure is the same in the drug group as it is in the placebo group versus the alternative that blood pressure is lower in the drug group. Allow a 5% chance of making a Type I error.

In Example 8.5, we found that the sum of the ranks for the group of 12 patients receiving the drug was 78.5. The alternative hypothesis states that, if the null hypothesis is false, the drug group will have lower blood pressures than the placebo group. Therefore, we should use 78.5 as R_1 and 12 as n_1 in Equation 8.3.

$$U = (n_1 \cdot n_2) + \frac{n_1 \cdot (n_1 + 1)}{2} - R_1 = (12 \cdot 8) + \frac{12 \cdot (12 + 1)}{2} - 78.5 = 95.5$$

We do not calculate U' in this example since we have a one-tailed alternative hypothesis and that hypothesis dictates which group should be considered as group 1.

Now we compare our calculated value to the value from Table B.6 associated with a one-tailed α of 0.05 and 8 and 12 observations in the two groups. That value is equal to 70. Since 95.5 is larger than 70, we reject the null hypothesis that the values of systolic blood pressure in the population are the same for the two treatment groups and accept, by elimination, the alternative hypothesis that systolic blood pressure in the population is lower for the group receiving the drug than for the group receiving the placebo.

SUMMARY

In Chapter 7, when we discussed procedures for a continuous dependent variable and a continuous independent variable, we investigated two procedures. These were correlation analysis and regression analysis. In Chapter 8, we discovered a method of correlation analysis designed for an ordinal dependent variable and an ordinal independent variable. That procedure involved estimation and inference for Spearman's correlation coefficient. We learned that there is no commonly used method of regression analysis specifically designed for an ordinal dependent variable and an ordinal independent variable.

Spearman's correlation coefficient is calculated from data converted to ranks. Those data can be ordinal or continuous in their natural scale. When a Spearman's correlation coefficient is used to describe the strength of association between two continuous variables, some of the assumptions of the continuous variable correlation coefficient (called Pearson's correlation coefficient) are circumvented. Those assumptions concern the nature of the distributions of the variables. Another assumption of Pearson's correlation coefficient, that the relationship between the variables is linear, is also changed. Rather than assume a linear relationship between the variables on their natural (continuous) scale, we assume a linear relationship on an ordinal scale. This is much easier to achieve since it involves only a consistency in ordering.

To calculate Spearman's correlation coefficient, values of the dependent and independent variables are ranked separately, and the squared difference between the ranks of those two variables (d^2) is determined for each individual. Then Equation 8.1 can be used to calculate Spearman's correlation coefficient.

$$r_s = 1 - \frac{6 \cdot \Sigma d_i^2}{n^3 - n} \qquad (8.1)$$

That method of calculation assumes that there are no tied ranks. If there are tied ranks, Equation 8.2 should be used to calculate Spearman's correlation coefficient.

$$r_s = \frac{\dfrac{n^3 - n}{6} - \Sigma d_i^2 - \Sigma T_X - \Sigma T_Y}{\sqrt{\left[\dfrac{n^3 - n}{6} - (2 \cdot \Sigma T_X)\right] \cdot \left[\dfrac{n^3 - n}{6} - (2 \cdot \Sigma T_Y)\right]}} \tag{8.2}$$

where

$\Sigma T_X = \Sigma(t_X^3 - t_X)/12$

$\Sigma T_Y = \Sigma(t_Y^3 - t_Y)/12$

t_X = the number of tied ranks in each group of tied ranks among ranks of values of the independent variable

t_Y = the number of tied ranks in each group of tied ranks among ranks of values of the dependent variable

Inference for Spearman's correlation coefficient when the null hypothesis is that the population's Spearman's correlation coefficient is equal to some value other than zero is not commonly encountered in the health research literature and involves a somewhat complicated procedure. If we wish to test the null hypothesis that the population's Spearman's correlation coefficient is equal to zero, however, inference involves comparison of the sample's estimate of Spearman's correlation coefficient with a value in Table B.5.

When we have an ordinal dependent variable and a nominal independent variable, our interest is in comparing the two groups of dependent variable values defined by the two values of the nominal independent variable. When we considered a continuous dependent variable and a nominal independent variable in Chapter 7, we estimated the difference between means. In contrast, we make no estimates of the difference between the groups when we have an ordinal dependent variable. Therefore, point and interval estimation are not often used when the dependent variable is ordinal.

The method of statistical inference that we discussed in this chapter for an ordinal dependent variable and a nominal independent variable was the Mann-Whitney U procedure. We use this procedure to test the null hypothesis that the dependent variable is the same in the two groups. The Mann-Whitney U statistic is calculated from the number of observations in each of the two groups and the sum of the ranks in one group (referred to as "group 1"). That calculation was described in Equation 8.3:

$$U = (n_1 \cdot n_2) + \frac{n_1 \cdot (n_1 + 1)}{2} - R_1 \tag{8.3}$$

The choice of the group that has its sum of ranks used in Equation 8.3 is arbitrary, but that choice will affect the value of the Mann-Whitney U statistic. We can find out what the value of U would have been if we had picked the other group by using Equation 8.4:

$$U' = (n_1 \cdot n_2) - U \tag{8.4}$$

When we are considering a two-tailed alternative hypothesis, the appropriate value of the Mann-Whitney U statistic is the larger of U and U'. For a one-tailed hypothesis, the appropriate Mann-Whitney U statistic is calculated by choosing group 1 to be the group that is hypothesized to have the lower sum of ranks. The appropriate Mann-Whitney U value calculated from the observations in the sample is compared to a value in Table B.6 to complete statistical inference.

| || PRACTICE PROBLEMS

8.1 Blood pressure measurements were recorded for a sample of ten patients in Problem 7.1. Estimate the population's Spearman's correlation coefficient for those measurements and compare it to Pearson's correlation coefficient estimated in Problem 7.1.

8.2 In a study of the relationship between maternal age (years) and infant birth weight (grams), records of 25 term deliveries were examined. The following data were collected.

Maternal Age (years)	Birth Weight (grams)
31	3,609
27	3,831
19	3,110
24	3,373
32	4,115
37	3,740
19	2,527
21	2,869
30	3,392
28	3,319
18	2,532
22	2,860
31	3,452
17	2,484
39	3,507
26	3,094
30	3,740
24	3,368
21	2,842
19	3,010
33	3,938
26	3,289
23	3,240
27	3,115
25	3,609

Estimate the population's Spearman's correlation coefficient that measures the strength of the association between maternal age and infant birth weight from these observations. Test the null hypothesis that there is no association between maternal age and birth weight in the population versus the alternative hypothesis that there is an association. Allow a 5% chance of making a Type I error.

8.3 For the observations in Problem 7.2, test the null hypothesis that there is no difference in the distribution of grade point averages for medical students given assertiveness training and those not receiving such training. As an alternative hypothesis, consider that there is a difference in the distribution of grade point averages. Do not assume that the means from all possible samples have a Gaussian distribution. Allow a 5% chance of making a Type I error.

8.4 In a study of a treatment for diabetic retinopathy, 16 patients were randomly selected to receive either an experimental drug or a placebo. After a period of time, their visual acuity was measured and the following results observed.

Treatment	Visual Acuity
Drug	20/30
Drug	20/50
Placebo	20/50
Drug	20/40
Placebo	20/100
Drug	20/50
Placebo	20/40
Placebo	20/200
Drug	20/50
Drug	20/100
Placebo	20/100
Drug	20/50
Placebo	20/50
Placebo	20/100
Drug	20/30
Placebo	20/200

Test the null hypothesis that visual acuity is the same regardless of treatment versus the alternative hypothesis that the drug improves visual acuity. Allow a 5% chance of making a Type I error.

CHAPTER 9

Nominal Dependent Variables

In this chapter, we will examine statistical techniques for analyzing data sets that contain a nominal dependent variable and one independent variable. In addition to the procedures described here, a nominal dependent variable and one independent variable can be analyzed using procedures for a nominal dependent variable and more than one independent variable, which will be described in Chapter 12.

Recall that a nominal variable can consist only of dichotomous data. That is to say, a nominal variable can have only one of two values for each individual observation. We must, however, distinguish between a nominal variable and nominal data. Nominal data can have more than two possible values. When nominal data have more than two potential categories, more than one nominal variable must be used to represent those data. If that situation exists for the data of primary interest (i.e., the dependent variable), we need to consider a multivariate (rather than a univariate) statistical procedure. With one exception, in which a multivariate method involves a simple extension of a univariate procedure (discussed later in this chapter), we will not examine multivariate methods in *Statistical First Aid*.

CONTINUOUS INDEPENDENT VARIABLE

In Chapter 7, we found that when we have a continuous dependent variable and a continuous independent variable, we are interested in how values of the dependent variable are associated with the various values of the independent variable. We discussed two general types of procedures to study this association. The first was correlation analysis, in which we were interested in estimating the strength of the association between the dependent and independent variables. The second was regression analysis, in which we were interested in estimating the straight line that mathematically describes the relationship between those two variables in the population from which the sample was drawn.

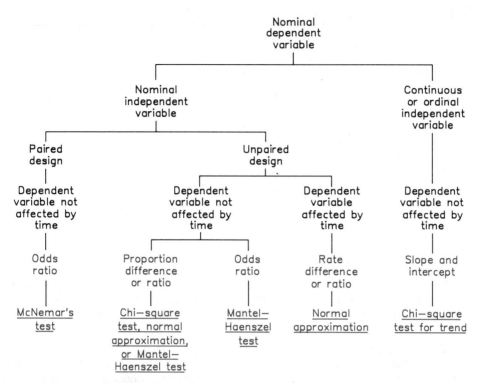

FLOWCHART 7 Bivariable analysis of a nominal dependent variable. Point estimates are indicated in red. Statistical procedures are in red and underlined.

When we have a nominal dependent variable and a continuous independent variable, we also are interested in how values of the dependent variable are associated with the various values of the independent variable. There are a number of statistical procedures available to calculate something similar to a correlation coefficient for a nominal dependent variable. None of these, however, is commonly encountered in the health research literature, and they will not be discussed in *Statistical First Aid*.

There also are a number of procedures to estimate the parameters of a mathematical formula that can be used to describe the relationship between a nominal dependent variable and a continuous independent variable. The most commonly used of these is called the **chi-square test for trend.** In a moment, we will look at what a chi-square test is. First, let us consider what we mean by a trend.

In regression analysis, we examined a straight-line relationship between a continuous dependent variable and a continuous independent variable. This straight line describes a particular type of relationship in which the dependent variable is assumed to change in a constant direction and to a constant degree with changes in values of the independent variable. In general, a trend implies that one variable changes in a constant direction relative to another. It does not necessarily imply, however, that the degree of change is constant.

With a continuous dependent variable, we were interested in how the mean of the dependent variable changed relative to values of the independent variable. The slope of the regression equation told us two things about how the mean of the dependent variable changed. First, the sign of the slope told us the direction of the relationship: a positive slope indicated a direct relationship, and a negative slope indicated an inverse relationship. Second, the numeric value of the slope told us the degree to which the mean of the dependent variable changed for each unit change in the value of the independent variable. With continuous dependent variables, we were always interested in estimating both the direction and the degree of change in the mean of the dependent variable.

When we have a nominal dependent variable, we are interested in how probabilities[1] change relative to values of the independent variable. We have two choices in investigating that relationship with a nominal dependent variable and a continuous independent variable. One choice is to specify the degree to which probabilities change for each unit change in the value of the independent variable (as we do for continuous dependent variables). The other choice is to examine the direction of the trend without specifying the degree of change (i.e., we could determine the sign of the slope without estimating its numeric value).

Investigation of a trend allows us to ignore the degree of change in dependent variable values, but it does not require us to do so. To take full advantage of the information in a continuous independent variable, we should examine this degree of change.[2] To examine the degree of change, we need to specify a mathematical relationship between the dependent and independent variables. In regression analysis for continuous dependent variables, we most often assumed that the mathematical relationship was a straight line. In a parallel procedure for nominal dependent variables, we make this same assumption. That is to say, we assume that the probability of the event addressed by the nominal dependent variable changes to a constant degree with each unit change in the value of the independent variable.

ESTIMATION   In Equation 7.7, we looked at the straight-line equation that told us how values of a continuous dependent variable (in the population) change relative to values of the independent variable. The corresponding relationship for a nominal dependent variable is shown in Equation 9.1.

$$\theta = \alpha + \beta X \tag{9.1}$$

---

[1]Recall from Chapter 6 that a probability is the measure that we most commonly use to summarize a collection of observations of nominal data. Each observation, however, can have only one of two values (e.g., "yes" or "no").

[2]When we ignore the degree of change in probabilities corresponding to changes in values of the independent variable, we are ignoring the size of the intervals between values of that variable. That is tantamount to conversion of the independent variable from a continuous scale to an ordinal scale. We will introduce such a procedure in the portion of this chapter that examines ordinal independent variables.

As in Equation 7.7, α in Equation 9.1 is the intercept. Here, the intercept indicates the probability of the event addressed by the dependent variable when the independent variable is equal to zero. β in Equation 9.1 is the slope. The slope tells us the magnitude of the change in the probability of the event (i.e., the value of the dependent variable) for each unit change in the value of the independent variable.

The first thing we need to do in this chi-square test for trend is to estimate the population's values of the slope and intercept in Equation 9.1. As in regression analysis for continuous dependent variables, those estimates are symbolized by the letter b (for the slope) and the letter a (for the intercept).

$$\hat{p} = a + bX \qquad (9.2)$$

In regression analysis for a continuous dependent variable, the slope is estimated by dividing the sum of cross products by the sum of squares of the independent variable (from Equation 7.10, $b = \Sigma(Y_i - \overline{Y})(X_i - \overline{X})/\Sigma(X_i - \overline{X})^2$). We use a similar procedure for nominal dependent variables in Equation 9.3:

$$b = \frac{\Sigma n_i(p_i - \overline{p})(X_i - \overline{X})}{\Sigma n_i(X_i - \overline{X})^2} \qquad (9.3)$$

where

n_i = number of observations corresponding to the ith value of the independent variable

p_i = observed probability of the event corresponding to the ith value of the independent variable

$\overline{p}$ = overall probability of the event (ignoring values of the independent variable

At first, Equation 9.3 might appear to be somewhat different from the method we use to estimate the slope for a continuous dependent variable (Equation 7.10). The numerator of Equation 9.3, however, is exactly the same as the sum of cross products of a continuous dependent variable. It only appears to be different from the sum of cross products for continuous dependent variables because of the difference between a single observation of continuous versus nominal data. Each observation of a nominal variable can consist of one of only two possible nominal values (e.g., "yes" or "no"). Nominal information can be placed on a scale of measurement only when it is summarized over a collection of observations. Then, the nominal variable is expressed as a probability. In Equation 9.3, we have used probabilities corresponding to each value of the independent variable as summary measurements for the nominal dependent variable. This implies that we have several (n_i) observations of the dependent variable for each value of the independent variable. Since each probability represents n_i observations of the dependent variable for each value of the independent variable, we multiply each difference between the summary measurement and the overall probability of the event by n_i. The denominator of Equation 9.3 is also exactly the same as the sum of squares of the independent variable that is in the denominator of Equation 7.10. Here, the differences between each value of the independent variable and the mean of the independent variable are multiplied by n_i for the same reason that the components of the sum of cross products were multiplied by n_i in the numerator.[3]

We will take a look at an example of estimating the slope for a nominal dependent variable in a moment, but first let us examine how the intercept is estimated. Notice that estimation of the intercept for a nominal dependent variable (Equation 9.4) uses the same procedure that was used for a continuous dependent variable (Equation 7.12), with the overall probability of the event ($\bar{p}$) substituted for the mean of the dependent variable.

$$a = \bar{p} - b\,\overline{X} \qquad\qquad (9.4)$$

Example 9.1 In a clinical trial of a treatment for coronary heart disease, 100 patients hospitalized for myocardial infarction were randomized at discharge to receive one of five dosages of an experimental drug. At the end of a five-year study period, the following five-year risks of death were observed:

Dose (mg)	Number of Patients	Number of Deaths	Five-Year Risk
5	20	10	0.50
10	20	8	0.40
15	20	6	0.30
20	20	7	0.35
25	20	5	0.25
	100	36	

Estimate the parameters of the straight line that describes the relationship between dose and the five-year risk of death in the population from which the sample was drawn.

We first need to estimate the overall probability of death. To do that, we divide the total number of deaths among all persons in the study (regardless of dose) by the total size of the sample.

$$\bar{p} = \frac{\Sigma\,a_i}{\Sigma\,n_i} = \frac{36}{100} = 0.36$$

Next, we need to estimate the mean of the independent variable (dose). When we estimate this mean, we need to remember that n_i observations have been made for each numeric value of the independent variable. Thus, the following calculation appears to be somewhat different from the way we usually calculate the sample's estimate of the population's mean (Equation 3.1). We can

---

[3]For each value of the independent variable, there are n_i observations with that value. Multiplying each difference between a value of the independent variable and the mean of the independent variable is easier than adding up all the differences for each observation.

think about this calculation as a weighted average of the dose, with the number of persons receiving each dose used as the weights.

$$\overline{X} = \frac{\Sigma\, n_i X_i}{\Sigma\, n_i} = \frac{(20 \cdot 5) + (20 \cdot 10) + \cdots + (20 \cdot 25)}{20 + 20 + \cdots + 20} = \frac{1500}{100} = 15 \text{ mg}$$

Then, we calculate the values that we will need to estimate the slope. This is easiest to do in a table. First, let us calculate the sum of squares for the independent variable.

Patients (n_i)	Dose (X_i)	$X_i - \overline{X}$	$(X_i - \overline{X})^2$	$n_i(X_i - \overline{X})^2$
20	5	−10	100	2,000
20	10	−5	25	500
20	15	0	0	0
20	20	5	25	500
20	25	10	100	2,000
	100	0		5,000

Thus, the sum of squares for the independent variable is equal to 5,000 mg². Now, we can calculate the sum of cross products.

Patients (n_i)	$X_i - \overline{X}$	Risk (p_i)	$p_i - \overline{p}$	$(p_i - \overline{p})(X_i - \overline{X})$	$n_i(p_i - \overline{p})(X_i - \overline{X})$
20	−10	0.50	0.14	−1.40	−28.00
20	−5	0.40	0.04	−0.20	−4.00
20	0	0.30	−0.06	0.00	0.00
20	5	0.35	−0.01	−0.05	−1.00
20	10	0.25	−0.11	−1.10	−22.00
	0		0		−55.00

Now, we are ready to use Equation 9.3 to estimate the slope of the straight line we will use to represent the relationship between risk and dose.

$$b = \frac{\Sigma\, n_i(p_i - \overline{p})\,(X_i - \overline{X})}{\Sigma\, n_i(X_i - \overline{X})^2} = \frac{-55.00}{5,000} = -0.011$$

The intercept of the straight line describing the relationship between risk and dose is estimated using Equation 9.4.

$$a = \bar{p} - b\overline{X} = 0.36 - (-0.011 \cdot 15) = 0.525$$

Thus, the formula for the straight line describing risk of death as a function of dose is estimated to be the following:

$$\hat{p} = 0.525 - 0.011\,X$$

INFERENCE   In Chapter 7, when we were interested in testing the overall regression relationship, we tested the omnibus null hypothesis. For a continuous dependent variable, the omnibus null hypothesis was tested by examining the ratio of the regression mean square (the explained variation of the dependent variable divided by its degrees of freedom) and the residual mean square (the unexplained variation of the dependent variable divided by its degrees of freedom). That ratio is known as the F ratio (Equation 7.22).

In the chi-square test for trend, we also examine a ratio of measures of dispersion to test the omnibus null hypothesis that there is no trend in probabilities associated with values of the independent variable. That ratio contains a value parallel to the regression sum of squares[4] in its numerator (Equation 9.5).

$$\text{Regression sum of squares} = \Sigma\, n_i (\hat{p}_i - \bar{p})^2 \qquad (9.5)$$

In the denominator of the ratio in the chi-square test for trend, we use a value that is not exactly parallel to the residual mean square of regression analysis for continuous dependent variables. Rather, we use an estimate of the total variation of the nominal dependent variable.[5] To estimate the total variation of the dependent variable, we need to remember that the dependent variable is nominal. In Chapter 6, we learned that the variance of a nominal variable assumed to come from a binomial distribution is a function of the point estimate and its complement.[6] Therefore, the ratio that we consider in the chi-square test for trend is equal to the regression sum of squares divided by the overall probability of the event times its complement (Equation 9.6).

$$\chi^2 = \frac{\Sigma\, n_i (\hat{p}_i - \bar{p})^2}{\bar{p}(1 - \bar{p})} \qquad (9.6)$$

A ratio of a sum of squares estimate and a variance has a **chi-square distribution**, rather than an F distribution (which is used for a ratio of two variance estimates).

---

[4]Because the regression mean square has one degree of freedom, the regression mean square and the regression sum of squares are numerically equal for one independent variable.

[5] This is really not very different from using the residual mean square in the denominator. Recall from Chapter 7 that, under the assumption that the null hypothesis is true, we expect the regression mean square, the residual mean square, and the total mean square to all be equal to the same value.

[6]In Equation 6.5, we examined the standard error for the sample's estimate of the probability of the event in the population. Like the standard error for the mean, Equation 6.5 consists of the square root of the data's variance divided by the sample size. Thus, the variance of nominal data is equal to $p(1 - p)$.

Remember that the F distribution is like the Student's t distribution in that it allows us to take the effect of chance into account in estimating the population's variance of data. The F distribution differs from the Student's t distribution in that the F distribution is able to take chance into account for two different estimates of the variance of data in the population (one in the numerator and one in the denominator). It does that by assigning degrees of freedom to each of the estimates. In the ratio for the chi-square test for trend (Equation 9.6), we also have two estimates of variation. The estimate in the numerator has one degree of freedom (like the regression mean square in Chapter 7). For the estimate in the denominator, we do not have to take chance into account; that estimate can be derived by knowing only the point estimate of the overall probability.[7]

Rather than use the F distribution to test the omnibus null hypothesis for a nominal dependent variable and a continuous independent variable, we use a new distribution: the chi-square distribution (Table B.7).[8] The chi-square distribution is another member of the Gaussian family that, like the Student's t distribution, is composed of various specific distributions, each defined by a certain number of degrees of freedom. Also like the Student's t distribution, the chi-square distribution is an extension of the standard normal distribution. A chi-square value corresponding to one degree of freedom and a particular α is equal to the square of a standard normal deviate with $\alpha/2$ in each tail.[9] We will discuss the implications of chi-square values with more than one degree of freedom when we look at nominal independent variables later in this chapter. For now, let us recognize that the ratio in Equation 9.6 is a chi-square value with one degree of freedom, which is exactly equal to the square of a (two-tailed) standard normal deviate.

Example 9.2   Test the null hypothesis that there is no trend in risk of death with dosage (versus the alternative hypothesis that there is a trend) for the observations in Example 9.1. Allow a 5% chance of making a Type I error.

To test this null hypothesis, we first calculate estimated values of the dependent variable and the squared differences between those estimated values and the observed values. These calcula-

---

[7]Another way to express this is to say that we have an infinite number of degrees of freedom in the denominator.

[8]Actually, we could consider the ratio in Equation 9.6 to be an F ratio with one degree of freedom in the numerator and infinite degrees of freedom in the denominator.

[9]To understand the relationship between the chi-square and standard normal distributions, let us first recall from Chapter 7 that the square root of an F ratio with one degree of freedom in the numerator is equal to a Student's t value, with degrees of freedom equal to the degrees of freedom in the denominator of the F ratio. Thus, the square root of the ratio in Equation 9.6 is a Student's t value with infinite degrees of freedom. Now, recall from Chapter 4 that a Student's t value with infinite degrees of freedom is the same as a standard normal deviate. Therefore, the square root of the ratio in Equation 9.6 is a standard normal deviate.

tions appear in the following table:

Patients (n_i)	Dose (X_i)	Risk (p_i)	$\hat{p}_i$	$\hat{p}_i - \bar{p}$	$n_i(\hat{p}_i - \bar{p})^2$
20	5	0.50	0.470	0.110	0.2420
20	10	0.40	0.415	0.055	0.0605
20	15	0.30	0.360	0.000	0.0000
20	20	0.35	0.305	−0.055	0.0605
20	25	0.25	0.250	−0.110	0.2420
100				0	0.6050

Then, we use Equation 9.6 to calculate the chi-square value.

$$\chi^2 = \frac{\Sigma\, n_i(\hat{p}_i - \bar{p})^2}{\bar{p}(1 - \bar{p})} = \frac{0.6050}{0.36 \cdot 0.64} = 2.626$$

To complete the test of the null hypothesis that there is no trend in the population, we find the chi-square value from Table B.7 that corresponds to one degree of freedom and an α of 0.05. That value is 3.842. Since our calculated chi-square (2.626) is less than 3.842, we do not reject the null hypothesis.

ORDINAL INDEPENDENT VARIABLE

With an ordinal independent variable and a nominal dependent variable, we are interested in the trend in probabilities with increasing relative values (i.e., ranks) of the independent variable. Unless we are willing to assign sizes to the intervals between relative values of the ordinal independent variable, however, we cannot describe the relationship between the dependent and independent variables with the slope and intercept of a straight line. Here, an analysis of trend is not concerned with a constant amount of change in values of the dependent variable. We can perform inference only by testing the null hypothesis that the probabilities in the population do not tend to increase (or decrease) as categories of the ordinal independent variable increase in relative value.

A good statistical test for trend for a nominal dependent variable and an ordinal independent variable is **Bartholomew's test.** The procedures used to conduct Bartholomew's test are rather complex and require special statistical tables. Because of this complexity and the infrequency with which we encounter Bartholomew's test in the health research literature, we will not discuss details of this method in *Statistical First Aid*.

NOMINAL INDEPENDENT VARIABLE

A nominal independent variable has the effect of dividing values of the dependent variable into two groups between which we want to compare estimates of the population's parameters. When the dependent variable is also nominal, the parameter estimates that we compare are often either probabilities or rates. When comparing means in Chapter 7, we looked at the difference between the means of the dependent variable in the two groups defined by values of the nominal independent variable. When comparing probabilities or rates, we can look either at the difference between those probabilities or rates or at their ratio.

ESTIMATION   Point estimates of differences or ratios of probabilities or rates are calculated by using the difference or ratio of the sample's estimates of those probabilities or rates. In general, differences between probabilities are examined more often than their ratios except when those probabilities are measures of disease frequency (i.e., prevalence or risk). With measures of disease frequency, probabilities and rates are usually small. The difference between two small numbers is also a small number. Ratios of small numbers, on the other hand, can be large. For example, suppose that the risk of developing lung cancer during a certain period of time is 0.00001 if a person smokes and 0.000001 if a person does not smoke. The difference between those probabilities is 0.000009. That gives us a very different perspective on the risk of lung cancer among smokers compared to nonsmokers than if we examined the ratio of these two probabilities. That ratio is equal to ten. That implies that smokers are at ten times the risk of developing lung cancer than are nonsmokers!

Neither a difference nor a ratio of probabilities or rates is the better choice for all applications. Which we choose to reflect the relationship between two groups of nominal data depends on the question we are asking. If we are interested in the actual distinction between two groups of values of the nominal dependent variable, we should estimate the difference between probabilities or rates. For example, if we wish to determine the practicality of treating two diseases, we would want estimates that reflected both the efficacy of the treatments and the underlying frequencies of the diseases. In that application, we would be much more impressed with the treatment of a disease if the difference in the probabilities of recovery between those patients who were treated and those who were not treated were 0.01 than we would be for a disease with that difference equal to 0.00001 even if the ratios of those probabilities were the same for the two diseases.

Thus, differences between probabilities or rates reflect not only the relationship but also the magnitude of the probabilities or rates. We could use differences to compare treatment of two diseases in which the frequency of the diseases was of interest. If, on the other hand, we wish to determine only the efficacies of treating two diseases without regard to the frequencies of the diseases they treat, we would not want estimates that were affected by the underlying frequencies of those diseases. In that case, we would consider the treatment that is associated with ten times the probability of recovery among those patients who were treated compared to those

TABLE 9.1 A general 2 × 2 table for organizing observations of a nominal dependent variable and a nominal independent variable. The letters *a*, *b*, *c*, and *d* represent the frequencies (i.e., counts) for each combination of values of the variables. ■

		Independent Variable		
		Group 1	Group 2	
Dependent Variable	Event	a	b	$a + b$
	No Event	c	d	$c + d$
		$a + c$	$b + d$	n

who were not treated to be more efficacious than the treatment that is associated with only twice the probability of recovery among treated persons. This would be true even if the first treatment is for a rare disease and the second is for a common disease. Thus, we should use the ratio of probabilities or rates if we want to ignore the underlying frequencies.

When we have a nominal dependent variable and a nominal independent variable, we organize our observations in a particular way to prepare for analysis. This organization is called a **contingency table** or, more commonly, a **2 × 2 table** (pronounced "2 by 2" table). A 2 × 2 table contains two rows and two columns. Although it is not a rule that is consistently followed in the health research literature, it is a good idea to assign values of the dependent variable to the rows and values of the independent variable columns to help us keep track of which variable is which.[10] Table 9.1 shows a general 2 × 2 table.

With our observations arranged in a 2 × 2 table, calculating probabilities and their differences and ratios is rather straightforward. For example, the probability of the event in group 1 is

$$p(\text{event}|\text{group 1}) = \frac{a}{a + c}$$

and the probability of the event in group 2 is

$$p(\text{event}|\text{group 2}) = \frac{b}{b + d}$$

Thus, the difference between and the ratio of two probabilities can be expressed using the notation from a 2 × 2 table as shown in Equations 9.7 and 9.8.

$$p(\text{event}|\text{group 1}) - p(\text{event}|\text{group 2}) = \frac{a}{a + c} - \frac{b}{b + d} \qquad (9.7)$$

[10] We have chosen this arrangement to be consistent with graphic representation of the dependent and independent variables. Graphically, values of the dependent variable are always assigned to the vertical axis and values of the independent variable are always assigned to the horizontal axis.

$$\frac{p(\text{event}|\text{group 1})}{p(\text{event}|\text{group 2})} = \frac{\dfrac{a}{a+c}}{\dfrac{b}{b+d}} \tag{9.8}$$

Example 9.3 In the clinical trial of a treatment for coronary artery disease described in Example 9.1, 100 persons were given the experimental treatment, and 36 died within the study period. Suppose that another 100 persons were given the standard treatment, and, of those persons, 54 died within the same period of time. Ignoring the dose of the experimental treatment, compare the risk of dying with the experimental treatment to the risk of dying with the standard treatment.

First, let us organize these data in a 2 × 2 table.

		Treatment Group		
		New	Standard	
Survival Outcome	Died	36	54	90
	Survived	64	46	110
		100	100	200

The risks of death for those two treatment groups are:

$$p(\text{death}|\text{new}) = \frac{a}{a+c} = \frac{36}{100} = 0.36$$

$$p(\text{death}|\text{standard}) = \frac{b}{b+d} = \frac{54}{100} = 0.54$$

We could compare those risks either by examining their difference (RD = risk difference) or by examining their ratio (RR = risk ratio or relative risk). If we are interested in the relative efficacy of the new treatment compared to the standard treatment, the risk ratio (Equation 9.7) is probably the better choice since it is not influenced by the underlying risk of death in coronary artery disease patients.

$$\text{RR} = \frac{p(\text{death}|\text{new})}{p(\text{death}|\text{standard})} = \frac{\dfrac{a}{a+c}}{\dfrac{b}{b+d}} = \frac{0.36}{0.54} = 0.67$$

Thus, the risk of death in the time period studied for persons given the new treatment is two-thirds the risk of death for persons given the standard treatment.

If, rather than just the efficacy of the new treatment, we are interested in the practicality of that treatment, it would be better to examine the risk difference (Equation 9.8) than the risk ratio since the risk difference takes into account the underlying frequency of death among coronary artery disease patients.

$$RD = p\,(\text{death}\,|\,\text{new}) - p\,(\text{death}\,|\,\text{standard}) = \frac{a}{a+c} - \frac{b}{b+d} = 0.36 - 0.54 = -0.18$$

The risk difference tells us that, for every 100 patients treated with the new treatment, 18 more persons will survive during the time period studied than would have survived if they had been given the standard treatment.   ▭

In addition to probabilities and rates, nominal dependent variables can be expressed as **odds.** Odds are the number of observations that had the event divided by the number of observations that did not have the event (Equation 9.9).

$$\text{Odds} = \frac{\text{Number of observations with event}}{\text{Number of observations without event}} \tag{9.9}$$

Odds are not rates since they do not contain time in the denominator. Neither are odds probabilities since the numerator is not contained in the denominator. When the probability of an event is small, however, odds have a value that is very close to the value of the probability of the event. For example, if the probability of an event is 0.5, that implies that, for every two observations, one observation will have the event and the other observation will not. The odds for that event would be equal to $1/1$ or 1.0. If, on the other hand, the probability of an event is 0.05, then one out of every 20 observations would have the event and the remaining 19 of those 20 observations would not. The odds of that event would be equal to $1/19$ or 0.053.

We did not consider odds in Chapter 6 when we were discussing univariable samples with a nominal dependent variable because odds are used in health research only to compare nominal dependent variables between groups. Then the odds of an event in the two groups are compared only as a ratio. The **odds ratio** is an important estimate of the relationship between two groups of nominal variables for several reasons. To the statistician, odds ratios are attractive because they have statistical properties that make analysis easier. To the health researcher, odds ratios are attractive because they are less affected by certain types of bias[11] and because they are the only sensible way to compare nominal dependent variables in case-control studies, as we will soon see.

A **case-control study** is a very useful approach to studying common characteristics (which we will call risk factors) and their relationships to rare diseases. In this type of study, the researcher identifies a certain number of persons with the disease (the cases) and a certain number of persons without the disease (the controls). Since disease status defines the groups to be compared, the independent variable in a case-control study is an indicator of whether a person is a case or a control. In case-control studies, the researcher always determines the numbers of cases and controls to be included. Thus, case-control studies always use purposive sampling.

Once cases and controls have been identified, the researcher measures the frequency of some characteristic (or risk factor) for those cases and controls. Since the

[11]The sample's odds ratio is an unbiased estimate of the population's odds ratio under the condition of nondifferential (i.e., the same in both groups) selection bias. Under that same condition, the sample's estimates of differences and ratios of probabilities and rates are biased estimates of the population's corresponding values.

TABLE 9.2 A 2 × 2 table for observations from a case-control study. Here, disease status is represented by the independent variable, and the presence or absence of some characteristic (called a risk factor) is represented by the dependent variable. ■

		Disease Groups		
		Cases	Controls	
Risk Factor	Present	a	b	$a + b$
	Absent	c	d	$c + d$
		$a + c$	$b + d$	n

frequency of the risk factor is what is being determined here, the dependent variable in a case-control study represents the presence or absence of that risk factor. At first, this might seem to be backwards since, as health professionals, we are primarily interested in disease frequency, not presence or absence of some risk factor. It is important to recognize, however, that the data represented by the dependent variable must be randomly sampled from the population. In a case-control study, only the presence or absence of the risk factor meets this criterion. In Table 9.2, we show observations from a case-control study arranged in a 2 × 2 table.

The odds ratio for a case-control study is the odds of exposure among cases divided by the odds of exposure among controls. Equation 9.10 shows the odds ratio (OR) calculated using 2 × 2 table notation.

$$\text{OR} = \frac{\dfrac{a}{c}}{\dfrac{b}{d}} = \frac{ad}{bc} \tag{9.10}$$

Example 9.4 Suppose that we conducted a case-control study of the relationship between consumption of a particular food preservative and stomach cancer. In this study, we identified 100 persons with stomach cancer and 100 persons without stomach cancer and asked them about their consumption of food containing the preservative. Among those persons with stomach cancer, 25 ate foods containing the preservative. Among those persons without stomach cancer, 14 ate foods containing the preservative. Compare the odds of consumption of the preservative between cases and controls.

First, let us organize these data in a 2 × 2 table.

		Disease Group		
		Cases	Controls	
Risk Factor	Preservative	25	14	39
	No Preservative	75	86	161
		100	100	200

The appropriate way to compare the frequencies of preservative consumption among cases and controls is with the odds ratio. Using Equation 9.10:

$$OR = \frac{\dfrac{a}{c}}{\dfrac{b}{d}} = \frac{ad}{bc} = \frac{25 \cdot 86}{75 \cdot 14} = 2.05$$

Thus, the odds of being exposed to this preservative are 2.05 times higher for persons in this sample with stomach cancer than for persons without stomach cancer.

If we wanted to estimate probabilities from observations in a case-control study, we could only calculate the probabilities of having the risk factor for cases and for controls since the frequency of the risk factor is the only variable that has been randomly sampled. Probabilities of having the risk factor, however, are not really of interest to us. Rather, we would like to compare estimates of the probabilities of having the disease for persons who have the risk factor relative to persons who do not have the risk factor. Unfortunately, we cannot estimate probabilities of having the disease from case-control data since the researcher has determined how many cases and how many controls were included in the sample.

With odds, we have a similar limitation in case-control studies. We would like to compare the odds of having the disease between persons with and without the risk factor, but we can only estimate the odds of having the risk factor for cases and controls for the same reason that we are limited to estimating probabilities of having the risk factor. When we compare odds in an odds ratio, however, we find that the ratio of the odds for having the risk factor is identical to the ratio of odds for having the disease. To prove that this is true, Equation 9.11 shows us the ratio of the odds of disease.

$$OR_{\text{Disease}} = \frac{\dfrac{a}{b}}{\dfrac{c}{d}} = \frac{ad}{bc} = OR_{\text{Exposure}} \tag{9.11}$$

Thus, we would calculate the same odds ratio for a case-control study that we would calculate for a cohort study (in which exposure status or presence of a risk factor is represented by the independent variable and disease status is represented by the dependent variable) or a randomized clinical trial. It does not matter which variable is the dependent variable and which is the independent variable; the odds ratio will have exactly the same value (this is not true for the ratio of probabilities). In addition, when we are studying a rare disease, the odds ratio is very close in value to the ratio of probabilities of having the disease. These features make the odds ratio an attractive way to compare nominal dependent variable values between groups defined by a nominal independent variable.

PAIRED DESIGN   In Chapter 4, we examined what was called a paired sample for a continuous dependent variable. These paired data were analyzed using a univariable procedure since only one value (the difference between the measurements) was necessary to summarize the data for each individual. This type of data incorporating a nominal dependent variable is not very common in health research (although we examined such a data set in Example 6.5). Rather, when we refer to a paired sample for nominal variables, we usually are referring to something more complex than a paired sample of continuous data.

When we have a paired design for a nominal dependent variable and a nominal independent variable, we measure two nominal variables (such as the presence or absence of a risk factor and the presence or absence of a disease) for each individual in the study, and for each individual there is another, identical individual for whom that same pair of variables is measured. Thus, a paired sample in this context refers to the observation of both paired data (as in a paired sample of a continuous variable described in Chapter 4) and paired variables (like any bivariable data set). For example, consider a randomized clinical trial in which we compare the frequency of cure (dependent variable) for two treatment groups (independent variable). For each individual in this clinical trial, we will determine values for both of those nominal variables (thus, we have paired variables). Now, suppose that we identify pairs of individuals in our study that are, say, the same age and gender. This pairing of individuals results in paired data.[12]

Nominal data from a paired sample are organized in a type of 2 × 2 table, but the table for a paired sample is quite different from the 2 × 2 tables we have examined for unpaired samples. For one thing, the frequencies in the table are the number of *pairs* of individuals rather than the number of individuals themselves.[13] Another difference between paired and unpaired 2 × 2 tables is that rows and columns in the paired 2 × 2 table are distinguished by categories of the independent variable rather than columns representing the independent variable and rows representing the dependent variable. The two columns (and the two rows) are identified by categories of the dependent variable in a paired 2 × 2 table. Table 9.3 illustrates a paired 2 × 2 table. Compare this table to the unpaired 2 × 2 table in Table 9.1.

Just as we did for unpaired samples, we can calculate a probability difference or probability ratio from paired data organized in a table such as Table 9.3. The probability difference and probability ratio are calculated differently using data arranged in a paired 2 × 2 table than when they are calculated using data arranged in an unpaired 2 × 2 table (but the values of the estimates and their interpretation are the same regardless of which method is used). The method of estimating the probability ratio from data arranged in a paired 2 × 2 table is shown in Equation 9.12, and the method for estimating the probability difference from a paired 2 × 2 table is shown in Equation 9.13.

---

[12]Recall from Chapter 4 that paired data can consist of two measurements on the same or similar individuals. Because of the nature of nominal data (e.g., an individual usually can be cured only once), it is often impossible to make the same set of observations twice on the same individual. Thus, paired nominal data usually consist of similar individuals rather than two measurements on the same individual.

[13] This procedure of looking at the results of a pair of nominal observations is parallel to finding the differences between paired observations of continuous data.

TABLE 9.3 A 2 × 2 table for nominal data from a paired sample. The numbers in this table refer to pairs of individuals rather than the individuals themselves. Rows and columns are distinguished by categories of the independent variable (group 1/group 2). Categories of the dependent variable (event/no event) identify each particular column and each particular row. ■

		Group 2		
		Event	No Event	
Group 1	Event	a	b	$a + b$
	No Event	c	d	$c + d$
		$a + c$	$b + d$	n

$$\text{PR} = \frac{a + b}{a + c} \tag{9.12}$$

$$\text{PD} = \frac{b - c}{n} \tag{9.13}$$

where

$\quad n$ = number of pairs

$\quad \text{PR}$ = probability ratio

$\quad \text{PD}$ = probability difference

Example 9.5 In Example 9.3, we examined data from a clinical trial comparing the effects of a new and a standard treatment on survival among persons with coronary artery disease. We were told that 100 persons were randomized to receive the new treatment and 100 persons were randomized to receive the standard treatment. Now, let us suppose that pairs of subjects were identified on the basis of age and gender, and one member of each of the 100 pairs was randomized to receive the new treatment and the other to receive the standard treatment. The outcomes in each of those pairs might look like the following:

		Standard Treatment		
		Died	Survived	
New Treatment	Died	24	12	36
	Survived	30	34	64
		54	46	100

Estimate the population's probability ratio and probability difference from those paired data.

Using Equation 9.12, we can estimate the probability ratio:

$$\text{PR} = \frac{a + b}{a + c} = \frac{36}{54} = 0.67$$

Note that this probability ratio is exactly the same as the probability ratio we obtained from the unpaired data in Example 9.3. Now, let us use Equation 9.13 to estimate the population's probability difference.

$$PD = \frac{b - c}{n} = \frac{-18}{100} = -0.18$$

That probability difference also is exactly equal to the one we calculated in Example 9.3.   ▯

In addition to probability ratios and differences, we can calculate an estimate of the population's odds ratio from paired nominal data. Unlike probability ratios and differences which are the same whether calculated from paired or unpaired 2 × 2 tables, odds ratios estimated from data that are obtained using a paired method of sampling are biased (i.e., they deviate from the truth in a predictable direction) if they are calculated without taking the paired method of sampling into account (using the data arranged in an unpaired 2 × 2 table). The correct way to estimate the population's odds ratio is to use Equation 9.14 on data arranged in a paired 2 × 2 table.

$$OR = \frac{b}{c} \qquad\qquad (9.14)$$

Example 9.6 From the paired data in Example 9.5, estimate the population's odds ratio. Compare this estimate to the odds ratio estimate that we would have calculated from the unpaired data in Example 9.3.

To estimate the population's odds ratio from the paired data in Example 9.5, we use Equation 9.14:

$$OR = \frac{b}{c} = \frac{12}{30} = 0.40$$

Note. This ratio is less than one, indicating that the odds of dying with the new treatment are less than the odds of dying on the old treatment. If we had arranged the 2 × 2 table in Example 9.5 differently (i.e., with the rows representing the standard treatment and the columns representing the new treatment), we would have obtained an odds ratio of $1/0.40 = 2.50$.

Now, let us use Equation 9.10 to estimate (incorrectly) the population's odds ratio from the unpaired data in Example 9.3.

$$OR = \frac{\dfrac{a}{c}}{\dfrac{b}{d}} = \frac{ad}{bc} = \frac{36 \cdot 46}{54 \cdot 64} = 0.48$$

Note that the odds ratio estimate calculated from the unpaired data (0.48) is different than the odds ratio estimate calculated from the paired data (0.40). Thus, we should use the method in Equation 9.14 when we have a paired sample of nominal data to avoid a biased estimate of the population's odds ratio.

INFERENCE Statistical methods to test inferences about a nominal dependent variable divided into groups by a nominal independent variable utilize the same procedures for differences and ratios. The most common null hypotheses that we are interested in testing about a nominal dependent variable and a nominal independent variable are that a difference is equal to zero or that a ratio is equal to one. Both of those null hypotheses are true under the same condition. That condition is met when the probabilities, rates, or odds are the same in the two groups specified by values of the independent variable. Thus, the same statistical test addresses both null hypotheses simultaneously.

There are several statistical procedures that can be used to test the null hypothesis that the difference between two probabilities is equal to zero or that the ratio of probabilities or odds is equal to one. Let us begin to examine the most popular of these by looking at a normal approximation for the difference between two probabilities. This test is similar to the Student's t procedure described in Chapter 7 for a continuous dependent variable in that we divide the difference between the observed and hypothesized differences by the standard error of the difference.

Calculation of the standard error for the difference between two probabilities also has some similarities to the standard error for the difference between two means. Recall from Chapter 7 that the standard error for the difference between two means is equal to the square root of the summed variances of the distributions of all possible samples' estimates of those means (Equation 7.26). Similarly, the standard error for the difference between two probabilities (in range of 0.05 to 0.95) is equal to the square root of their summed variances. The standard error for the difference between two probabilities also has some similarity to the standard error for a single probability. We learned in Chapter 6 that the standard error of all possible samples' estimates of a population's probability is equal to the square root of the probability times its complement divided by the sample's size (Equation 6.5). The standard error for the difference between two probabilities also is a function of the point estimates of those probabilities.

The fact that the standard error for the difference between two probabilities is calculated from the estimates of probabilities themselves has two effects on the method we use to test hypotheses about that difference. First, it implies that we do not need to penalize ourselves for the effect of chance in estimating the population's variance of data. Thus, as in the normal approximation to the binomial, we convert the difference between two probabilities to a standard normal deviate rather than a Student's t value (Equation 9.15).

$$z = \frac{(p_1 - p_2) - (\theta_1 - \theta_2)}{SE_{p_1 - p_2}}$$ (9.15)

The second effect of having the standard error for the difference between two probabilities a function of the probabilities themselves is that the probabilities that are used in calculating the standard error are dictated by the null hypothesis rather than by the point estimates of those probabilities. For the null hypothesis that the difference is equal to zero, we assume that both groups have the same probability (represented by $\bar{p}$) in the population when performing inference. The reason for this assumption here is that, if the null hypothesis is true, then the probabilities in the population are equal. Recall from Chapter 3 that statistical inference is performed under the assumption that the null hypothesis is true.[14] Thus, the standard error for the difference between two probabilities is calculated as in Equation 9.16 when the null hypothesis states that the probabilities are equal in the population from which the sample was drawn. Our best guess at the value of the probability in the population is a weighted average of the probability estimates, with the number of observations in each group used as the weights:

$$ SE_{p_1 - p_2} = \sqrt{\frac{\bar{p}(1 - \bar{p})}{n_1} + \frac{\bar{p}(1 - \bar{p})}{n_2}} \tag{9.16} $$

where $\bar{p}$ = weighted average of the two probability estimates, with the number of observations in each group used as the weights. Specifically:

$$ \bar{p} = \frac{(p_1 \cdot n_1) + (p_2 \cdot n_2)}{n_1 + n_2} $$

Example 9.7 Using the observations in Example 9.3 (assuming that this is an unpaired experiment), test the null hypothesis that the risk of death in the group given the new treatment is the same as the risk in the group given the standard treatment. As an alternative, consider that the risks are not equal. Allow a 5% chance of making a Type I error.

In Example 9.3, we found that the risk of death among the 100 persons on the new treatment was 0.36 and that risk among the 100 persons given the standard treatment was 0.54. The first step in testing the null hypothesis that these risks are equal in the population is to calculate a weighted average of the sample's two estimates of the risk.

$$ \bar{p} = \frac{(p_1 \cdot n_1) + (p_2 \cdot n_2)}{n_1 + n_2} = \frac{(0.36 \cdot 100) + (0.54 \cdot 100)}{100 + 100} = 0.45 $$

Next, we use that weighted average of the sample's estimates of the risk of death in Equation 9.16 to estimate the standard error for the difference in risks.

$$ SE_{p_1 - p_2} = \sqrt{\frac{\bar{p}(1 - \bar{p})}{n_1} + \frac{\bar{p}(1 - \bar{p})}{n_2}} = \sqrt{\frac{0.45(1 - 0.45)}{100} + \frac{0.45(1 - 0.45)}{100}} = 0.0704 $$

[14]It is not assumed that the population's probabilities are equal in interval estimation since interval estimation does not involve any assumptions about the null hypothesis. Thus, the standard error in interval estimation for a nominal dependent variable and a nominal independent variable is different from the standard error for inference. This implies that the test-based confidence interval method described in Chapter 3 will not give us the same confidence interval to compare probabilities that we could obtain using a more exact method (although it will usually be close). We will not discuss these more exact methods in *Statistical First Aid*.

Then, we use Equation 9.15 to convert our observed risk difference to a standard normal deviate.

$$z = \frac{(p_1 - p_2) - (\theta_1 - \theta_2)}{SE_{p_1 - p_2}} = \frac{(0.36 - 0.54) - 0}{0.0704} = 2.56$$

From Table B.1, we find that a standard normal deviate with an area of $0.05/2 = 0.025$ in each tail is equal to 1.96. Since our calculated standard normal deviate (2.56) is greater than 1.96, we reject the null hypothesis and accept, by elimination, the alternative hypothesis stating that the probabilities are not equal in the population from which the sample was drawn.   ⊟

    With the procedure that we have just examined for the difference between two probabilities, it is necessary to distinguish between the dependent and independent variables. A more common statistical procedure for two nominal variables tests a more generalized null hypothesis about the relationship between the variables that does not rely on a distinction between the dependent and independent variables (at least in its method of calculation). The null hypothesis in that procedure is that the two variables represent independent events.

    By independent, we mean the same thing that was implied by independence between events in Chapter 1. Recall from Chapter 1 that the definition of independent events is that the probability of their intersection is equal to the product of their individual, unconditional probabilities (the multiplication rule of probability theory). In a 2×2 table, an unconditional probability refers to the probability of obtaining an observation in a particular row regardless of which column the observation is in (or in a particular column regardless of which row). Thus, in the context of a 2×2 table, independence means that the probability of an observation in any cell (a **cell** is where a specific row and column intersect in the 2×2 table) is equal to the probability associated with that row times the probability associated with that column. For example, if the variables represent independent events, the probability of being in group 1 and having the event represented by the dependent variable (the cell containing a in Table 9.1) would be equal to the overall probability of being in group 1 times the overall probability of having the event. These overall probabilities are called **marginal probabilities** since they are calculated from the row and column totals that appear in the margins (i.e., outside the cells) of the 2×2 table.

    To test the null hypothesis that the dependent and independent variable values are independent of one another, we first determine the values we would expect to see in the 2×2 table if the null hypothesis were true. We calculate the probability of making an observation in any particular cell by multiplying the corresponding marginal probabilities. Since a 2×2 table itself contains frequencies (i.e., counts) rather than probabilities, we multiply the expected probability by the total number of observations (i.e., the number in all the cells combined) to determine the number of observations we would expect to observe in each cell if the null hypothesis were true. As an illustration of how these expected values are calculated, Equation 9.17 shows the method of determining the number of observations that we would expect to observe in the a cell of a 2×2 table if the null hypothesis were true.

$$E_a = \frac{a+b}{n} \cdot \frac{a+c}{n} \cdot n = \frac{(a+b) \cdot (a+c)}{n} \qquad (9.17)$$

where

E_a = number of observations in the a cell of a 2×2 table that would be expected if the null hypothesis of independence between the variables were true

n = total number of observations ($n = a + b + c + d$)

Notice in Equation 9.17 that the calculation of the expected number in a cell of the 2×2 table can be algebraically simplified to be equal to the product of the marginal frequencies (corresponding to the cell in which we are interested) divided by the total number of observations. Table 9.4 shows how to calculate the expected frequencies for each of the cells of a 2×2 table using this simplification.

To test the null hypothesis that the dependent and independent variables are independent of each other, we compare the frequencies that we actually observed with those that we would have expected to observe if the null hypothesis were true. If we make that comparison by squaring the difference between the frequency we observed and the frequency we expect for a particular cell and dividing by the frequency we expect, then the sum of those values for all four cells of the 2×2 table is equal to a **chi-square** statistic (Equation 9.18).

$$\chi^2 = \sum \frac{(O_i - E_i)^2}{E_i} \qquad (9.18)$$

where

O_i = observed frequency in a particular cell of the 2×2 table
E_i = expected frequency in a particular cell of the 2×2 table

As we discussed earlier in this chapter, the chi-square distribution is an extension of the standard normal distribution. Like the Student's t distribution, the chi-square distribution is characterized by degrees of freedom. Unlike the Student's t distribu-

---

TABLE 9.4 Calculation of the frequencies expected in each cell of a 2×2 table under the assumption that the dependent and independent variables are independent of each other. The expected frequencies are equal to the product of corresponding marginal frequencies divided by the total number of observations. ■

		Independent Variable		
		Group 1	Group 2	
Dependent Variable	Event	$\dfrac{(a+b) \cdot (a+c)}{n}$	$\dfrac{(a+b) \cdot (b+d)}{n}$	$a+b$
	No Event	$\dfrac{(c+d) \cdot (a+c)}{n}$	$\dfrac{(c+d) \cdot (b+d)}{n}$	$c+d$
		$a+c$	$b+d$	n

tion, however, the number of degrees of freedom in the chi-square distribution does not reflect the effect of chance in estimating the population's variance of data. This is not necessary for the chi-square distribution since it is used only for combinations of binomial distributions. Rather, degrees of freedom in the chi-square distribution reflect the amount of information contained in the calculation of a chi-square value. This distinction is more clear if we compare how Student's t values change with increasing degrees of freedom to how chi-square values change. Notice in Table B.2 that Student's t values decrease (approaching standard normal deviates) as the degrees of freedom increase. This reflects the decreasing influence of chance on estimation of the population's variance of data. Chi-square values, on the other hand, increase (starting as the square of standard normal deviates) as the degrees of freedom increase (Table B.7). This reflects the fact that a chi-square value with more degrees of freedom contains more information and, thus, is expected to be a larger number for a particular probability of making a Type I error.

Degrees of freedom in the chi-square distribution reflect the amount of information that goes into calculating the chi-square value. If we look at Equation 9.18, we might think that there are four separate pieces of information in that calculation. In fact, there is only one piece of information that we are using four times. That value is the squared difference between what we observe and what we expect. For each of the four cells, that difference is equal to the same value (we will see in Example 9.8 that all four squared differences are $9^2 = 81$).

Thus, the chi-square value calculated in Equation 9.18 has one degree of freedom. To further understand why that is the case, we first need to understand that the chi-square test assumes that the marginal probabilities are "fixed." That is to say, when using the chi-square distribution on a 2×2 table, we are assuming that we have observed one 2×2 table from a collection of all possible 2×2 tables with the same marginal frequencies. Now, we can look at the degrees of freedom in a 2×2 table another way. Imagine a 2×2 table in which the marginal frequencies are given but none of the cell frequencies are known. How many cell frequencies would we need to know to fill out the rest of the table? To demonstrate to yourself that we need to know only one cell frequency before the cell frequencies of all four cells are determined, take a look at Table 9.5. Pick any value (equal to ten or less) for the frequency of the event in Group 1 (i.e., the a cell). Notice that now you can derive the rest of the values in the 2×2 table by subtraction. Thus, the 2×2 table, with the marginal frequencies known, contains only one piece of information or, in other words, one degree of freedom.

In Table B.7, only one-tailed α values appear at the top of the table. This reflects the fact that the chi-square distribution is an expansion of the *square* of the standard normal distribution. The square root of a chi-square value with one degree of freedom associated with an area of α in one tail is, thus, equal to a standard normal deviate with an area of $\alpha/2$ in each tail (i.e., a two-tailed standard normal deviate). When the null hypothesis of independence is true, we expect, on the average, to obtain a chi-square

---

TABLE 9.5 Demonstration that a 2 × 2 table contains only one piece of information when the marginal frequencies are fixed (i.e., known). Once you choose a value for the *a* cell, the values of the remaining three cells can be determined by subtraction from the marginal frequencies.

		Independent Variable		
		Group 1	Group 2	
Dependent Variable	Event	*a*	?	10
	No Event	?	?	90
		50	50	100

---

value of zero. When the null hypothesis is not true, we expect to obtain a chi-square value greater than zero.[15] Thus, chi-square values are one-tailed even though deviations from independence can be in either direction.

Example 9.8   Test the null hypothesis that there is no association between (i.e., that there is independence of) the type of treatment and the risk of death in the population from which the observations in Example 9.3 were drawn. Allow a 5% chance of making a Type I error.

In Example 9.3, we were given the following 2 × 2 table.

		Treatment Group		
		New	Standard	
Survival Outcome	Died	36	54	90
	Survived	64	46	110
		100	100	200

The first step in testing this null hypothesis is calculation of the values we would have expected to observe in this 2 × 2 table if the null hypothesis were true. Those expected values are calculated using the procedure shown for the *a* cell in Equation 9.17.

$$E_a = \frac{(a + b) \cdot (a + c)}{n} = \frac{90 \cdot 100}{200} = 45$$

$$E_b = \frac{(a + b) \cdot (b + d)}{n} = \frac{90 \cdot 100}{200} = 45$$

---

[15]Squaring either a negative or a positive number with a given (absolute) value results in the same positive number. Thus, values from the chi-square distribution (with one degree of freedom) cannot distinguish between the two tails of the standard normal distribution.

$$E_c = \frac{(c + d) \cdot (a + c)}{n} = \frac{100 \cdot 100}{200} = 55$$

$$E_d = \frac{(c + d) \cdot (b + d)}{n} = \frac{110 \cdot 100}{200} = 55$$

It is helpful to include those expected frequencies in the 2 × 2 table. We have enclosed them in brackets in the following table.

		Treatment Group		
		New	Standard	
Survival Outcome	Died	36 {45}	54 {45}	90
	Survived	64 {55}	46 {55}	110
		100	100	200

Now, we can calculate the chi-square value using Equation 9.18.

$$\chi^2 = \sum \frac{(O_i - E_i)^2}{E_i} = \frac{(36 - 45)^2}{45} + \frac{(54 - 45)^2}{45} + \frac{(64 - 55)^2}{55} + \frac{(46 - 55)^2}{55} = 6.545$$

From Table B.7, we find that a chi-square value corresponding to an α of 0.05 and one degree of freedom is equal to 3.841. Since our calculated chi-square value (6.545) is greater than the value from Table B.7, we reject the null hypothesis that treatment and outcome are independent and accept, by elimination, the alternative hypothesis that these variables are not independent (i.e., they are associated) in the population from which the sample was drawn.

Thus far, we have examined two apparently different approaches to 2 × 2 table data. Actually, the normal approximation between two probabilities and the chi-square test for independence are different only in the methods of calculation. Testing the null hypothesis that the variables are independent is really the same as a two-tailed test of the null hypothesis that the probabilities are equal. We can convince ourselves of this by comparing the square root of the chi-square value we found in Example 9.8 to the standard normal deviate we found in Example 9.7. The square root of 6.545 is equal to 2.56, which is exactly the value of the standard normal deviate calculated in Example 9.7. So, we have done nothing new with the chi-square test that we could not do with the normal approximation to the difference between probabilities testing the null hypothesis that the probabilities are equal in the population that was sampled.

If these tests are identical, why do we study both? We study the normal approximation for the difference between probabilities because, in some ways, it is more flexible than the chi-square test. Specifically, the normal approximation allows testing a null hypothesis other than equality of the probabilities. In addition, the normal approximation for the difference between probabilities allows a one-tailed alternative hypothesis. We study the chi-square test because it is so commonly used in health research statistics. There are two reasons for the popularity of the chi-square test. First, many people believe that calculation of the chi-square value is easier than calculation of the standard normal deviate (as in Equation 9.15). A more important reason is that the chi-square procedure can easily be expanded to analyze several nominal dependent variables and/or several nominal independent variables. Instead of 2×2 tables, data sets that contain several dependent and/or independent variables are organized in $R \times C$ tables (R stands for the number of rows and C stands for the number of columns). Calculation of a chi-square value for an $R \times C$ table follows the same procedures we have examined for 2×2 tables. The resulting chi-square value has $(R - 1) \cdot (C - 1)$ degrees of freedom.[16]

The chi-square value calculated from a 2×2 table has one degree of freedom, reflecting the fact that we need to know the frequency in only one cell to be able to determine the frequencies in the other three cells (if the marginal frequencies are known). In other words, most of the information used in calculation of the chi-square value is redundant. Thus, it seems as if we should be able to examine just one of the four cells and draw the same conclusion that we can draw from examining all four cells. In fact, another type of statistical test does examine the null hypothesis that the variables are independent by looking at just one of the four cells. The calculated test statistic in this procedure is a standard normal deviate, but it is conventional to use the symbol χ_{M-H} rather than z to represent it. The M-H subscript refers to the names of the developers of this procedure (Mantel and Haenszel), and the test statistic is called the **Mantel-Haenszel chi**.[17] The Mantel-Haenszel procedure uses a standard normal deviate rather than a chi-square value. Thus, one-tailed as well as two-tailed alternative hypotheses can be considered.

The Mantel-Haenszel chi is calculated by subtracting the value we would expect for a particular cell (if the null hypothesis were true) from the value we actually observed and, then, dividing by the standard error of that difference. It does not matter which cell frequency we use to calculate the Mantel-Haenszel chi, but the frequency in the upper left of the 2×2 table (the a cell) is customarily selected. Equation 9.19 shows how the Mantel-Haenszel chi is calculated. Notice that the value that we expect for the cell frequency is the same as the expected value we calculated for that cell using the chi-square procedure.

$$\chi_{M-H} = \frac{a - \dfrac{(a + b) \cdot (a + c)}{n}}{\sqrt{\dfrac{(a + b) \cdot (c + d) \cdot (a + c) \cdot (b + d)}{n^2 \cdot (n - 1)}}} \tag{9.19}$$

[16]Strictly speaking, calculation of a chi-square for an $R \times C$ table is a multivariate procedure when the number of rows is greater than two. Under this condition, we have more than one dependent variable.

[17]Mantel and Haenszel actually developed this test statistic for the special purpose of multivariable analysis. We present it in the form that it takes when there is only one independent variable. In Chapter 12, we will look at this statistic again in the context in which it was originally presented.

Example 9.9   Test the null hypothesis that there is no association between type of treatment and risk of death for the observations in Example 9.3, using the Mantel-Haenszel chi procedure. As an alternative hypothesis, consider that there is an association, without specifying the direction of the deviation from independence (i.e., use a two-tailed alternative hypothesis). Allow a 5% chance of making a Type I error.

Using Equation 9.19, we find the following standard normal deviate, assuming that the null hypothesis is correct.

$$\chi_{M-H} = \frac{a - \dfrac{(a+b)\cdot(a+c)}{n}}{\sqrt{\dfrac{(a+b)\cdot(c+d)\cdot(a+c)\cdot(b+d)}{n^2\cdot(n-1)}}} = \frac{36 - \dfrac{90\cdot 100}{200}}{\sqrt{\dfrac{90\cdot 110\cdot 100\cdot 100}{200^2\cdot(200-1)}}} = 2.552$$

To test the null hypothesis that treatment and outcome are independent, we compare our calculated value (2.552) to the value from Table B.1 that corresponds to an area of $0.05/2 = 0.025$ in each tail of the standard normal distribution (1.96). Since the calculated value is greater than 1.96, we reject the null hypothesis that there is no association between these variables and accept, by elimination, the alternative hypothesis that there is an association in the population. ▱

The conclusion we draw in Example 9.9 is the same as the one we encountered in Example 9.8. In both cases, we rejected the null hypothesis. The value of the Mantel-Haenzsel chi, however, is not exactly equal to the square root of the chi-square value in Example 9.8 (the square root of 6.545 is equal to 2.558). The reason for this difference is that both the Mantel-Haenszel chi and the chi-square are normal approximations, but they are slightly different approximations.[18]

Both the Mantel-Haenszel procedure and the chi-square test (as well as the equivalent test in Equation 9.15) test the null hypothesis that the dependent and independent variables in a 2 × 2 table are independent. This is the same as testing the null hypothesis that the difference between two probabilities is equal to zero or the null hypothesis that the ratio of two probabilities is equal to one. It is also the same as testing the null hypothesis that the odds ratio is equal to one. Each of these statistical procedures is appropriate for unpaired 2 × 2 table data. If the data are paired, however, we should use a different statistical procedure to test hypotheses about probabilities and odds. This procedure for paired nominal data is called **McNemar's test.**

Like the test for independence between variables for unpaired nominal data, McNemar's test calculates a chi-square statistic with one degree of freedom that is based on a normal approximation for the difference between probabilities. McNemar's test is different from the chi-square test of independence in that the method of calculating McNemar's chi-square uses data arranged in a paired 2 × 2 table (as in

---

[18] Under most circumstances, the approximation used in the Mantel-Haenszel method is a slightly better approximation.

Table 9.3). Equation 9.20 shows how McNemar's chi-square is calculated from paired data.

$$\chi^2 = \frac{(b - c)^2}{b + c} \tag{9.20}$$

Example 9.10   For the paired data in Example 9.5, test the null hypothesis that the risk ratio is equal to one in the population from which the sample was drawn versus the alternative hypothesis that the risk ratio is not equal to one. Allow a 5% chance of making a Type I error.

Since these data are paired, we use McNemar's test and calculate a chi-square as in Equation 9.20.

$$\chi^2 = \frac{(b - c)^2}{b + c} = \frac{(12 - 30)^2}{12 + 30} = 7.714$$

From Table B.7, we find that a chi-square corresponding to an α of 0.05 and one degree of freedom is equal to 3.841. Since our calculated chi-square value (7.714) is greater than the value from Table B.7, we reject the null hypothesis that treatment and outcome are independent and accept, by elimination, the alternative hypothesis that these variables are not independent in the population.

Note that the chi-square value that we calculated in this example is larger than the chi-square value that we calculated in Example 9.8 (6.545) when we analyzed these data as if they were not paired. McNemar's test should result in a larger chi-square value (and, thus, have greater statistical power) if the data are collected utilizing pairs of individuals who share characteristics that are strong determinants of the outcome.

So far, we have considered inference for probabilities and odds. To test the null hypothesis that the difference between two rates is equal to zero or that their ratio is equal to one in the population from which the sample was drawn, we need to use a different method. The statistical procedure for rates (i.e., incidences) is similar to, but not the same as, the Mantel-Haenszel procedure. This procedure for incidences also calculates a standard normal deviate by subtracting the expected frequency of the event in one of the groups (assuming that the incidences are the same in both groups) from the observed frequency and dividing by the standard error of that difference. The procedure for incidences, however, uses the follow-up time (person-years) as part of the calculation of the expected value (Equation 9.21). That expected value is calculated by multiplying the total number of events observed by the proportion of the total follow-up time associated with that group. In other words, we assume that, if the null hypothesis is true, the number of events we will observe in a particular group is only a function of how long we look for events in that group.

$$\chi = \frac{a - \left[(a + b) \cdot \dfrac{py_1}{py_{total}}\right]}{\sqrt{\dfrac{(a + b) \cdot (py_1) \cdot (py_2)}{py_{total}^2}}} \tag{9.21}$$

where

a = number of events in group 1
b = number of events in group 2
py_1 = number of person-years of follow-up in group 1
py_2 = number of person-years of follow-up in group 2
py_{total} = total number of person-years of follow-up

Example 9.11   Suppose that, in a cohort study of senile cataracts, we followed a group of persons with diabetes for a total of 120 person-years and group of persons without diabetes for a total of 150 person-years. Among the persons with diabetes, 12 senile cataracts developed. Among the persons without diabetes, 10 senile cataracts were observed. Test the null hypothesis that the incidence of cataracts in the population is the same for these two groups. As an alternative hypothesis, consider that the incidences are not the same. Allow a 5% chance of making a Type I error.

To test this hypothesis, we can compare the number of cataracts actually observed in one of the groups with the number we would expect if the incidence of cataracts were the same among persons with diabetes as among persons without diabetes. We will arbitrarily choose the group of persons with diabetes to calculate a standard normal deviate. Then, using Equation 9.21, we get the following result:

$$\chi = \frac{a - \left[(a + b) \cdot \dfrac{py_1}{py_{total}}\right]}{\sqrt{\dfrac{(a + b) \cdot (py_1) \cdot (py_2)}{py_{total}^2}}} = \frac{12 - \left[(12 + 10) \cdot \dfrac{120}{270}\right]}{\sqrt{\dfrac{(12 + 10) \cdot 120 \cdot 150}{270^2}}} = 0.95$$

We compare that result with a standard normal deviate from Table B.1 corresponding to an area of $0.05/2 = 0.025$ in each tail. That standard normal deviate is equal to 1.96. Since 0.95 is less than 1.96, we do not reject the null hypothesis.

In each of the procedures we have described for a nominal dependent variable and a nominal independent variable, we have used a continuous distribution (i.e., the Gaussian distribution) to approximate a distribution for data that are not continuous. Some statisticians suggest that approximations of a continuous distribution with bivariable nominal data should include a correction for the discontinuity of distributions of discrete data.[19] The most common method of correction is to subtract one half from the absolute value of each difference between an observed value and an expected value (this is called the **Yates correction**). Not all statisticians are convinced that such corrections are necessary. Because of this controversy and because these corrections are likely to detract from our understanding of the basic statistical procedures, we have not

[19] Distributions of discrete (i.e., nominal or ordinal) data allow calculation of probabilities for a limited number of specific values. For example, we can calculate the probability of observing 10 out of 100 persons with a disease or of observing 11 out of 100 persons with that disease. We cannot, however, calculate the probability of observing a number of cases of disease between 10 and 11. Thus, we say that distributions of discrete data are discontinuous.

included continuity corrections in the equations presented in *Statistical First Aid*. If they are used, they will have the effect of decreasing the calculated test statistic by a small amount.

||| SUMMARY

Many of the statistical procedures that we have examined in this chapter for a nominal dependent variable and one independent variable are very similar to the procedures described in Chapter 7 for bivariable data sets containing a continuous dependent variable. An example is the chi-square test for trend which involves estimation of a straight line to describe probabilities as a function of a continuous independent variable.

$$\hat{p} = a + b X \qquad (9.2)$$

Estimation of the slope of the straight line in trend analysis is accomplished by dividing the sum of cross products by the sum of squares for the independent variable. Although the notation is slightly different for a nominal dependent variable, the principle is the same as regression analysis for a continuous dependent variable.

$$b = \frac{\Sigma\, n_i(\hat{p}_i - \bar{p})\,(X_i - \overline{X})}{\Sigma\, n_i(X_i - \overline{X})^2} \qquad (9.3)$$

Estimation of the intercept in trend analysis relies on the fact that the straight line will pass through the point corresponding to the mean of both variables just as in estimation of the intercept for a continuous dependent variable.

$$a = \bar{p} - b\overline{X} \qquad (9.4)$$

Testing the omnibus null hypothesis in trend analysis for a nominal dependent variable and a continuous independent variable is similar to the F test in regression analysis in that inference in trend analysis involves examination of a ratio of two estimates of the variation of data represented by the dependent variable. In regression analysis, the F ratio is calculated by dividing the explained variation (the regression mean square) by the unexplained variation (the residual mean square). In trend analysis, we divide the explained variation by the total variation. The reason for this difference between regression analysis and trend analysis is that the total variation of a nominal dependent variable is a function of the point estimates and, therefore, is not subject to separate effects of chance. The ratio in trend analysis has a distribution that is the square of the standard normal distribution. The square of the standard normal distribution is represented by the chi-square distribution with one degree of freedom.

$$\chi^2 = \frac{\Sigma\, n_i(\hat{p}_i - \bar{p})^2}{\bar{p}(1 - \bar{p})} \qquad (9.6)$$

The distinction between the terms "regression analysis" and "trend analysis" is that regression analysis implies estimation of the magnitude of the change in values of the dependent variable for each unit change in the value of the independent variable, while trend analysis implies that values of the dependent variable change as values of the independent variable change, without necessarily specifying the magnitude of that change. When we have a nominal dependent variable and a continuous independent variable, we use procedures for analysis of trend that also estimate the magnitude of the change in values of the dependent variable. This is not true of trend analysis for a nominal dependent variable and an ordinal independent variable. In that case, we examine the tendency of values of the dependent variable to change as values of the independent variable change. The method introduced in this chapter for trend analysis when the independent variable is ordinal is called Bartholomew's test. Because of the complexity of the procedures involved in Bartholomew's test, we did not describe them.

Another parallel between bivariable data sets that contain a continuous dependent variable and those that contain a nominal dependent variable can be seen when the independent variable is nominal. In both cases, the nominal independent variable has the effect of dividing values of the dependent variable into two groups. Similar to comparing means of a continuous dependent variable between two groups, comparison of probabilities between two groups of nominal dependent variable values can be accomplished by examining the difference between those probabilities.

Means are always compared by examining their difference. Estimates of nominal dependent variable values (e.g., probabilities) can be compared by examining their difference or by examining their ratio. A ratio of nominal dependent variable estimates allows us to consider the relative, rather than absolute, distinction between two groups. Differences can be used to compare probabilities or rates. Probabilities and rates also can be compared as a ratio.

Another ratio that can be used to compare values of a nominal dependent variable between two groups is the odds ratio. The odds ratio is equal to the odds of the event represented by the dependent variable in one group divided by the odds of that event in the other group. Odds are equal to the number of observations in which the event occurred divided by the number of observations in which the event did not occur.

$$\text{OR} = \frac{\frac{a}{c}}{\frac{b}{d}} = \frac{ad}{bc} \tag{9.10}$$

The difference and ratios that we have examined thus far assume that two nominal variables are measured for each individual and that only the values of those variables indicate any relationship among the individuals in a set of observations. In another type of data set for a nominal dependent variable and a nominal independent variable, individuals are paired based on characteristics thought to be associated with values of the dependent variable. In this paired sample, one member of the pair has one value of the nominal independent variable, and the other member of the pair has the other value of the independent variable.

Paired nominal data are arranged in a 2 × 2 table that is different from the type of 2 × 2 table used to organized unpaired nominal data. Ratios and differences between probabilities are calculated from a paired 2 × 2 table using different formulas from those used for an unpaired 2 × 2 table, but the point estimates are the same regardless of which formula is used. That is not true for odds ratios, which must be estimated using the formula for paired data if the data are paired (Equation 9.14):

$$\text{OR} = \frac{b}{c} \tag{9.14}$$

Statistical inference for nominal dependent and independent variables uses the same statistical procedures to test the most common null hypothesis about differences as is used to test the most common null hypothesis about ratios. Those null hypotheses are that the difference is equal to zero and that the ratio is equal to one. If one of those null hypotheses is true, then both are true, since they both imply that the nominal dependent variable estimates in the two groups are equal.

Thus, we need only one test of inference for probabilities (and odds) and one test for rates. In this chapter, we presented three alternative methods to test null hypotheses about probabilities. The reason for presenting three alternative methods is that all three are commonly encountered in the health research literature. The first method involves conversion of the difference between probabilities to a standard normal deviate.

$$z = \frac{(p_1 - p_2) - (\theta_1 - \theta_2)}{SE_{p_1 - p_2}} \tag{9.15}$$

The standard error for that difference is calculated using a weighted average of the point estimates of the probability of the event in the population.

$$SE_{p_1 - p_2} = \sqrt{\frac{\bar{p}(1 - \bar{p})}{n_1} + \frac{\bar{p}(1 - \bar{p})}{n_2}} \tag{9.16}$$

Another method, known as the chi-square test, is based on the 2×2 table. In this approach, observed frequencies for the four combinations of dependent and independent variable values are compared to what we would expect if the probability of the event were the same for each of the two groups. Calculation of expected values is based on the multiplication rule of probability theory.

$$E_a = \frac{a + b}{n} \cdot \frac{a + c}{n} \cdot n = \frac{(a + b) \cdot (a + c)}{n} \tag{9.17}$$

Observed and expected frequencies are compared for each cell of the 2×2 table. Their sum is a chi-square value with one degree of freedom.

$$\chi^2 = \sum \frac{(O_i - E_i)^2}{E_i} \tag{9.18}$$

The results of those two methods of inference are exactly the same with the chi-square value being the square of the standard normal deviate. The popularity of the chi-square test is due, in part, to its ability for expansion to consider more than one dependent and/or independent variable.

The chi-square test uses redundant information since only one cell of a 2×2 table needs to be known to know all four cells (if the marginal frequencies are known). The third procedure we examined for probabilities and odds uses only one cell of the 2×2 table. This procedure is a slightly different normal approximation, known as the Mantel-Haenszel test.

$$\chi_{M-H} = \frac{a - \frac{(a + b) \cdot (a + c)}{n}}{\sqrt{\frac{(a + b) \cdot (c + d) \cdot (a + c) \cdot (b + d)}{n^2 \cdot (n - 1)}}} \tag{9.19}$$

For statistical inference on paired nominal data, we calculate a chi-square statistic using a special method known as McNemar's test.

$$\chi^2 = \frac{(b - c)^2}{b + c} \tag{9.20}$$

To test the null hypothesis that the difference between rates is equal to one or that the ratio of rates is equal to one, we use a method that is similar to the Mantel-Haenszel procedure.

$$\chi = \frac{a - \left[(a + b) \cdot \dfrac{py_1}{py_{total}}\right]}{\sqrt{\dfrac{(a + b) \cdot (py_1) \cdot (py_2)}{py_{total}^2}}} \qquad (9.21)$$

||| PRACTICE PROBLEMS

9.1 Suppose that we are interested in the relationship between the length of time a patient has had hypertension and the probability that the patient also has diabetes. To investigate this, we examine medical records for a sample of 2,000 persons diagnosed as having hypertension and record the number of years since hypertension was diagnosed and the presence or absence of the diagnosis of diabetes. Suppose we make the following observations:

Years Since Diagnosis	Number with Hypertension	Number with Diabetes
1	306	0
2	314	2
3	321	2
4	264	3
5	215	2
6	248	4
7	179	3
8	153	3

Mathematically describe the linear relationship between the length of time since the diagnosis of hypertension and the probability of having diabetes. Test the omnibus null hypothesis that no linear relationship exists between those variables in the population versus the alternative that a relationship does exist. Allow a 5% chance of incorrectly concluding that a relationship exists.

9.2 An investigator has a study hypothesis that one particular form of senile dementia is associated with a 75% or greater reduction in cerebral blood flow due to arteriosclerosis. To investigate this possibility, she identifies 150 persons with this form of dementia and 150 persons of approximately the same age without dementia in a geriatric practice. Then, she determines whether or not each of those 300 persons also has reduced cerebral blood flow. Suppose that the following results are observed:

		Dementia	
		Cases	Controls
Reduced Cerebral Blood Flow	Present	51	47
	Absent	99	103
		150	150

Calculate a point estimate that best summarizes the relationship between this form of dementia and reduced cerebral blood flow (due to arteriosclerosis) from these sample observations.

9.3 For the population from which the observations in Problem 9.2 were derived, test the hypothesis that the odds ratio is equal to one versus the alternative that it is not equal to one. Allow a 5% chance of making a Type I error.

9.4 Suppose that, in the study described in Problem 9.2, each case was paired with a control of the same age and gender and the following relationships among those pairs were observed.

		Controls		
		Present	Absent	
Cases	Present	30	21	51
	Absent	17	82	99
		47	103	150

Estimate the odds ratio and test the null hypothesis that the odds ratio in the population is equal to one. As an alternative hypothesis, consider that the odds ratio is not equal to one. Allow a 5% chance of making a Type I error.

9.5 A group of researchers believe they have a new treatment that will reduce the death rate among persons with AIDS. To examine this treatment, they randomize 100 persons with AIDS to receive the new treatment and 100 persons with AIDS to receive standard therapy. Then, they follow those 200 persons for a total of five years and make the following observations.

Time Period (years)	Number Surviving at End	
	Treated	Untreated
0–1	91	92
1–2	82	81
2–3	74	71
3–4	67	60
4–5	60	51

Test the null hypothesis that the rates of death are the same in these two groups versus the alternative that the rates of death are different. Allow a 5% chance of making a Type I error.

9.6 It is suspected that two different organisms (gonorrhea and chlamydia) causing a sexually transmitted disease have a tendency to occur together in the same individual more often than would be expected by chance. To examine that suspicion, 100 persons with the sexually transmitted disease were cultured for those organisms. It was found that half of those persons were infected with gonorrhea (with or without chlamydia) and 75 were infected with chlamydia (with or without gonorrhea). Forty-two persons were infected with both gonorrhea and chlamydia. Test the hypothesis that the probability of being infected with gonorrhea is independent of infection with chlamydia. Allow a 5% chance of making a Type I error.

PART FOUR

Understanding Multivariable Analysis

If there is one thing on which we can all agree it is the fact that the science of health and disease is complex. Few diseases have a single cause. There are few measurements that we can make on individuals that are not related to other characteristics of those individuals. To do justice to this complexity, our analyses of data from health research should take these interrelationships into account. This can be done by considering more than one independent variable. When we have a data set with more than one independent variable, we call it a multivariable data set. The methods we use to analyze those data are multivariable procedures.

Usually, we conduct statistical analyses with one variable of primary interest. We know that this variable is the dependent variable. We also know that independent variables define conditions under which we wish to make estimates of or test inferences about that dependent variable. Those conditions are defined for one of two reasons. The first reason is that we wish to examine the relationship between the dependent variable and the independent variable. For example, in data from clinical trials, we have nominal independent variables that specify treatment groups. Our interest in analyzing those data is to compare values of the dependent variable between the treatment groups. So far in *Statistical First Aid,* every example and practice problem has considered independent variables with the purpose of examining the relationship between the dependent and independent variables.

As we learn about multivariable procedures, we will be able to expand the things we can do in statistical analyses. For instance, we previously recognized that nominal data with more than two potential categories must be represented by more than one nominal variable. However, we have not yet learned how to analyze data with more than one independent variable. Also, we will have the ability to examine the relationship between the dependent variable and one or more independent variables, while taking into account or controlling for the effects of other characteristics. For example, when we looked at the relationship between arteriosclerosis and senile dementia in Practice Problem 9.2, we were told that cases and controls were of approximately the same age. The reason for such a statement is that both senile dementia and arteriosclerosis are related to age. If we paid no attention to the ages of cases compared to controls in that problem, we might see an apparent relationship between dementia and arteriosclerosis simply because the cases were older than the controls. In other words, our observations would have been biased in favor of seeing a relationship even if one did not exist.[1] This particular type of bias is called **confounding.** Controlling for the effects of confounding is the second reason for including independent variables in an analysis.

There are two ways to control for the effects of confounding in health research. One way is by designing our research to make confounding unlikely. At the beginning of a study, we may utilize a variety of methods to increase the likelihood of a similar distribution of an important characteristic between groups. For example, in Practice Problem 9.2, we selected controls to have the same age distribution as the cases. In a clinical trial, we randomly assign different treatments to individuals to reduce, but not eliminate, the possibility that the characteristics of the persons receiving one treatment are different from the characteristics of persons receiving another treatment in ways that influence their outcome. Often, however, it is not possible to design a study in such a way that confounding is avoided. Even randomization leaves open the possibility that groups will be different in ways that influence their outcome. For example, even though we randomize persons to one or another mode of treatment in a clinical trial, it is possible that, by chance, persons receiving one treatment might end up being more severely ill than persons receiving the other treatment. Thus, we need another way to control for the effects of confounding. That other way involves the method we choose to analyze our data.

Therefore, the second reason that we are interested in multivariable procedures is their usefulness in reducing the influence of confounding as part of our statistical analysis. As we will see in Chapter 10, the association between one independent variable and the dependent variable in multivariable analysis is evaluated after taking into account the relationships between other independent variables and the dependent variable. This is accomplished by representing characteristics that could lead to confounding as independent variables in a multivariable procedure. In that way, confounding is taken into account in the process of analyzing the relationship between the characteristics of interest and the dependent variable.

---

[1]Bias can also keep us from seeing a relationship that actually does exist between two variables.

CHAPTER 10

Continuous Dependent Variables

In our discussion of bivariable procedures in Chapters 7, 8, and 9, each chapter was divided into three sections according to the type of data represented by the single independent variable. In multivariable data sets, we have more than one independent variable. All those independent variables might represent data of the same type or of different types. Thus, this and subsequent chapters will contain four sections. Three of those sections will discuss procedures for independent variables all representing data of a particular type, and one section will discuss procedures for data sets containing independent variables representing data of more than one type. The potential for having statistical procedures that involve independent variables representing data of more than one type is also reflected in Flowchart 8.

CONTINUOUS INDEPENDENT VARIABLES

When we discussed analysis of a continuous dependent variable and a continuous independent variable in Chapter 7, we considered two general types of analyses: correlation analysis and regression analysis. Correlation analysis was concerned with estimating the strength of the association between the dependent and independent variables. Regression analysis was concerned with estimating the parameters of a straight line mathematically describing the association between the dependent and independent variables. If we have a naturalistic sample (i.e., the distribution of values of the independent variable are a random sample of their distribution in the population), then either correlation analysis or regression analysis are appropriate. If, on the other hand, we have a purposive sample (i.e., the distribution of values of the independent variable in the sample are determined by the researcher), only regression analysis is appropriate.

When we have more than one continuous independent variable, we also have a choice between correlation analysis and regression analysis. That choice is also

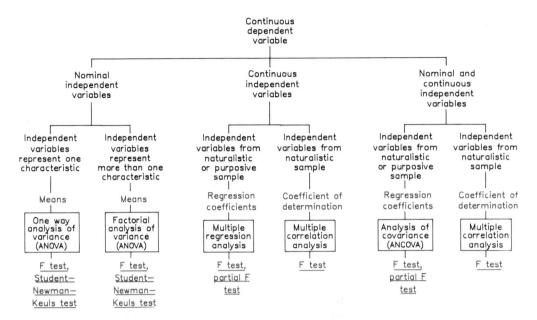

FLOWCHART 8 Multivariable analysis of a continuous dependent variable. Point estimates are indicated in red. Statistical procedures are indicated in red and underlined. Common names for a general class of statistical procedures appear in boxes.

governed, in part, by whether we have a naturalistic or a purposive sample. Only if all the continuous independent variables have been randomly sampled so that their distributions in the sample are representative of their distributions in the population can we interpret the results of multivariable correlation analysis. Thus, the methods of sampling each of the independent variables in a multivariable data set need to be examined, for it is possible that some of the variables have been sampled naturalistically, while others have been sampled purposively. For example, suppose that we were interested in examining the relationship between the dose of a particular drug (an independent variable) and diastolic blood pressure (the dependent variable). If we were to take a random sample of hypertensive patients for this study, we could consider patient characteristics such as age and gender to be sampled naturalistically. Dose, on the other hand, would be assigned by the researcher and, therefore, be from a purposive sample. Multiple correlation analysis would be improper in this case since the distribution of doses in the sample is not the result of a naturalistic sample.[1]

The procedures for correlation and regression analyses with more than one independent variable are extensions of the procedures we discussed in Chapter 7 for a

---

[1] It is uncommon in health research to find a collection of independent variables in which *all* of them have been sampled naturalistically.

single continuous independent variable. We have bad news and good news about those extended procedures. The bad news is that those procedures become quite complex as more independent variables are considered. The good news is that we will not discuss the computational details of those procedures. It is our impression that the ability to understand what is going on in multivariable correlation or regression analysis is not sufficiently improved by examining the details of calculation to warrant exposure to their complexity. These calculations are rarely performed by hand (except by graduate students in statistics). Rather, multivariable correlation and regression analyses rely on calculations performed by computer programs. However, those computer programs do not tell us how to interpret the results of those analyses properly. In our discussion of multivariable correlation and regression analyses, we will be concerned with interpretation of the results that we would encounter if we used a computer program to analyze a continuous dependent variable and more than one continuous independent variable.

CORRELATION ANALYSIS

ESTIMATION   In **multiple correlation analysis,** we are interested in the association between the dependent variable and all the independent variables considered simultaneously. When we had a single independent variable, the relationship between the dependent and independent variables assumed in correlation analysis was a linear one (i.e., represented by a straight line). In multiple correlation analysis, we think of the independent variables as a linear combination. In other words, the effects of each of the independent variables are added together. This is an extension of the idea of a straight line. We can think of this graphically for two continuous independent variables for which a linear combination is represented by a flat plane. Imagining a graphic representation of the relationship between a continuous dependent variable and more than two independent variables is impossible for most of us. Therefore, we must rely on mathematic, rather than graphic, representations to appreciate how independent variables in combination are associated with the dependent variable in multiple correlation analysis. That mathematic representation is discussed in the subsection on regression analysis (Equation 10.2). Just as in correlation analysis for single dependent and independent variables (which we will call simple correlation analysis), there is a close relationship between multiple correlation analysis and multiple regression analysis for a dependent variable and more than one independent variable.

In simple correlation analysis, we calculate r, the sample's estimate of the population's correlation coefficient ρ. We use these same symbols for the multiple correlation coefficient. We also interpret the value of the multiple correlation coefficient in the same way that we interpret the simple correlation coefficient: Namely, we square the multiple correlation coefficient to calculate the coefficient of determination (sometimes called the **coefficient of multiple determination** to distinguish it from the coefficient of determination in simple correlation analysis). In multiple correlation analysis, the coefficient of determination estimates the proportion of variation of the dependent variable associated with the *entire collection* of independent variables considered simultaneously. We will see how to interpret the coefficient of multiple determination in Example 10.1.

INFERENCE   Often, we are interested in testing the null hypothesis that the multiple correlation coefficient or coefficient of multiple determination is equal to zero. As in the case of a single independent variable, this null hypothesis can be tested by examining the F ratio used to test the omnibus null hypothesis in regression analysis. We will see this in Example 10.1.

REGRESSION ANALYSIS

ESTIMATION   In Chapter 7, we learned that regression analysis for a continuous dependent variable and one continuous independent variable involved estimation of the parameters of an equation describing a straight line. That relationship in the population was as follows (from Equation 7.7):

$$Y = \alpha + \beta X \tag{10.1}$$

In **multiple regression analysis,** we are concerned with estimating the coefficients of an equation that is an expanded version of Equation 10.1, with the inclusion of all the independent variables (Equation 10.2).

$$Y = \alpha + \beta_1 X_1 + \beta_2 X_2 + \cdots + \beta_j X_j + \cdots + \beta_k X_k \tag{10.2}$$

where

X_j = the jth independent variable in a collection of k independent variables
β_j = the "slope" or regression coefficient for the jth independent variable in a collection of k independent variables

In bivariable regression analysis (when we have one independent variable) the intercept (α) is the value of the dependent variable when the independent variable is equal to zero. In multiple regression analysis, α is the value of the dependent variable when *all* the independent variables are equal to zero. The sample's estimate of α is symbolized by the letter a and is often referred to as the "constant" by computer programs for multiple regression analysis.

In bivariable regression analysis, β was the slope of the straight line. The slope indicated how much values of the dependent variable changed for each unit change in values of the independent variable. β_j has this same meaning for the jth independent variable in multiple regression analysis (i.e., it indicates how much values of the dependent variable change for each unit change in values of the jth independent variable. We most often refer to β_j as a **regression coefficient,** rather than as a slope, in multiple regression analysis. The reason for this is that the word "slope" makes us think of a two-dimensional graphic representation of a straight-line relationship between a dependent variable and the independent variable. Since it is impossible to imagine a multidimensional graphic representation of the relationship between a dependent variable and several independent variables, referring to β_j as a "slope" has lost its usefulness in multiple regression analysis. We symbolize the sample's estimate of β_j by b_j, as we did in bivariable regression analysis.

Although we will not examine the actual methods of calculation in multiple regression analysis, it will greatly aid our ability to interpret the results of this type of analysis if we understand the basic process. Since multiple regression analysis is an extension of bivariable regression analysis, let us first refresh our memories about the approach we use when we have a continuous dependent variable and a single continuous independent variable. Recall from Chapter 7 that the method of least squares is used to select values of the slope and intercept in bivariable regression analysis. That method is designed to minimize the sum of the squared differences between observed values of the dependent variable and the corresponding values of the dependent variable estimated from the regression equation. The sum of those squared differences between observed and estimated values is also known as the residual sum of squares $[\Sigma(\Upsilon_i - \hat{\Upsilon}_i)^2]$.[2]

Multiple regression analysis relies on an extension of the least squares procedure that was used in bivariable regression analysis. Parallel to the least squares procedure in bivariable analysis, the purpose of the least squares procedure in multiple regression analysis is to choose a value for each of the regression coefficients so that the residual sum of squares is as small as possible. This procedure is probably easier to appreciate if we explain what is happening in multiple regression analysis in mathematical language. To do that, we first need to understand that the mathematical procedures in multiple regression analysis are concerned with two types of regression equations that contain different collections of the independent variables in a data set. The first collection includes all the independent variables. The regression equation that includes all the independent variables we call the **full model.** A regression equation that contains fewer than all the independent variables we call a **reduced model.** The particular reduced model we want to consider here is one that includes all the independent variables except the independent variable for which we wish to estimate a regression coefficient.

---

[2]Remember from Chapter 7 that the total sum of squares estimates the total variation in data represented by the dependent variable, ignoring the independent variable. The residual sum of squares estimates the variation in data represented by the dependent variable that is left over after we have explained some of the variation by taking into account values of the independent variable. That explained variation in data represented by the dependent variable is estimated by the regression sum of squares. The residual sum of squares and the regression sum of squares added together equal the total sum of squares. Thus, as the method of least squares seeks to minimize the residual sum of squares, it must, by necessity, seek to maximize the regression sum of squares.

If we were analyzing a data set that contained four independent variables, the full model would include all four of those independent variables (Equation 10.3).

$$\hat{Y}_F = a + b_1 X_1 + b_2 X_2 + b_3 X_3 + b_4 X_4 \qquad (10.3)$$

Now, when we are interested in estimating the regression coefficient for, say, the third independent variable, the reduced model would be the regression equation in Equation 10.3 but without the third independent variable (as shown in Equation 10.4).

$$\hat{Y}_R = a + b_1 X_1 + b_2 X_2 + b_4 X_4 \qquad (10.4)$$

In the least squares approach to multiple regression, a regression coefficient for a particular independent variable is selected so that the difference between the regression sum of squares for the dependent variable estimated by the full model and the regression sum of squares for the dependent variable estimated by the reduced model is as large as possible. That implies that the relationship between a particular independent variable and the dependent variable in multiple regression is not the same as the relationship would be between those two variables in bivariable regression. What actually is being examined in multiple regression is the relationship between a particular independent variable and the variation in the dependent variable that is not explained by the other independent variables (i.e., the residual variation of the reduced model). This method of estimating regression coefficients has important implications that must be considered when interpreting those estimates or when performing statistical inference. We will think more about how this method of selecting regression coefficients affects our interpretation of individual regression coefficients in a moment, but let us first take a look at inference in multiple regression analysis.

INFERENCE   In multiple regression analysis, statistical inference relies on estimating the same sources of variation of data represented by the dependent variable that we discussed in bivariable regression analysis. In Chapter 7, we found that we can think about three sources of variation: the total, regression, and residual variation. The methods of estimating those three sources of variation are nearly the same in multiple regression analysis as the methods described for bivariable regression analysis. The only difference is in the degrees of freedom for the residual mean square and the regression mean square.

In bivariable regression analysis, the residual mean square was estimated by dividing the residual sum of squares $[\Sigma(Y_i - \hat{Y}_i)^2]$ by the sample's size (n) minus two. The reason we subtracted two from the sample's size was that we needed to estimate the intercept and the slope to estimate values of the dependent variable when determining the residual sum of squares. In multiple regression, we need to estimate the intercept and k regression coefficients (where k is the number of independent variables) to estimate a value of the dependent variable. Thus, the number of residual

TABLE 10.1 The three sources of variation of data represented by the dependent variable in regression analysis (expanded version of Table 7.1 to allow application to both bivariable and multiple regression analyses).

Source	Degrees of Freedom	Sum of Squares	Mean Square
Total	$n - 1$	$\Sigma(Y_i - \overline{Y})^2$	$s_Y^2 = \dfrac{\Sigma(Y_i - \overline{Y})^2}{n - 1}$
Residual	$n - (k + 1)$	$\Sigma(Y_i - \acute{Y}_i)^2$	$s_{Y\mid X}^2 = \dfrac{\Sigma(Y_i - \acute{Y}_i)^2}{n - (k + 1)}$
Regression	k	$\Sigma(\acute{Y}_i - \overline{Y})^2$	$s_{\text{reg}}^2 = \dfrac{\Sigma(\acute{Y}_i - \overline{Y})^2}{k}$

degrees of freedom is equal to $n - (k + 1)$. Since k is equal to one in bivariable regression analysis, $n - (k + 1)$ is the same as $n - 2$.

If the number of residual degrees of freedom changes in multiple regression analysis, so must the regression degrees of freedom. This is because the residual degrees of freedom plus the regression degrees of freedom must equal the total degrees of freedom (which always equals $n - 1$ regardless of the number of independent variables). That implies that the number of regression degrees of freedom in multiple regression analysis is equal to $(n - 1) - [n - (k + 1)]$, which is equal to k (the number of independent variables).[3] The degrees of freedom, sum of squares, and mean square calculations expanded for use in multiple regression analysis are summarized in Table 10.1.

To test individual null hypotheses about the intercept and the regression coefficients in multiple regression, we can use the standard errors of these estimates (if they are provided by the computer program we are using) to convert the point estimate of the intercept or any particular regression coefficient to a Student's t statistic, as was described in Chapter 7 for bivariable regression analysis (Equations 7.20 and 7.21). However, a test of the null hypothesis that the intercept is equal to zero or that a particular regression coefficient is equal to zero in the population is usually included in the output from a multiple regression analysis computer program. Frequently, an F value, rather than a Student's t value, is the test statistic reported. If we took the square root of those F values, we would get the Student's t value resulting from a test of the null hypothesis that the regression coefficient (or intercept) is equal to zero in the population. The fact that many computer programs report the F rather than the

---

[3]Recall that the regression degrees of freedom in bivariable regression analysis were equal to one. This reflects the fact that we have only one independent variable in bivariable analysis.

Student's t value is a reflection of a different way to test the null hypothesis that a particular regression coefficient is equal to zero. Although either method of testing that null hypothesis gives us the same result, conducting the F ratio method reminds us of how the role of a particular independent variable in multiple regression analysis is evaluated.

Recall from our previous discussion of the least squares procedure in multiple regression that estimates of regression coefficients are calculated so that the difference in the explained variation in data represented by the dependent variable is as large as possible between the full and reduced models. To calculate the F ratio used to test the null hypothesis that a particular regression coefficient is equal to zero we use information from both of those models. This particular F ratio is called a **partial F ratio.** The partial F ratio has in its numerator the amount that our ability to estimate values of the dependent variable is increased by inclusion of a particular independent variable in the full regression model. Specifically, the amount that our ability to estimate values of the dependent variable increases is equal to the regression sum of squares from the full model minus the regression sum of squares from the reduced model. The partial F ratio contains in its numerator that difference between regression sums of squares divided by the difference in the regression degrees of freedom (equal to one when the reduced model has one fewer independent variables than does the full model). The denominator of the partial F ratio contains the residual mean square for the full model (Equation 10.5).

$$F = \frac{\dfrac{\text{Regression sum of squares}_{\text{Full}} - \text{Regression sum of squares}_{\text{Reduced}}}{\text{Regression degrees of freedom}_{\text{Full}} - \text{Regression degrees of freedom}_{\text{Reduced}}}}{\dfrac{\text{Residual sum of squares}_{\text{Full}}}{\text{Residual degrees of freedom}_{\text{Full}}}} \qquad (10.5)$$

Thus, tests of individual null hypotheses about regression coefficients using the partial F ratio employ the same principle that is used to estimate those coefficients. Specifically, the abilities of the full and reduced models to explain variation in data represented by the dependent variable are compared.

In addition to testing null hypotheses about the intercept and slope in bivariable regression analysis, we calculated an F ratio with the regression mean square in the numerator and the residual mean square in the denominator (Equation 7.22). This F ratio was used to test the omnibus null hypothesis which states that the population's regression equation does not help to explain variation in data represented by the dependent variable. In multiple regression, we can calculate an F ratio with the regression mean square (from the full model) in the numerator and the residual mean square (from the full model) in the denominator. This F ratio is also used in multiple regression analysis to test the omnibus null hypothesis (Equation 10.6).

$$F = \frac{\text{Regression mean square}_{\text{Full}}}{\text{Residual mean square}_{\text{Full}}} \qquad (10.6)$$

In multiple regression analysis, the omnibus null hypothesis states that the *entire collection* of independent variables does not help to explain variation in data represented by the dependent variable. Thus, we can use partial F ratios calculated as in Equation 10.5 to test null hypotheses about individual regression coefficients, or we can use the omnibus F ratio to test a null hypothesis about all the regression coefficients simultaneously.

Equation 10.6 is the same as the F ratio that was used in bivariable regression analysis to test the omnibus null hypothesis (Equation 7.22). Recall from Chapter 7 that the F ratio in bivariable regression also tests the null hypotheses that the coefficient of determination (and, therefore, the correlation coefficient) is equal to zero and that the slope is equal to zero in the population. Like the F ratio in bivariable regression analysis, the omnibus F ratio in multiple regression analysis also tests the null hypothesis that the coefficient of multiple determination (and, therefore, the multiple correlation coefficient) is equal to zero in the population. The omnibus F ratio in multiple regression analysis, however, does not test hypotheses about individual regression coefficients. In fact, it is possible in multiple regression analysis to reject the omnibus null hypothesis without being able to reject any of the null hypotheses that the regression coefficients are equal to zero (we will see this in Example 10.1).

To examine further how to interpret the results of multiple regression analyses, let us take a look at a particular type of multiple regression called a **polynomial regression.** Polynomial regression analysis is a form of multiple regression analysis in which all the independent variables are multiples of one continuous variable (Equation 10.7).

$$Y = \alpha + \beta_1 X + \beta_2 X^2 + \cdots + \beta_j X^j + \cdots + \beta_k X^k \qquad (10.7)$$

The purpose of polynomial regression is to describe a relationship between a dependent variable and an independent variable that is not a straight line. Each polynomial regression equation is said to have a specific **order** identified by the highest multiple of the independent variable that is included. A first-order polynomial is the same as a straight line. A second-order polynomial includes the independent variable (X) and its square (X^2). A third-order polynomial includes the independent variable (X), its square (X^2), and its cube (X^3). For each multiple of the independent variable that is added to the polynomial regression equation, one change in direction of the slope is possible. With a first-order polynomial (i.e., a straight line), the slope is a constant for all values of the independent variable. With a second-order polynomial, there is a constant change in the slope as the value of the independent variable increases, thus producing a constantly changing curve. The complexity of curves possible with higher-order polynomials is illustrated in Example 10.1.

The utility of polynomial regression analysis in practice is to allow examination of a **curvilinear** (i.e., not a straight line) relationship between a continuous dependent variable and a continuous independent variable. It is useful to us as students of statistics because it provides a transition between bivariable and multiple regression analyses. Polynomial regression has all the analytic and interpretational features of multiple regression, but we are able to investigate what is happening graphically since each independent variable in the regression equation is really a function of a single variable.

Example 10.1 Suppose that we wanted to conduct an experiment to investigate the relationship between the dose of a particular drug and the change in diastolic blood pressure experienced by hypertensive patients. As a pilot study, we randomly select 10 hypertensive patients from some population of interest and randomize each to a different dose of the drug in 5 mg intervals from 5 mg to 50 mg. Imagine that we observed the following results:

Dose	Blood Pressure Change
5	0.5
10	0.5
15	0.6
20	1.5
25	1.3
30	5.2
35	5.8
40	14.3
45	18.7
50	41.0

Describe the change in blood pressure as a function of the dose of the drug.

In Chapter 7, we learned how to estimate a straight line to describe a continuous dependent variable as a function of a continuous independent variable. Rather than go through the exercise of making the necessary calculations by hand, let us take this opportunity to look at the way a computer program might present the results of regression analysis. The following is designed to be typical of the type of output we can expect from most popular programs for statistical analysis.

$$RSQ = 0.67241 \qquad F = 16.42091 \qquad P = 0.00367$$

SOURCE	DF	SUM OF SQS	MEAN SQ
REGRESSION	1	1,009.575	1,009.57528
RESIDUAL	8	491.849	61.48109

VARIABLE	B	SE B	F	P
DOSE	0.69964	0.17265	16.421	0.004
(CONSTANT)	−10.30000	5.35641	6.698	0.091

Let us take a moment to see what this computer program is telling us. In the first line, we find out that the coefficient of determination (RSQ) is equal to 0.67241. That implies that 67.241% of the variation in the change in blood pressure is associated with the dose of the drug.[4] Also, we are told in that line that the F ratio (F) for the test of the omnibus null hypothesis is equal to 16.42091 and that a value so extreme represents an area of 0.00367 in the F distribution (i.e., $P = 0.00367$). Therefore, we can reject the omnibus null hypothesis that variation in blood pressure changes is not associated with dose in the population if we are willing to take at least a 0.367% chance of making a Type I error.

The first table in this computer output gives us the degrees of freedom (DF), sum of squares (SUM OF SQS), and mean square (MEAN SQ) for the explained variation (REGRESSION) and the unexplained variation (RESIDUAL) of data represented by the dependent variable. We are not given the total sum of squares or total degrees of freedom for variation of data represented by the dependent variable, but we can calculate the total sum of squares by adding the regression and residual sums of squares, and we can calculate the total degrees of freedom by adding the regression and residual degrees of freedom.

The next table in this computer output shows the sample's estimates (B) of the slope and intercept. In this computer program, the intercept is referred to as the CONSTANT. Also, this table gives us the standard error (SE B) for the slope and the intercept and the P-value (P) obtained by testing the null hypothesis that the population's value for the slope or intercept is equal to zero. That result is given as a partial F ratio (F).

If we examined only the information in this computer output, we might be satisfied that a straight line describes how changes in blood pressure are related to dose of the drug. There are two reasons we might draw that conclusion. First, we are able to reject the omnibus null hypothesis and the null hypothesis that the slope is equal to zero in the population from which the sample was drawn. Second, we are able to explain more than two-thirds of the variation in blood pressure changes (in the sample) by knowing the dose ($R^2 = 0.67241$). These results tell us that a straight line does a fairly good job at estimating the change in blood pressure from knowledge of the dose. Those results do not tell us, however, that estimation using a straight line is the best we can do. To begin to evaluate further how well we have done in explaining the relationship between change in blood pressure and dose, let us take a look at a scatterplot of these observations and the regression line.

---

[4]Remember that we need to interpret the coefficient of determination with caution when we do not have a naturalistic sample. We cannot conclude that 67.241% of the variation in the dependent variable is associated with the independent variable in the population from which the sample was drawn. We can, however, say that 67.241% of the variation in the dependent variable *in the sample* is associated with the independent variable.

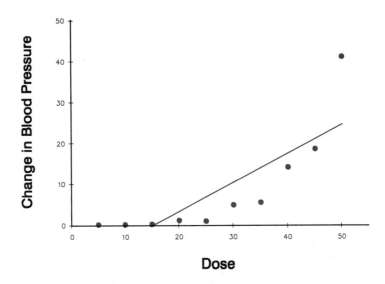

From the scatterplot, we can see that the relationship between dose and blood pressure change is really a curve rather than a straight line. We will use polynomial regression analysis to describe that curvilinear relationship mathematically and, thus, "fit" the data better. The next step is to add the square of the dose (DOSE2) as the second independent variable in the regression equation. When we do that, we get the following results from our computer program.

$$RSQ = 0.92692 \qquad F = 44.40828 \qquad P = 0.00011$$

SOURCE	DF	SUM OF SQS	MEAN SQ
REGRESSION	2	1,391.736	695.86779
RESIDUAL	7	109.688	15.66978

VARIABLE	B	SE B	F	P
DOSE	−1.17203	0.38889	9.083	0.020
DOSE2	0.03403	6.891−03*	24.388	0.002
(CONSTANT)	8.41667	4.65581	3.628	0.114

*This is computer shorthand for 6.891 times 10^{-3} or 0.006891.

There are a number of interesting things that we notice as we examine this computer output. Perhaps most impressive, the coefficient of determination has increased substantially (from 0.67241 to 0.92694). Remember that the coefficient of determination in multiple regression addresses the ability of the entire collection of independent variables to account for the variability of data represented by the dependent variable. The only difference between this second-order polynomial equation and the equation for a straight line is the addition of the square of dose. Thus, the difference between these coefficients of determination indicates that adding the square of the independent variable was able to account for an additional 25.453% of the variation of data represented by the dependent variable in the sample.

By making another comparison between the results of the first-order polynomial (i.e., straight line) analysis and the results of this second-order polynomial analysis, we can see how the partial F ratio testing the null hypothesis that the regression coefficient for the square of dose is equal to zero is derived using Equation 10.5. Let us take a moment to examine how that partial F ratio is calculated.

The numerator of the partial F ratio tells us how much our ability to estimate values of the dependent variable increases in the full model compared to the reduced model. If we want to test the null hypothesis that the coefficient for the square of dose is equal to zero in the population, the full model would include dose and the square of dose and the reduced model would include only dose. Thus, we subtract the regression sum of squares from the regression model that includes only dose (1,009.575 from the first computer output) from the regression sum of squares from the regression model that includes both dose and the square of dose (1,391.736 from the second computer output). Then, we divide that difference in the regression sums of squares by the difference in the degrees of freedom. The full model has two degrees of freedom since it includes two independent variables (dose and the square of dose). The reduced model has only one degree of freedom since it includes dose as the only independent variable. The difference between those degrees of freedom is equal to one.

The denominator of the partial F testing the null hypothesis that the regression coefficient for the square of dose is equal to zero in the population contains the residual sum of squares from the full model divided by its degrees of freedom. This is the residual mean square from the second computer output (15.66978). With this information, we can calculate the partial F testing the null hypothesis that the coefficient for the square of dose is equal to zero.

$$F = \frac{\dfrac{\text{Regression sum of squares}_{\text{Full}} - \text{Regression sum of squares}_{\text{Reduced}}}{\text{Regression degrees of freedom}_{\text{Full}} - \text{Regression degrees of freedom}_{\text{Reduced}}}}{\dfrac{\text{Residual sum of squares}_{\text{Full}}}{\text{Residual degrees of freedom}_{\text{Full}}}}$$

$$= \frac{1{,}391.736 - 1{,}009.575}{15.66978} = 24.388$$

Notice that this partial F is exactly the same as the one that appears in the second computer output for the square of dose. That partial F is associated with a P-value of 0.002. In other words, we can reject the null hypothesis that this coefficient is equal to zero in the population if we are willing to take a 0.2% chance of making a Type I error. Including the square of dose seems to be important in estimation of blood pressure.

A look at a scatterplot that includes the second-order polynomial curve shows us why we are better able to estimate values of the dependent variable with this polynomial regression equation than we were with a straight line.

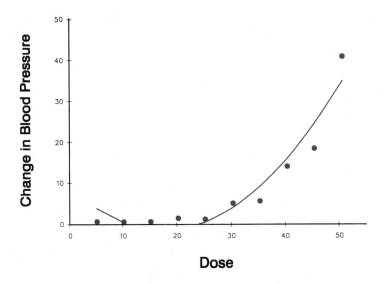

So, the second-degree polynomial is a better fit to these data than was the first-degree polynomial (straight line). To learn if adding more multiples of dose will continue to increase our ability to estimate values of the dependent variable, let us examine computer output and scatterplots for some higher-order polynomial regression analyses.

For the third-order polynomial regression equation, we add the cube of dose (DOSE3):

$$RSQ = 0.97497 \qquad F = 77.91770 \qquad P = 0.00003$$

SOURCE	DF	SUM OF SQS	MEAN SQ
REGRESSION	3	1,463.850	487.94992
RESIDUAL	6	37.574	6.26238

VARIABLE	B	SE B	F	P
DOSE	1.15354	0.72808	2.510	0.164
DOSE2	−0.06682	0.03004	4.949	0.068
DOSE3	1.222−03	3.602−04	11.515	0.015
(CONSTANT)	−4.69333	4.85678	0.934	0.371

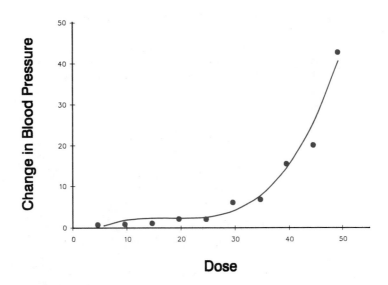

For the fourth-order polynomial regression equation, we add the fourth multiple of dose (DOSE4):

RSQ = 0.98526   F = 83.57509   P = 0.00009

SOURCE	DF	SUM OF SQS	MEAN SQ
REGRESSION	4	1,479.299	369.82468
RESIDUAL	5	22.125	4.42506

VARIABLE	B	SE B	F	P
DOSE	−1.54133	1.56676	0.968	0.370
DOSE2	0.13040	0.10853	1.444	0.283
DOSE3	−4.167−03	2.900−03	2.064	0.210
DOSE4	4.900−05	2.622−05	3.491	0.121
(CONSTANT)	5.81667	6.95032	0.700	0.441

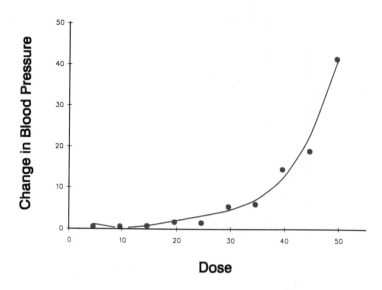

With each higher order of the polynomial equation, the coefficient of determination is higher. That implies that the more independent variables included in a multiple regression equation, the greater the proportion of the variation in data represented by the dependent variable that will be explained (in the sample) by the collection of independent variables. This will always be the case. We might ask ourselves, however, how important is the difference between the coefficient of determination in the third-order polynomial equation (0.97497) and the coefficient of determination in the fourth-order polynomial equation (0.98526). There are a number of ways we might address that question. First, we notice that the coefficient of determination changes by only 0.01029 between those two orders. We might consider this too small a difference to be of concern.

Alternatively, we can ask whether or not there is a statistically significant increase in our ability to estimate values of the dependent variable between the third and fourth orders. That is tantamount to asking if the fourth multiple of the independent variable is associated with a regression coefficient in the population that is equal to zero. We can test that null hypothesis by examining the partial F ratio associated with the fourth multiple of dose in the fourth-order polynomial. In this example, that F ratio is equal to 3.491 with a corresponding P-value of 0.121. Thus, we are unable to reject the null hypothesis that the regression coefficient associated with the fourth multiple of dose is equal to zero in the population (if we were unwilling to take a 12.1% chance of making a Type I error). The third-order polynomial seems to be our simplest best guess at the relationship between changes in blood pressure and dose in the population from which the sample was drawn.

So far, we have examined only polynomial regression as our first example of a multiple regression analysis. Even though polynomial regression equations include multiples of a single variable, we can use them to begin to understand some of the general principles of multiple regression analysis. Soon we will take a look at other types of multiple regression equations that include a variety of independent variables. Before we do that, however, there is one more very important principle that we can learn from polynomial regression analysis.

A feature of all multivariable procedures is that the relationship between each independent variable and the dependent variable is evaluated while taking into account the variability of the dependent variable that is associated with all the other independent variables. This is done in multiple regression by calculating a partial F ratio. Other multivariable methods use procedures that are based on similar calculations.

The consequence of this method of examining each particular independent variable after removing variability associated with all the other independent variables is that any ability to explain variability of the dependent variable that is shared among two or more independent variables is not credited to any of the independent variables. This apparently illogical circumstance is the result of how inference is conducted for each of the independent variables (see Equation 10.5). Forgetting this feature of multivariable procedures can lead to serious misinterpretation of the results of data analysis. Thus, it is crucial that we understand the relationships among the independent variables to evaluate their relationships with the dependent variable in multivariable analyses.

This sharing of information about the variability of the dependent variable between two (or more) independent variables is called **multicollinearity.** When multicollinearity exists between two independent variables in multiple regression analysis, the two partial F ratios that test whether the regression coefficients for those two independent variables are each equal to zero in the population will be "less significant" (i.e., have larger P-values) than if the relationships between the dependent variable and each of those two independent variables were evaluated individually in bivariable regression analyses.

We can see multicollinearity occurring in the relationship between the change in blood pressure and the dose of the drug in Example 10.1. When dose was evaluated in a bivariable regression analysis (i.e., the first-order polynomial equation), the partial F ratio associated with a test of the null hypothesis that the regression coefficient for dose is equal to zero in the population was equal to 16.421 and associated with a P-value of 0.004. When the square of dose was added to create the second-order polynomial equation, the partial F ratio testing that same null hypothesis was 9.083 associated with a P-value of 0.020. When the cube of dose is added to create the third-order polynomial equation, we are unable to reject the null hypothesis (with an α of 0.05) that the regression coefficient for dose is equal to zero in the population ($F = 2.510$, $P = 0.164$). The fourth-order polynomial demonstrates an extreme result in which there is so much multicollinearity among the independent variables that tests of the null hypothesis that the regression coefficient is equal to zero in the population cannot be rejected for any of the independent variables. Such observation of changes in the statistical significance of partial F ratios is, by definition, the best way to detect the presence of multicollinearity.

Multicollinearity is very common in polynomial regression analysis since the independent variables share quite a bit of their information about values of the dependent variable. This phenomenon of multicollinearity, however, is not confined to polynomial regression analysis, as we can see in the next example, which demonstrates how the principles we illustrated with polynomial regression can be applied to multivariable regression with more than one continuous independent variable..

Example 10.2 Suppose that we were to take a sample of twelve nutritionally deficient children who attend a certain clinic. For each of those children, we measure their weight, and height and determine their age. Imagine that we observe the following results:

Weight (lb)	Height (in.)	Age (yr)
64	57	8
71	59	10
53	49	6
67	62	11
55	51	8
58	50	7
77	55	10
57	48	9
56	42	10
51	42	6
76	61	12
68	57	9

Examine the relationship of weight to height and age.

Here, we are primarily interested in the weight of the children in the population which was sampled and how their weight is related to their height and to their age. Thus, we are interested in estimating the parameters of the following multiple regression equation:

$$\text{Weight} = \alpha + (\beta_1 \cdot \text{Height}) + (\beta_2 \cdot \text{Age})$$

With these twelve observations, we get the following computer output:

RSQ = 0.77999   F = 15.95235   P = 0.00110

SOURCE	DF	SUM OF SQS	MEAN SQ
REGRESSION	2	692.823	346.41130
RESIDUAL	9	195.427	21.71415

VARIABLE	B	SE B	F	P
HEIGHT	0.72204	0.26081	7.665	0.022
AGE	2.05013	0.93723	4.785	0.056
(CONSTANT)	6.55305	10.94483	0.358	0.564

From that multiple regression analysis, we estimate that knowing height and age allows us to account for 77.999% of the variation in children's weight (at least in the sample). Further, we are able to reject the null hypothesis that the regression coefficient for height is equal to zero in the population (with an α of 0.05). However, we are not able to reject the null hypothesis that the regression coefficient for age is equal to zero in the population. That does not imply that age is unrelated to weight. Rather, our inability to reject the null hypothesis that the regression coefficient for age is equal to zero might be due to shared information about weight by age and height. To evaluate this possibility, we need to examine bivariable regression analyses for each of the independent variables separately.

The first bivariable regression analysis that we will examine is one in which age is the only independent variable. In that analysis, we observe the following results:

RSQ = 0.59262   F = 14.54698   P = 0.00341

SOURCE	DF	SUM OF SQS	MEAN SQ
REGRESSION	1	526.393	526.39286
RESIDUAL	10	361.857	36.18571

VARIABLE	B	SE B	F	P
AGE	3.64286	0.95512	14.547	0.003
(CONSTANT)	30.57143	8.61371	12.597	0.005

For height as the only independent variable, we observe the following results:

RSQ = 0.66301   F = 19.67486   P = 0.00126

SOURCE	DF	SUM OF SQS	MEAN SQ
REGRESSION	1	588.923	588.92252
RESIDUAL	10	299.327	29.93275

VARIABLE	B	SE B	F	P
HEIGHT	1.07223	0.24173	19.675	0.001
(CONSTANT)	6.18985	12.84875	0.232	0.640

Thus, we can reject the null hypothesis that the regression coefficient for age is equal to zero in the population in a bivariable regression analysis, but we cannot reject that null hypothesis in a multiple regression analysis when height is included as the other independent variable. That implies that age and height share information that can be used to estimate weight. In other words, age and height are multicollinear. That multicollinearity affects the level of statistical significance of partial F ratios (and the value of the coefficient estimates) for each of the independent variables in multiple regression analysis. In this example, notice that the partial F ratio for height is associated with a smaller area (i.e., a smaller probability) of the F distribution in the bivariable analysis ($F = 19.675, P = 0.001$) than in the multivariable analysis ($F = 7.665$, $P = 0.022$).

Multicollinearity can be good or bad, depending on what we are trying to accomplish in a multivariable procedure. In Example 10.2, if we were interested in the relationships between weight and height and between weight and age, the multivariable regression analysis would have been misleading (both height and age appear to be less associated with weight than they actually are). On the other hand, if we were interested in the relationship between weight and height, adjusting for (or independent of) the effect of age (or between weight and age, adjusting for the effect of height), the multiple regression analysis would have provided us with the information we wanted. Thus, whether we see multicollinearity as a desirable feature or as an impediment to interpretation depends on the question that we are asking. Multicollinearity is the mechanism by which multivariable analyses can examine the relationship between a dependent variable and some independent variables while controlling for the confounding effects of other independent variables. It is also the reason that certain independent variables might appear to be unrelated to the dependent variable even though a relationship exists.

A common, but not very useful, suggestion is that the degree of correlation (i.e., the size of the simple correlation coefficient) between two independent variables should be used as a measure of the degree of multicollinearity. Correlation between independent variables is a necessary, but not sufficient, indicator of how much the relationship between an independent variable and the dependent variable will be influenced by the presence of other independent variables in a multiple regression equation. Remember that multicollinearity results from information shared by independent variables that is used to estimate values of the dependent variable. Generally, only a portion of the information in an independent variable is associated with the dependent variable (otherwise, we could estimate values of the dependent variable without error). It is the correlation between the information in independent variables that is associated with the dependent variable that causes multicollinearity.

To illustrate how multicollinearity works, imagine that the three rectangles in the following diagrams (Figure 10.1) symbolize the variability in data represented by the dependent (Y) and two independent (X_1 and X_2) variables and that the areas where those rectangles overlap indicate shared information. Since the rectangles symbolizing the independent variables (X_1 and X_2) have the same amount of overlap with each other in all three of the diagrams, the degree of correlation between those independent variables is the same in each case. The amount of multicollinearity, however, is quite different. There is no multicollinearity in Figure 10.1(a) since the association between the independent variables (X_1 and X_2) and the dependent variable (Y) does not involve the area of overlap between the independent variables. In Figure 10.1(b), there is a moderate amount of multicollinearity since some, but not all, of the variability in data

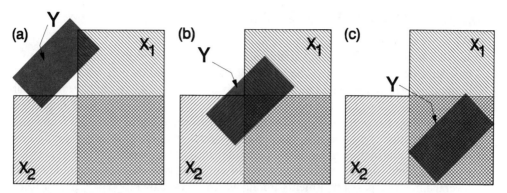

FIGURE 10.1 A diagrammatic representation of the relationship between two independent variables X_1 (▧) and X_2 (▨) and a dependent variable Y. Areas of overlap represent shared information between variables. In all three diagrams, the area of overlap between X_1 and X_2 (▨) is the same. The amount that Y overlaps the area of overlap between X_1 and X_2 indicates the degree of multicollinearity. Thus, that overlap results in (a) no, (b) moderate, and (c) complete multicollinearity.

represented by the dependent variable that is associated with the independent variables is in the area of overlap between the independent variables. On the other hand, multicollinearity is nearly complete in Figure 10.1(c) since nearly all the area representing variability of data represented by dependent variables is confined to the area of overlap of the independent variables.

The best way to evaluate the presence and degree of multicollinearity is to examine regression equations with and without each of the independent variables included in the equation (as we did in Example 10.2). If the estimate of a particular regression coefficient (or the P-value associated with a test of the null hypothesis that the particular regression coefficient is equal to zero in the population[5]) changes as another independent variable is included or excluded from a regression equation, we suspect that those two independent variables are multicollinear. The greater the degree of change, the greater the degree of multicollinearity.

ORDINAL INDEPENDENT VARIABLES

As in bivariable analysis of a continuous dependent variable, when we have ordinal independent variables, we generally convert values of the dependent variable to an ordinal scale and use the procedures described in Chapter 11, or we create a collection of nominal variables from the ordinal independent variables and use the procedures described in the next section of this chapter.

---

[5]P-values can change also as a result of increased precision in estimating values of the dependent variable or decreased degrees of freedom in the denominator of the partial F ratio as independent variables are added to a regression equation.

NOMINAL INDEPENDENT VARIABLES

When we discussed bivariable data sets consisting of a continuous dependent variable and a nominal independent variable in Chapter 7, we found that the nominal independent variable divided the values of the dependent variable into two groups between which we compared means. In multivariable analysis, we can have more than one nominal independent variable and, thus, more than two groups of dependent variable values to compare. For example, if we performed a clinical trial of treatments for hypertension, one nominal independent variable would allow us to specify only two treatment groups (e.g., an antihypertensive medication versus a placebo) between which we could compare blood pressures. In a multivariable data set, we could specify several different types of treatments among which to compare blood pressure measurements. Remember that, when we wish to identify more than two groups, we must have more than one nominal variable. Specifically, we need one fewer variable than the number of groups we wish to identify.

The most common way to compare several groups of dependent variable values is by comparing the means of the groups. The method of comparing those means is called **analysis of variance** or **ANOVA.** It might seem incongruous to call a method to compare means an analysis of *variance,* but the name of this procedure tells us that we compare means among groups of dependent variable values by examining sources of variation of the dependent variable. The null hypothesis tested in this procedure is, nonetheless, that the means of the groups are equal.

Since analysis of variance is concerned with sources of variation of data represented by the dependent variable, the first thing we should do is to find out what those sources of variation are. Our job is made easier by the fact that, in analysis of variance, we think about various sources of variation of data represented by the dependent variable that are parallel to the three sources of variation we considered in regression analysis.

First, let us consider the total variation of data represented by the dependent variable without taking into consideration the groups defined by values of the independent variables. This is called the **total sum of squares** (as it was in regression analysis). The total mean square is the total sum of squares divided by the total degrees of freedom (Equation 10.8) and is exactly the same as the sample's estimate of the variance of data represented by the dependent variable (s^2).

$$s^2 = \frac{\Sigma(\Upsilon_i - \overline{\Upsilon})^2}{n-1} = \frac{\text{Total sum of squares}}{\text{Total degrees of freedom}} = \text{Total mean square} \qquad (10.8)$$

To keep track of groups and observations within groups in analysis of variance, let us expand the terminology we use in our mathematical language a little bit. Let us say that we have m groups of dependent variable values corresponding to values of the $m - 1$ nominal independent variables, and we will keep track of the group we are considering with the subscript j. In other words, $\overline{\Upsilon}_j$ will be the mean of values of the dependent variable in the jth group. Within each group we have n_j observations of the dependent variable. Each observation, then, can be specified by Υ_{ij} which is the ith observation in the jth group. Using that terminology, the equation for estimation of the total mean square becomes:

$$\text{Total mean square} = \frac{\text{Total sum of squares}}{\text{Total degrees of freedom}} = \frac{\displaystyle\sum_{j=1}^{m}\sum_{i=1}^{n_j}(\Upsilon_{ij} - \overline{\Upsilon})^2}{\left(\displaystyle\sum_{j=1}^{m} n_j\right) - 1} \tag{10.9}$$

where

Υ_{ij} = the ith value of the dependent variable in the jth group
$\overline{\Upsilon}$ = the overall mean of values of the dependent variable
n_j = the number of observations in the jth group
m = the number of groups of values of the dependent variable
$\displaystyle\sum_{j=1}^{m}$ = the sum of all values of j from 1 to m
$\displaystyle\sum_{i=1}^{n_j}$ = the sum of all values of i from 1 to n_j

Equation 10.9 tells us that, to estimate the total sum of squares, we first square the difference between each observed value of the dependent variable and the mean of all values of the dependent variable and then add those squared differences for all the n_j observations in each group and for all the m groups. To calculate the total degrees of freedom, we add the number of observations in each group $(\Sigma\, n_j)$ and subtract one from that total. This terminology will help us communicate in mathematical language how to make the calculations used in analysis of variance. This will become more clear when we estimate the total mean square in Example 10.3, but first, let us examine the other sources of variation in analysis of variance.

In regression analysis, we divided the total variation into two components. One of these was called the residual sum of squares, which estimates the leftover variation of data represented by the dependent variable after taking the independent variable into account (i.e., the variation of data represented by the dependent variable corresponding to each value of the independent variable). The other was called the regression sum of squares, which estimates the variation of data represented by the dependent variable explained by the independent variable (i.e., the variation of the estimated values of the dependent variable among the values of the independent variable). In analysis of variance, we also divide the total variation into components. The **within sum of squares** estimates the variation of data represented by the dependent variable within each of the groups specified by values of the independent variables. The **between sum of squares** estimates the variation of the dependent variable from group to group.

In the Student's t test (see Chapter 7), we arrived at our best estimate of the population's variance of data represented by the dependent variable by making the assumption that the variance of data represented by the dependent variable in the population is the same regardless of group. Making that assumption, we combined the estimates of the variance of data in each of the groups. We did this by finding a weighted average of the estimates of the variance of data with degrees of freedom used as the weights. We do this again in analysis of variance. The weighted average of the estimates of the variance of data within each group is calculated as shown in Equation 10.10. In the Student's t procedure, we called this weighted average the pooled variance estimate. In analysis of variance, we call this the **within mean square.**

$$\text{Within mean square} = \frac{\text{Within sum of squares}}{\text{Within degrees of freedom}} = \frac{\sum_{j=1}^{m} \sum_{i=1}^{n_j} (Y_{ij} - \overline{Y}_j)^2}{\sum_{j=1}^{m} (n_j - 1)} \quad (10.10)$$

where $\overline{Y}_j$ = mean of values of the dependent variable in the jth group.

Like the pooled variance in the Student's t test, the within mean square is our best guess at the value of the variance of data represented by the dependent variable. This estimate is not influenced by the differences between the groups because separate

FIGURE 10.2 Graphic representation of two of the three sources of variation of systolic blood pressure (the dependent variable) in analysis of variance for three treatment groups (TX_1, TX_2, and TX_3). The total mean square (TMS) is the variance of systolic blood pressure ignoring treatment groups. The within mean square (WMS) is the variance of systolic blood pressure within each treatment group. The between mean squares is not illustrated, but it can be calculated by finding the difference between the total sum of squares and the within sum of squares and dividing by the number of groups minus one.

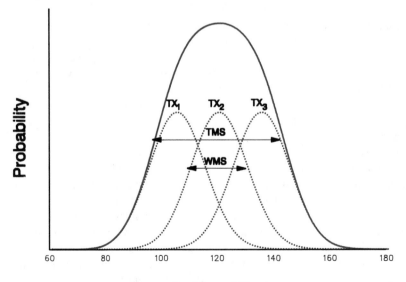

estimates of the variance are made for each group before those estimates are combined. This is not true of the total mean square since it is calculated for all the values of the dependent variable regardless of the groups specified by the independent variables. Thus, the value of the total sum of squares is a combination of the variation of data within the groups and the variation of data between the groups. This implies that we can estimate the variation of data between the groups by subtracting the within sum of squares from the total sum of squares. Then, the **between mean square** can be found by dividing by the difference between the total degrees of freedom and the within degrees of freedom (Equation 10.11).

$$\text{Between mean square} = \frac{\text{Between sum of squares}}{\text{Between degrees of freedom}} = \frac{\sum_{j=1}^{m} \sum_{i=1}^{n_j} (\overline{Y}_j - \overline{Y})^2}{m - 1} \tag{10.11}$$

$$= \frac{\text{Total sum of squares} - \text{Within sum of squares}}{\text{Total degrees of freedom} - \text{Within degrees of freedom}}$$

Thus, as illustrated in Figure 10.2 and summarized in Table 10.2, we have three sources of variation of the dependent variable in analysis of variance. The total mean square estimates the variance of data represented by the dependent variable values without taking into account the groups specified by the independent variables. The

TABLE 10.2 Methods of calculating the three sources of variation of data represented by the dependent variable in analysis of variance. ■

Source	Degrees of Freedom	Sum of Squares	Mean Square
Total	$\left(\sum_{j=1}^{m} n_j\right) - 1$	$\sum_{j=1}^{m} \sum_{i=1}^{n_j} (Y_{ij} - \overline{Y})^2$	$\dfrac{\sum_{j=1}^{m} \sum_{i=1}^{n_j} (Y_{ij} - \overline{Y})^2}{\left(\sum_{j=1}^{m} n_j\right) - 1}$
Within	$\sum_{j=1}^{m} (n_j - 1)$	$\sum_{j=1}^{m} \sum_{i=1}^{n_j} (Y_{ij} - \overline{Y}_j)^2$	$\dfrac{\sum_{j=1}^{m} \sum_{i=1}^{n_j} (Y_{ij} - \overline{Y}_j)^2}{\sum_{j=1}^{m} (n_j - 1)}$
Between	$m - 1*$	$\sum_{j=1}^{m} \sum_{i=1}^{n_j} (\overline{Y}_j - \overline{Y})^{2}*$	$\dfrac{\sum_{j=1}^{m} \sum_{i=1}^{n_j} (\overline{Y}_j - \overline{Y})^2}{m - 1}$

*This value is usually found by subtraction, as shown in Equation 10.11.

within mean square estimates the variance of data represented by the dependent variable within each of those groups. The between mean square estimates the variation of data from group to group.

Now that we understand the sources of variation in analysis of variance, let us take a look at an example of how to estimate those sources of variation in a data set that contains a continuous dependent variable and more than one nominal independent variable.

Example 10.3   Suppose we are interested in determining the minimum dose of a particular drug from four different manufacturers that would result in prophylaxis of migraine headaches among patients that experienced migraine headaches at least once per week. First, we randomize 40 patients to receive one of the drugs. Then, we increase the dose of the assigned drug each week until the patient reports a week without a migraine headache. The dose that the patient was taking that week is considered to be the minimum effective dose of that drug. Imagine that we make the following observations:

Drug 1 (mg)	Drug 2 (mg)	Drug 3 (mg)	Drug 4 (mg)
17	29	17	18
16	28	25	20
21	23	24	25
22	26	19	24
23	26	28	16
18	19	21	20
20	25	20	20
17	29	25	17
25	26	19	19
21	28	24	17
200	259	222	196

Estimate the three sources of variation of data represented by the dependent variable in the population from which those observations were selected.

First, we will find the total variation of the dependent variable. That is, we will calculate the variance of the minimum effective dose without considering which drug was being taken. To do that, we need to find the squared deviations between each of the observations and the overall mean, taking into account all the values of the dependent variable. That mean is equal to the following:

$$\overline{Y} = \frac{200 + 259 + 222 + 196}{10 + 10 + 10 + 10} = 21.9 \text{ mg}$$

Then, we calculate the squared deviations between that mean and each of the observations:

Drug 1	$(Y_{i1} - \overline{Y})^2$	Drug 2	$(Y_{i2} - \overline{Y})^2$	Drug 3	$(Y_{i3} - \overline{Y})^2$	Drug 4	$(Y_{i4} - \overline{Y})^2$
17	24.01	29	50.41	17	24.01	18	15.21
16	34.81	28	37.21	25	9.61	20	3.61
21	0.81	23	1.21	24	4.41	25	9.61
22	0.01	26	16.81	19	8.41	24	4.41
23	1.21	26	16.81	28	37.21	16	34.81
18	15.21	19	8.41	21	0.81	20	3.61
20	3.61	25	9.61	20	3.61	20	3.61
17	24.01	29	50.41	25	9.61	17	24.01
25	9.61	26	16.81	19	8.41	19	8.41
21	0.81	28	37.21	24	4.41	17	24.01
200	114.10	259	244.90	222	110.50	196	131.30

Using Equation 10.9, we calculate the total mean square.

$$\text{Total mean square} = \frac{\text{Total sum of squares}}{\text{Total degrees of freedom}} = \frac{\sum_{j=1}^{m} \sum_{i=1}^{n_j} (Y_{ij} - \overline{Y})^2}{\left(\sum_{j=1}^{m} n_j \right) - 1}$$

$$= \frac{114.10 + 244.90 + 110.50 + 131.30}{(10 + 10 + 10 + 10) - 1} = \frac{600.80}{39} = 15.405 \text{ mg}^2$$

Thus, the variance of the minimum effective dose without regard to the source of the drug is estimated to be 15.405 mg².

Next, let us estimate the variance of the minimum effective dose within each of the drug groups. That is, we will estimate the within mean square that is a weighted average of the variance of minimum effective dose for any particular drug. To prepare to calculate the within mean square, we calculate the means of the dependent variable values in each of the groups.

$$\overline{Y}_1 = \frac{200}{10} = 20.0 \text{ mg}$$

$$\overline{Y}_2 = \frac{259}{10} = 25.9 \text{ mg}$$

$$\overline{Y}_3 = \frac{222}{10} = 22.2 \text{ mg}$$

$$\overline{Y}_4 = \frac{196}{10} = 19.6 \text{ mg}$$

Now, for each group separately we calculate the squared differences between each of the observations in the group that received a particular drug and the mean of that particular group.

Drug 1	$(\Upsilon_{i1} - \overline{\Upsilon}_1)^2$	Drug 2	$(\Upsilon_{i2} - \overline{\Upsilon}_2)^2$	Drug 3	$(\Upsilon_{i3} - \overline{\Upsilon}_3)^2$	Drug 4	$(\Upsilon_{i4} - \overline{\Upsilon}_4)^2$
17	9.00	29	9.61	17	27.04	18	2.56
16	16.00	28	4.41	25	7.84	20	0.16
21	1.00	23	8.41	24	3.24	25	29.16
22	4.00	26	0.01	19	10.24	24	19.36
23	9.00	26	0.01	28	33.64	16	12.96
18	4.00	19	47.61	21	1.44	20	0.16
20	0.00	25	0.81	20	4.84	20	0.16
17	9.00	29	9.61	25	7.84	17	6.76
25	25.00	26	0.01	19	10.24	19	0.36
21	1.00	28	4.41	24	3.24	17	6.76
200	78.00	259	84.90	222	109.60	196	78.40

Then, we use Equation 10.10 to calculate the sample's estimate of the within mean square.

$$\text{Within mean square} = \frac{\text{Within sum of squares}}{\text{Within degrees of freedom}} = \frac{\sum_{j=1}^{m} \sum_{i=1}^{n_j} (\Upsilon_{ij} - \overline{\Upsilon}_j)^2}{\sum_{j=1}^{m} (n_j - 1)}$$

$$= \frac{78.00 + 84.90 + 109.60 + 78.40}{9 + 9 + 9 + 9} = \frac{350.90}{36} = 9.747 \text{ mg}^2$$

Thus, our estimate of the variance of minimum effective dose, taking the drug group into account, is equal to 9.747 mg^2.

Finally, let us estimate the variation in minimum effective dose that is due to the variations between groups. We use Equation 10.11 to estimate the between mean square.

$$\text{Between mean square} = \frac{\text{Between sum of squares}}{\text{Between degrees of freedom}}$$

$$= \frac{\text{Total sum of squares} - \text{Within sum of squares}}{\text{Total degrees of freedom} - \text{Within degrees of freedom}}$$

$$= \frac{600.80 - 350.90}{39 - 36} = 83.300 \text{ mg}^2$$

Thus, the variation of minimum effective dose that is due to variations among the drug groups is estimated to be 83.300 mg^2.[6]

___

[6]Remember that we must calculate the between mean square by subtracting the within sum of squares from the total sum of squares and dividing by the difference between the within and total degrees of freedom. We *cannot* calculate the between mean square by subtracting the within mean square from the total mean square. In this example, if we made the mistake of subtracting mean squares, we would have concluded that the between mean square is equal to $15.405 - 9.747 = 5.658$. This is far from the correct estimate of 83.300.

If, in the previous example, the mean effective doses (dependent variable) for each of the drug groups (independent variables) are equal to each other in the population from which the sample was drawn, then we would expect to see variation among our sample's estimates of the drug groups' means that is a reflection only of the variation of data in the population. In other words, we would expect the variation between different groups (as measured by the between mean square) to be equal to the variation within the groups (as measured by the within mean square) in our sample. Thus, we can test the null hypothesis that all the groups' means are equal by comparing the sample's estimate of the between mean square to the sample's estimate of the within mean square. This comparison is made as a ratio, and it is an F value (Equation 10.12).

$$F = \frac{\text{Between mean square}}{\text{Within mean square}} = \frac{\dfrac{\sum_{j=1}^{m} \sum_{i=1}^{n_j} (\overline{Y}_j - \overline{Y})^2}{m - 1}}{\dfrac{\sum_{j=1}^{m} \sum_{i=1}^{n_j} (Y_{ij} - \overline{Y}_j)^2}{\sum_{j=1}^{m} (n_j - 1)}} \qquad (10.12)$$

That F ratio has $m - 1$ (the number of groups minus one) degrees of freedom in the numerator and $\Sigma(n_j - 1)$ degrees of freedom in the denominator. The null hypothesis tested here, called the **omnibus null hypothesis,** is like the hypothesis in regression analysis that states that estimation of values of the dependent variable is not improved by knowing values of the independent variable(s). Also like in regression analysis, we expect that F ratio to be equal to one if the null hypothesis is true and greater than one if the null hypothesis is false. Thus, the alternative hypothesis is always one-tailed.

Example 10.4   Test the null hypothesis that the mean minimum effective doses of the drug from the four manufacturers are all equal, using the observations in Example 10.3. Allow a 5% chance of making a Type I error.

Using Equation 10.12 and the estimates of the between mean square and within mean square from Example 10.3, we find the following F ratio:

$$F = \frac{\text{Between mean square}}{\text{Within mean square}} = \frac{\dfrac{\sum_{j=1}^{m} \sum_{i=1}^{n_j} (\overline{Y}_j - \overline{Y})^2}{m - 1}}{\dfrac{\sum_{j=1}^{m} \sum_{i=1}^{n_j} (Y_{ij} - \overline{Y}_j)^2}{\sum_{j=1}^{m} (n_j - 1)}}$$

$$= \frac{83.30}{9.747} = 8.546$$

To test the omnibus null hypothesis, we compare this calculated F ratio to a value that corresponds to 3 degrees of freedom in the numerator, 36 degrees of freedom in the denominator, and an area of 0.05 in one tail. Table B.4 does not list 36 degrees of freedom. The F value for 3 and 35 degrees of freedom and an α of 0.05 is equal to 2.87. The F value for 3 and 40 degrees of freedom and an α of 0.05 is equal to 2.84. We can either use linear interpolation to estimate the F ratio corresponding to 3 and 36 degrees of freedom[7] ($F = 2.864$), or we can compare our calculated F ratio to the value from Table B.4 corresponding to the next fewer degrees of freedom in the numerator. Since the value we have calculated is larger than either of those values from Table B.4, we can reject the omnibus null hypothesis and accept, by elimination, the alternative hypothesis that not all the mean effective doses for the drug groups are equal to each other in the population from which the sample was drawn.

The alternative hypothesis for the omnibus null hypothesis is that the population's means of the groups specified by values of the independent variables are not all equal. Notice, however, that rejecting the null hypothesis in favor of the alternative hypothesis could imply that one of the groups' means is not equal to the other groups' means, that each of the groups' means is not equal to any of the other groups' means, or anything in between. Generally, this is not a very satisfactory answer in health research. Rather, we would like to know specifically which groups' means we can conclude are different from which other groups' means. Rejecting the omnibus null hypothesis cannot answer this question. To make specific comparisons between means, we need to use an additional statistical procedure after rejecting the omnibus null hypothesis. This statistical procedure is called a **posterior test** since it is performed after the omnibus null hypothesis has been rejected.[8]

A number of posterior tests are available to make comparisons between the means of two groups at a time (known as **pairwise comparisons**). All of these posterior tests have the feature of being designed to maintain the Type I error equal to α for the entire series of pairwise comparisons. The chance of making at least one Type I error among all of the pairwise comparisons is called the **experimentwise error rate.**[9] This is different from the chance of making a Type I error in a single comparison, which is known as the **testwise error rate.** A Student's t test has a testwise error rate of 0.05. If we used Student's t tests to compare each of the four means in Example 10.3 to each of the other means (making a total of six comparisons), the chance of making a Type I

---

[7]Using linear interpolation, we observe that 36 is four-fifths of the way between 40 and 35. The F ratio for 36 degrees of freedom is, then, taken to be a value four-fifths of the way between 2.84 and 2.87.

[8]The posterior test that we will describe here does not rely on rejection of the omnibus null hypothesis before it can be used. Some of the older posterior tests did rely on rejection of that null hypothesis to have appropriate statistical properties. Although it is not necessary to do so with modern posterior tests, we generally look for specific differences between groups' means only if we are able to reject the omnibus null hypothesis.

[9]We would like to reserve the word "rate" to refer to a value with the units of 1/time (like an incidence), but "rate" is commonly used here to refer to a probability rather than a true rate.

error in at least one of those comparisons would be 0.21 instead of 0.05. We say that the experimentwise error rate in performing six Student's t tests on four means is equal to 0.21.

One of the goals in designing statistical procedures is to keep the chance of making an error at a minimum. If it is possible to reduce the experimentwise error when comparing several group means, we should do so. It is important, however, that we recognize that there is generally a cost for reducing the probability of making a Type I error. That cost is usually increasing the probability of making a Type II error (i.e., reducing the power). An example of a posterior procedure that maintains an experimentwise Type I error rate equal to α is called the **Bonferroni method.** In that procedure, we conduct each of the pairwise comparisons (e.g., using the Student's t test) using a modified α value. For example, if we wished to compare four means with an experimentwise Type I error rate equal to 0.05, the Bonferroni method would direct us to make each comparison with a testwise α of 0.01. The cost of using the Bonferroni method, however, is quite high. It does not take many pairwise comparisons to require a testwise α so small that it becomes virtually impossible to reject null hypotheses in any of the pairwise comparisons. That is because reducing α increases β (the probability of making a Type II error). Because of its low statistical power, we do not recommend the Bonferroni method.

Another posterior test for making pairwise comparison among several means is called the **Student-Newman-Keuls** procedure. This test establishes an experimentwise Type I error rate equal to α without a substantial increase in the Type II error rate. It is able to do this, in part, due to the order in which means are compared. To prepare to conduct the Student-Newman-Keuls test, we array the group means from lowest to highest. The first comparison we make is between the highest mean and the lowest mean. If *and only if* we are able to reject the null hypothesis that the means of those two groups are equal in the population are we permitted by the Student-Newman-Keuls procedure to make further comparisons. If we are able to reject that null hypothesis, then we are permitted to make two more comparisons. Specifically, we can compare the lowest mean to the second highest mean and the second lowest mean to the highest mean. If either one of these comparisons results in rejection of the null hypothesis that the means are equal, then we can make comparisons of the next most extreme means (between those means) for which we were able to reject the null hypothesis. In general, to make any comparisons in the Student-Newman-Keuls procedure, we must be able to reject the null hypothesis for more extreme means before we can compare less extreme means within a specific interval of means. This protocol will be illustrated in Example 10.5.

Other than this protocol to select which means can be compared and the table we use to compare the results of our calculations, the Student-Newman-Keuls test is very much like the Student's t test that we discussed in Chapter 7. The standard error for the difference between two means in the Student-Newman-Keuls test is a function of the pooled variance of data represented by the dependent variable (which is equal to the within mean square from the analysis of variance procedure) and the number of observations in the two groups being compared. One way that this standard error differs from that used in the Student's t procedure is that the pooled variance of data is divided by two in the Student-Newman-Keuls procedure (Equation 10.13).

$$SE_{\overline{Y}_1 - \overline{Y}_2} = \sqrt{\frac{s_p^2}{2} \cdot \left(\frac{1}{n_1} + \frac{1}{n_2} \right)} \tag{10.13}$$

The observed difference between two means is converted to a standard value from a distribution called the q distribution. Table B.8 provides values of the q distribution. The q distribution is like the Student's t distribution, but it includes a fourth parameter.[10] That parameter is the number of means that are in the interval being compared (including the two means actually being compared). We use the letter k to symbolize this parameter. The value of k for the first pairwise comparison is equal to the total number of groups, since the first comparison we make is between the highest and the lowest means. As the means being compared become less extreme, the value of k is reduced. This parameter is not used in any calculations. Rather, k is used to find the appropriate q statistic in Table B.8 for comparison with our calculated value of q. The calculated value of q is obtained by using a formula that is the same as the one used to calculate a Student's t statistic (see Equation 7.31):

$$q = \frac{(\overline{Y}_1 - \overline{Y}_2) - (\mu_1 - \mu_2)}{SE_{\overline{Y}_1 - \overline{Y}_2}} \tag{10.14}$$

Since the Student-Newman-Keuls test is designed only to test the null hypothesis that the means of two groups are equal in the population from which the sample was drawn (i.e., that the difference between the population's means is equal to zero), Equation 10.14 can be simplified to the following:

$$q = \frac{\overline{Y}_1 - \overline{Y}_2}{SE_{\overline{Y}_1 - \overline{Y}_2}} \tag{10.15}$$

Example 10.5   Test the null hypothesis that the difference between means of minimum effective dose is equal to zero in the population which was sampled for each pair of means in Example 10.3. Allow an experimentwise Type I error rate of 5%.

First, we rank the means in ascending order.

Drug 4	Drug 1	Drug 3	Drug 2
19.6	20.0	22.2	25.9

---

[10]Remember that the three parameters of the Student's t distribution are the mean ($=0$), the variance ($=1$), and degrees of freedom.

Since all the groups in this example have the same number of observations, the standard errors for all the comparisons will be equal to the same value. We use Equation 10.13 to find that value.

$$SE_{\bar{Y}_1 - \bar{Y}_2} = \sqrt{\frac{s_p^2}{2} \cdot \left(\frac{1}{n_1} + \frac{1}{n_2}\right)} = \sqrt{\frac{9.747}{2} \cdot \left(\frac{1}{10} + \frac{1}{10}\right)} = 0.987 \text{ mg}$$

Then, we can begin to make our pairwise comparisons. The following table summarizes that process. Since 36 degrees of freedom is not listed in Table B.8, we have used linear interpolation to find $q_{0.05,36,k}$ (this is calculated by adding 4/10 of the difference between the q value for 40 degrees of freedom and the q value for 30 degrees of freedom to the q value for 40 degrees of freedom). Notice in the following table that we first compare the most extreme means and, then, we compare less extreme means if and only if we are able to reject the null hypothesis. Also notice how the value of k is reduced as we examine less extreme means.

Compare Drugs	Difference	SE	q	k	$q_{0.05,36,k}$	Reject H_0?
4 and 2	6.3	0.987	6.38	4	3.813	Yes
4 and 3	2.6	0.987	2.63	3	3.460	No
1 and 2	5.9	0.987	5.98	3	3.460	Yes
4 and 1	This comparison is not examined (Drug 4 vs. Drug 3 not rejected).					
1 and 3	This comparison is not examined (Drug 4 vs. Drug 3 not rejected).					
3 and 2	3.7	0.987	3.75	2	2.870	Yes

In this case, we were unable to reject the null hypothesis that the mean effective doses for drugs 4 and 3 are equal in the population from which the sample was drawn. Following the protocol for the Student-Newman-Keuls procedure, we did not make further comparisons between the means of those two drugs. Rather, we conclude that, not only are we unable to reject the null hypothesis for drug 4 versus drug 3, but we are also unable to reject that null hypothesis for drug 4 versus drug 1 and drug 1 versus drug 3. Failure to follow this protocol will cause the Student-Newman-Keuls procedure to have an experimentwise error rate greater than α.

The particular kind of analysis of variance that we have discussed so far is more specifically called a **one-way analysis of variance.** This is the most straightforward type of analysis of variance. A one-way analysis of variance is defined as a set of data in which we have three or more groups of values of the dependent variable, all of which represent categories of a single **factor** or characteristic. For instance, in the previous examples, we had four groups of minimum effective dose measurements. Each group was defined by a drug from a different manufacturer, but all the groups represented drugs. Thus, those groups represented categories of a single factor: drugs.

When we have a collection of nominal independent variables that define groups of values of the dependent variable made up of more than one factor or characteristic, we analyze these data with an analysis of variance procedure for a **factorial analysis of variance.** To see what we imply by a data set in which the independent variables specify more than one factor or characteristic, let us take a look at an example.

Example 10.6   Suppose that we were interested in evaluating a treatment for herpes labialis versus a placebo. In this study, we identify three student health clinics that agree to serve as sources of patients with these lesions. A supply of the treatment and the placebo is given to each clinic and they are asked to randomize the prescriptions using a method to ensure that six patients receive the treatment and six receive the placebo. The patients are asked to call the clinic on the day that the lesion disappears. Imagine that we observe the following number of days until healing is complete for those patients.

Clinic A		Clinic B		Clinic C	
Placebo	Treatment	Placebo	Treatment	Placebo	Treatment
13	10	13	7	17	19
20	14	10	8	23	12
18	17	18	15	17	11
15	9	15	12	20	15
12	14	11	14	14	16
16	16	14	11	18	18

These data represent two factors. One factor specifies clinics, and it contains three categories (A, B, and C). The other factor specifies treatment, and it contains two categories (placebo and treatment).

Analysis of groups of dependent variable values that represent more than one factor is not substantially different from analysis of groups that represent one factor. The only difference we see between one-way and factorial analyses of variance is that in factorial analysis of variance we can separate the components of the between sum of squares, which measures the variation of values of the dependent variable between groups. These components represent variation in values of the dependent variable associated with each factor. We will not discuss the mechanics of calculating values for these components in *Statistical First Aid*; however, let us take a look at how the results of factorial analysis of variance can be interpreted.

We can think of the same three sources of variation of data represented by the dependent variable in factorial analysis of variance that we considered in one-way analysis of variance. In fact, the total, within, and between sums of squares, degrees of freedom, and mean squares are calculated in factorial analysis in the same way that they are calculated in one-way analysis of variance. However, there are additional sums of squares, degrees of freedom, and mean squares that are calculated in factorial analysis of variance. These are all components of what we have previously referred to as the between variation.

The between sum of squares estimates the amount of variation in data represented by the dependent variable that is due to differences in values of the dependent variable between the groups. If we have more than one factor, the between sum of squares is composed of variation between groups within each of the factors. The process of separating the components of the between sums of squares corresponding to each particular factor is known as **partitioning** the between sum of squares. Example 10.7 demonstrates what we imply by this process of partitioning the between sum of squares.

Example 10.7   Let us take a look at a computer output estimating the sources of variation of data represented by the dependent variable for the observations in Example 10.6.

Source of Variation	Degrees of Freedom	Sum of Squares	Mean Square
Total	35	459.00	13.11
Within	30	286.67	9.56
Between	5	172.33	34.47
Clinics	2	112.67	56.33
Treatments	1	58.78	58.78

In that output, we see three sources of variation in days until healing (dependent variable) that are familiar to us from our discussion of one-way analysis of variance. Those sources of variation are the total, within, and between variation. Each of those have the same value that they would have if we thought of the data in Example 10.6 as a one-way analysis of variance with six categories of a single factor or characteristic. In factorial analysis of variance, however, we recognize that the variation between the six groups of values of the dependent variable is partially due to variation in days until healing among the three clinics and partially due to variation in days until healing between the two treatments. Those components of the between variation have been calculated in this computer output. The sum of squares for clinics estimates how much variation in days until healing there is in the population among clinics, and the sum of squares for treatments estimates the variation in days until healing between the two treatments.

The estimates of the variation in data represented by the dependent variable between categories of a particular factor are called the estimates of **main effects.** The estimates of main effects are components of the variation between all the groups without regard to factors (i.e., the between variation). In our example, there is a main effect of clinics and a main effect of treatments. Since these are components of the between variation, we should be able to add the sums of squares for the main effects and get the between sum of squares and add the degrees of freedom for the main effects and get the between degrees of freedom. If we look at the results in Example 10.7, we can see that these main effects sums of squares and degrees of freedom do not add up to be equal to the between sum of squares and degrees of freedom. The reason they do not is that we have failed to consider one more source of variation of data represented by the dependent variable.

The main effects mean squares estimate the average variation in data represented by the dependent variable between categories of a particular factor. Looking only at main effect mean squares would assume that the differences between the category means within a factor are the same for each of the categories of the other factors. In our example of a treatment for herpes labialis, exclusive use of the mean square for clinics (reflecting differences between the mean days until cure for the three clinics) would have to assume that the relationship between those means for the placebo compared to the treatment is the same for all three clinics. In other words, we would have to assume that patients from different clinics might have different mean times until the lesion disappears, but the degree to which the treatment is more efficacious than the placebo is the same, on the average, for all patients. We would have to make that same assumption to interpret the treatment main effect mean square as an indicator of the difference between the placebo and treatment means.

If the relationship between the efficacies of the two treatments is not the same among the three clinics, we say that there is an **interaction** between treatment and clinics.[11] Thus, another component of the between variation is the interaction variation. The larger the interaction mean square, the more the relationship among categories of one factor differs between the categories of the other factor.

Example 10.8 Let us look at a computer output in which the variation due to the interaction between clinics and treatments for the observations in Example 10.6 is calculated.

Source of Variation	Degrees of Freedom	Sum of Squares	Mean Square
Total	35	459.00	13.11
Within	30	286.67	9.56
Between	5	172.33	34.47
Clinics	2	112.67	56.33
Treatments	1	58.78	58.78
Interaction	2	0.89	0.44

[11] A less commonly used synonym for "interaction" is "**effect modification**," which appears mostly in epidemiologic literature.

TABLE 10.3 Tests of inference in a factorial analysis of variance. ■

Null Hypothesis	F Ratio
The means of the dependent variable values in all the groups are equal in the population.	Omnibus F ratio: $F = \dfrac{\text{Between mean square}}{\text{Within mean square}}$
The means of the dependent variable values in the categories of a particular factor are equal in the population.	Main effects F ratio: $F = \dfrac{\text{Main effect mean square}}{\text{Within mean square}}$
The relationship between the means of the dependent variable values among the categories of one factor are the same regardless of the category of another factor.	Interaction F ratio: $F = \dfrac{\text{Interaction mean square}}{\text{Within mean square}}$

When we have a factorial analysis of variance, we can test the omnibus null hypothesis that all the groups' means are equal just as we did for a one-way analysis of variance. Specifically, the omnibus null hypothesis is tested by examining the F ratio with the between mean square in the numerator and the within mean square in the denominator. In addition, we can calculate F ratios to test null hypotheses that the means between categories within a particular factor are equal. Those **main effects F ratios** have the mean square for the main effect in the numerator and the within mean square in the denominator.[12] We also can calculate an F ratio to test the null hypothesis that there is no interaction between the main effects. This **interaction F ratio** has the interaction mean square in the numerator and the within mean square in the denominator. These tests of inference are summarized in Table 10.3.

If we are able to reject the null hypothesis that the means of values of the dependent variable in the categories of a particular factor are equal in the population, we would like to assume that there are differences between at least some of those means. Conversely, if we are unable to reject that null hypothesis, we would like to believe that there is insufficient evidence for differences between any of those means. However, if we also are able to reject the null hypothesis that there is no interaction

---

[12]Here, we are assuming that the categories are chosen by the researcher. This is most often the case in health research.

between the factors, then those tests for main effects become difficult to interpret. The reason for this difficulty is that rejection of the null hypothesis that there is no interaction suggests that the relationship between means of categories of one factor is not consistent for all categories of another factor in the population. If we cannot assume that there is consistency, we cannot use tests of hypotheses for main effects to examine the relationships among means of categories of a single factor. We usually assume that there is consistency when we are unable to reject the hypothesis of no interaction.[13] This ability or inability to assume consistency will become important when we examine how to make pairwise comparisons among means following factorial analysis of variance. Before we look at pairwise comparisons, however, let us take a look at an example of statistical inference in a factorial ANOVA.

Example 10.9 Test the null hypotheses that the mean number of days until cure for the three clinics are all equal in the population from which the sample in Example 10.6 was derived. Test the null hypothesis that the mean number of days until cure for the two treatments are equal in that population. Test the null hypothesis that there is no interaction between clinics and treatments for those same data. In all tests of inference, allow a 5% chance of making a Type I error.

To test the null hypotheses that the mean number of days until cure for the three clinics are all equal in the population, we divide the mean square for clinics by the within mean square.

$$F = \frac{\text{Clinic mean square}}{\text{Within mean square}} = \frac{56.33}{9.56} = 5.90$$

The mean square for clinics has 2 degrees of freedom, and the within mean square has 30 degrees of freedom. Therefore, we can evaluate our calculated F ratio by comparing it to the value from Table B.4 corresponding to an α of 0.05, 2 degrees of freedom in the numerator, and 30 degrees of freedom in the denominator. That F value is equal to 3.32. Since our calculated F ratio (5.90) is larger than 3.32, we reject the null hypothesis.

To test the null hypotheses that the mean number of days until cure for the two treatments are equal in the population, we divide the mean square for treatments by the within mean square.

$$F = \frac{\text{Treatment mean square}}{\text{Within mean square}} = \frac{58.78}{9.56} = 6.15$$

The mean square for treatments has 1 degree of freedom, and the within mean square has 30 degrees of freedom. Therefore, we need to compare our calculated F ratio to the value from

---

[13]Note that assuming that there is consistency among means of categories of one factor for all categories of another factor is tantamount to assuming that the null hypothesis is true when we are unable to reject the null hypothesis. This is a dangerous practice since our chance of making a mistake depends on the statistical power of the test. It is conventional to follow this practice, however, when determining our ability to interpret tests of inference for main effects. The reason for this convention is that there is no better method available for deciding that there is no interaction between factors in the population.

Table B.4 corresponding to an α of 0.05, 1 degree of freedom in the numerator, and 30 degrees of freedom in the denominator. That F value is equal to 4.17. Since our calculated F ratio (6.15) is larger than 4.17, we reject the null hypothesis.

To test the null hypotheses that the mean number of days until cure for the two treatments have the same relationship in all three clinics (i.e., that there is no interaction between treatment and clinic) in the population, we divide the interaction mean square by the within mean square.

$$F = \frac{\text{Interaction mean square}}{\text{Within mean square}} = \frac{0.44}{9.56} = 0.05$$

The mean square for the interaction has 2 degrees of freedom, and the within mean square has 30 degrees of freedom. Therefore, we can evaluate our calculated F ratio for the interaction by comparing it to the value from Table B.4 corresponding to an α of 0.05, 2 degrees of freedom in the numerator, and 30 degrees of freedom in the denominator. That F value is equal to 3.32. Since our calculated F ratio (0.05) is smaller than 3.32, we do not reject the null hypothesis. Thus, we assume that the relationship between treatments is consistent for all clinics, and the relationship among clinics is the same for both treatments in the population.

If a factor has more than two categories and we are able to reject the null hypothesis that all the means for categories of that factor are equal, we probably will want to use a posterior test procedure to determine which of the means are different from each other. In this application, we can use the Student-Newman-Keuls procedure described for a one-way analysis of variance.

There are two ways in which we can use the Student-Newman-Keuls test when we have a factorial analysis of variance. If we have not rejected the null hypothesis that an interaction does not exist between the factors, we can compare the means for each category within a particular factor in a separate Student-Newman-Keuls test. We can then conduct other Student-Newman-Keuls tests for the means for categories of other factors if we desire. If, on the other hand, we have rejected the null hypothesis of no interaction between the factors, we should perform a single Student-Newman-Keuls test on all the groups' means (for all categories of all factors) rather than on means for categories of a single factor.

We have looked at two designs in analysis of variance: the one-way design and the factorial design. There are many other analysis of variance designs to account for a great variety of relationships among the independent variables defining groups of dependent variables. Few of these are commonly used in health research. One exception is a design called a **repeated measures** analysis of variance. This design is useful when measurements of the dependent variable are taken more than once for each individual. For example, a repeated measures analysis of variance could be used to analyze data from a clinical trial of various methods of controlling blood pressure when blood pressure is measured at regular times during treatment. The details of repeated measures designs will not be discussed in *Statistical First Aid*.

MIXED INDEPENDENT VARIABLES

The most frequently encountered data set in health research contains a mixture of continuous and nominal independent variables. The method used to analyze a continuous dependent variable and a mixture of nominal and continuous independent variables is called **analysis of covariance** or **ANCOVA.** Analysis of covariance is often a feature available in computer programs that perform analysis of variance. In that application, analysis of covariance allows us to take into account the confounding effects of a continuous independent variable, while comparing means of groups specified by other (nominal) independent variables. Analysis of covariance also can be thought of as a type of regression analysis. In that application, a continuous independent variable is used to estimate values of the dependent variable in the same way it is used in regression analysis. The nominal independent variable(s) in this regression application can be thought of as a way to separate data to create two (or more) different regression lines (one for each of the two categories of the nominal independent variable) to be compared. How analysis of covariance can perform both of these functions will become clear as we investigate further a regression analysis that includes continuous and nominal independent variables.

To include a variable in regression analysis, it must have a number that expresses its value. The first problem we encounter with nominal independent variables is that they are not numeric but rather consist of two named conditions (yes/no). We solve this problem by creating **indicator variables**[14] from the nominal variables. The most common way to create an indicator variable is to assign a value of one to observations in which the nominal event is observed (i.e., "yes" = 1) and a value of zero to observations in which the event is not observed (i.e., "no" = 0).[15] For example, if we had a nominal variable that indicated whether or not a person received the treatment (versus a placebo) in a clinical trial, an indicator variable could be created that would have the value of one if the persons received the treatment and the value of zero if the persons received the placebo. Equation 10.16 shows a regression model that includes such an indicator variable.

$$Y = \alpha + (\beta_1 \cdot X) + (\beta_2 \cdot I) \qquad (10.16)$$

where

X = continuous independent variable
I = indicator variable created from a nominal independent variable

To see how we can interpret a regression equation that contains an indicator variable as a way to compare two regression equations, let us assume that we are

[14]Indicator variables are sometimes called "dummy" variables. We do not use this term since it tends to give the false impression that these variables are not very important.

[15]The choice of which category is assigned the value of one and which is assigned the value of zero is arbitrary. The only differences in the regression equation will be in the sign of the regression coefficient associated with the indicator variable and the value of the intercept. The interpretation of the regression analysis will be the same regardless of that choice.

estimating the coefficients in Equation 10.16 for a study of diastolic blood pressure (DBP) and its relationship to dose of an antihypertensive agent. Imagine that the nominal variable in our data set is gender. To construct a regression equation like Equation 10.16, we need to create an indicator variable for gender. Let us do that by assigning a value of one to the indicator variable for women and a value of zero for men. Then, for men the regression equation estimated in the sample is:

$$\text{DBP} = a + (b_1 \cdot \text{Dose}) + (b_2 \cdot 0) = a + (b_1 \cdot \text{Dose}) \qquad (10.17)$$

Since the value of the indicator variable is zero for men, the regression coefficient for the indicator term drops out of the equation, and we are left with an equation for a straight-line relationship between diastolic blood pressure and dose. Now, let us see what happens to that equation when the indicator variable is equal to one (as it is for women in this example).

$$\text{DBP} = a + (b_1 \cdot \text{Dose}) + (b_2 \cdot 1) = (a + b_2) + (b_1 \cdot \text{Dose}) \qquad (10.18)$$

When the indicator variable is equal to one, then the coefficient for the indicator variable remains in the regression as a constant (i.e., it does not change as values of the continuous independent variable change). We have rearranged the regression equation in Equation 10.18 to illustrate that, because the regression coefficient times one is equal to a constant, its value can be added to the value of the intercept (which is also a constant). Like Equation 10.17, Equation 10.18 describes a straight line. The difference between the two straight lines is that the intercept in Equation 10.17 is equal to a and the intercept in Equation 10.18 is equal to $a + b_2$. Thus, the regression coefficient for an indicator variable that has the values of one and zero tells us how much the intercepts differ between regression equations for the nominal states (such as male and female) represented by the indicator variable.

When we have nominal independent variables in a regression analysis that have been converted to indicator variables, we often create another type of variable by multiplying an indicator variable by another (continuous or nominal) independent variable. The product of an indicator variable and another independent variable is called an **interaction**. Equation 10.19 shows us a regression equation in a population that includes an interaction between a continuous and a nominal independent variable.

$$Y = \alpha + (\beta_1 \cdot X) + (\beta_2 \cdot I) + (\beta_3 \cdot X \cdot I) \qquad (10.19)$$

To see what an interaction implies in regression analysis, let us take another look at the example of diastolic blood pressure and its relationship to dose and gender. For men, the regression equation becomes:

$$\text{DBP} = a + (b_1 \cdot \text{Dose}) + (b_2 \cdot 0) + (b_3 \cdot \text{Dose} \cdot 0) = a + (b_1 \cdot \text{Dose}) \qquad (10.20)$$

Since the regression equation for men has a value of zero for the indicator variable, both the indicator variable and its interaction with dose drop out of Equation 10.20.

Even with the addition of the interaction term, the relationship between dose and diastolic blood pressure remains a straight line. This does not happen, however, when the value of the indicator variable is one, as it is for women in Equation 10.21.

$$\text{DBP} = a + (b_1 \cdot \text{Dose}) + (b_2 \cdot 1) + (b_3 \cdot \text{Dose} \cdot 1) = (a + b_2) + [(b_1 + b_3) \cdot \text{Dose}] \quad \text{(10.21)}$$

The interaction term becomes equal to its regression coefficient (b_3) times dose. Since the regression coefficient for dose (b_1) times dose is added to the regression coefficient for the interaction times dose, we can combine those regression coefficients as shown in Equation 10.21. The slope of the regression equation for women is equal to $b_1 + b_3$. The equation is, however, still a straight line. Thus, the regression coefficient for the indicator variable tells us how much the intercepts of two straight lines differ, and the regression coefficient for the interaction tells us how much the slopes of those two straight lines differ. In general, analysis of covariance applied to regression analysis allows us to compare slopes (by examining regression coefficients for interactions) and intercepts (by examining regression coefficients for indicators) between categories specified by values of nominal variables.[16]

Thus, we can have regression equations that include only continuous independent variables or a mixture of nominal (i.e., indicator) and continuous independent variables. We also can have regression equations that include only nominal (indicator) variables. Suppose that instead of knowing the dose of the antihypertensive drug in our example, we knew only whether a person received the drug or a placebo. Then, we would have two indicator variables. One of those indicator variables (I_1) would be equal to one when a person had received the drug and equal to zero when a person had received the placebo. The other indicator variable (I_2) would be equal to one for a woman and equal to zero for a man. Equation 10.22 shows a regression equation with those two indicator variables and their interaction.

$$\text{DBP} = a + (b_1 \cdot I_1) + (b_2 \cdot I_2) + (b_3 \cdot I_1 \cdot I_2) \quad \text{(10.22)}$$

Equation 10.22 can be used to estimate the mean diastolic blood pressure for four groups of persons defined by values of the independent variables. Let us take a look at those estimated values.

Men receiving the placebo:

$$\text{DBP} = a + (b_1 \cdot 0) + (b_2 \cdot 0) + (b_3 \cdot 0 \cdot 0) = a \quad \text{(10.23)}$$

Men receiving the drug:

$$\text{DBP} = a + (b_1 \cdot 1) + (b_2 \cdot 0) + (b_3 \cdot 1 \cdot 0) = a + b_1 \quad \text{(10.24)}$$

Women receiving the placebo:

$$\text{DBP} = a + (b_1 \cdot 0) + (b_2 \cdot 1) + (b_3 \cdot 0 \cdot 1) = a + b_2 \quad \text{(10.25)}$$

---

[16]If an interaction term is not included in a regression equation, that is tantamount to assuming that the slopes are identical in the groups.

Women receiving the drug:

$$\text{DBP} = a + (b_1 \cdot 1) + (b_2 \cdot 1) + (b_3 \cdot 1 \cdot 1) = a + b_1 + b_2 + b_3 \qquad (10.26)$$

From Equations 10.23 through 10.26, we can see that the intercept (a) gives us the mean diastolic blood pressure for men receiving the placebo. The regression coefficient for the indicator of treatment (b_1) tells us how much blood pressure changes for persons receiving the drug regardless of their gender. The regression coefficient for the indicator of gender (b_2) tells us how much the diastolic blood pressure changes for women regardless of which treatment they are receiving. The regression coefficient for the interaction (b_3) tells us how much more the diastolic blood pressure changes for women receiving the drug than would be expected by simply adding the treatment effect (b_1) to the gender effect (b_2).

Thus, a regression equation containing only nominal independent variables (or, rather, their corresponding indicator variables) allows us to compare means of the dependent variable (DBP) among groups defined by values of the independent variables (men/women and drug/placebo). That description sounds more like analysis of variance than it does regression analysis. In fact, Equation 10.22 is a regression analysis, but it is also a factorial analysis of variance![17]

The coefficients in Equation 10.22 correspond to the main effects and interaction that we would find in an analysis of variance applied to diastolic blood pressure divided into the four groups represented by Equations 10.23 through 10.26. A test of the null hypothesis that β_1 is equal to zero would give us exactly the same F ratio as we would obtain comparing the main effect of treatment (i.e., the treatment mean square) to the within mean square in analysis of variance. A test of the null hypothesis that β_2 is equal to zero would give us exactly the same F ratio as we would obtain comparing the main effect of gender (i.e., the gender mean square) to the within mean square in analysis of variance. A test of the null hypothesis that β_3 is equal to zero would give us exactly the same F ratio as we would obtain comparing the interaction mean square to the within mean square in analysis of variance.

If we included a continuous independent variable (e.g., age) in this example, we could then compare mean diastolic blood pressure for the drug versus the placebo group, or for men versus women, while taking into account the confounding effects of age. This would be an example of analysis of covariance as an extension of analysis of variance to include a continuous independent variable. The only difference between this application of analysis of covariance and analysis of covariance as an extension of regression analysis is the way in which we interpret the results. In the analysis of variance application, our main interest is in comparing means of the dependent variable for the groups specified by the nominal independent variables. In the regression application, our main interest usually is in the relationship between the dependent variable and the continuous independent variable. The equations that we use in these two applications, however, are identical.

[17]Analysis of variance relies on indicator variables defined differently than 0 and 1, but when we have only two categories for each factor, the results will be the same.

Therefore, we can think about regression analysis, analysis of variance, and analysis of covariance as the same statistical procedure, differing only in the types of data represented by the independent variables. In fact, all of the statistical procedures we have discussed in *Statistical First Aid* for continuous dependent variables are related in this way.[18]

||| SUMMARY

When we have a continuous dependent variable and more than one continuous independent variable, we can perform statistical procedures that are extensions of correlation analysis and regression analysis discussed in Chapter 7 for a single independent variable. For more than one independent variable, the procedures are called multiple correlation analysis and multiple regression analysis. Both of those procedures examine a linear combination of the independent variables multiplied by their corresponding slopes or regression coefficients.

$$Y = \alpha + \beta_1 X_1 + \beta_2 X_2 + \cdots + \beta_j X_j + \cdots + \beta_k X_k \tag{10.2}$$

where

X_j = the jth independent variable in a collection of k independent variables

β_j = the "slope" or regression coefficient for the jth independent variable in a collection of k independent variables

In analysis of multivariable data sets, we can think about the relationship of the dependent variable to each of the independent variables or about its relationship to the entire collection of independent variables. In multiple correlation analysis, however, only the association between the dependent variable and the entire collection of independent variables is considered. To interpret the multiple correlation coefficient or its square, the coefficient of multiple determination, as an estimate of the association in the population from which the sample was drawn, all the independent variables must be from a naturalistic sample. That is to say, their distributions in the sample must be the result of a random sample from their distributions in the population.

In multiple regression analysis, we also can examine the relationship between the dependent variable and the entire collection of independent variables. One way that we do this is to test the omnibus null hypothesis.

$$F = \frac{\text{Regression mean square}_{\text{Full}}}{\text{Residual mean square}_{\text{Full}}} \tag{10.6}$$

We can also examine each individual independent variable in multiple regression analysis. The relationship between the dependent variable and an individual independent variable in

---

[18]For instance, consider the following regression equation in which we have a single nominal independent variable.

$$\hat{Y} = a + (b \cdot I)$$

This is a regression equation that is also a Student's t test. If we take the square root of the F ratio for this regression equation, we will get exactly the same Student's t value that would be obtained by following the procedures in Chapter 7 for the Student's t test.

multiple regression analysis, however, is not necessarily the same as the relationship between those variables in bivariable regression analysis (i.e., when we have only one independent variable). The difference is that, in multiple regression analysis, we examine the relationship between an independent variable and the variability in data represented by the dependent variable that is not associated with the other independent variables. This procedure is reflected in the method used to test the null hypothesis that a particular regression coefficient is equal to zero in the population. This is done with a partial F ratio.

$$F = \frac{\dfrac{\text{Regression sum of squares}_{\text{Full}} - \text{Regression sum of squares}_{\text{Reduced}}}{\text{Regression degrees of freedom}_{\text{Full}} - \text{Regression degrees of freedom}_{\text{Reduced}}}}{\dfrac{\text{Residual sum of squares}_{\text{Full}}}{\text{Residual degrees of freedom}_{\text{Full}}}} \tag{10.5}$$

If two or more independent variables share information (i.e., if they are correlated) and, in addition, that shared information is the same as the information that they use to estimate values of the dependent variable, we say that we have multicollinearity. Multicollinearity can make estimation and inference for individual regression coefficients difficult. It also makes it possible to take into account the confounding effects of one or more independent variables, while examining the relationship between another independent variable and the dependent variable. Multicollinearity is a feature, not only of multiple regression analysis, but of all multivariable procedures.

Polynomial regression is a special type of multiple regression in which all the independent variables are multiples of a single continuous variable. Polynomial regression is used to describe a curvilinear relationship between the dependent variable and the independent variable. For each multiple of the continuous independent variable included in a polynomial regression equation, the slope can have one change in direction. The best polynomial regression equation for a particular dependent variable and a particular independent variable is usually taken to be the one in which the inclusion of an additional multiple of the independent variable would not allow rejection of the null hypothesis that the coefficient associated with that multiple is equal to zero in the population.

When we have more than one nominal independent variable, we are able to specify more than two groups of dependent variable values. The means of the dependent variable values for those groups are compared using analysis of variance procedures. Analysis of variance involves estimating three sources of variation of data represented by the dependent variable. The variation of the dependent variable without regard to independent variable values is called the total sum of squares. The total mean square is equal to the total sum of squares divided by the total degrees of freedom.

$$\text{Total mean square} = \frac{\text{Total sum of squares}}{\text{Total degrees of freedom}} = \frac{\displaystyle\sum_{j=1}^{m}\sum_{i=1}^{n_j} (\Upsilon_{ij} - \overline{\Upsilon})^2}{\left(\displaystyle\sum_{j=1}^{m} n_j\right) - 1} \tag{10.9}$$

The best estimate of the population's variance of data represented by the dependent variable is found by taking a weighted average (with degrees of freedom as the weights) of the estimates of the variance of data within each group of values of the dependent variable. This estimate is called the within mean square.

$$\text{Within mean square} = \frac{\text{Within sum of squares}}{\text{Within degrees of freedom}} = \frac{\sum\limits_{j=1}^{m} \sum\limits_{i=1}^{n_j} (Y_{ij} - \overline{Y}_j)^2}{\sum\limits_{j=1}^{m} (n_j - 1)} \tag{10.10}$$

The within sum of squares is one of two portions of the total sum of squares. The remaining portion describes the variation among the group means. This is called the between sum of squares. The between sum of squares divided by its degrees of freedom (the number of groups minus one) gives us the average variation among group means called the between mean square.

$$\text{Between mean square} = \frac{\text{Between sum of squares}}{\text{Between degrees of freedom}} = \frac{\sum\limits_{j=1}^{m} \sum\limits_{i=1}^{n_j} (\overline{Y}_j - \overline{Y})^2}{m - 1}$$

$$= \frac{\text{Total sum of squares} - \text{Within sum of squares}}{\text{Total degrees of freedom} - \text{Within degrees of freedom}} \tag{10.11}$$

We can test the omnibus null hypothesis that the means of the dependent variable in all the groups specified by independent variable values are equal in the population from which the sample was drawn by comparing the between mean square and the within mean square. This is done by calculating an F ratio. If the omnibus null hypothesis is true, that ratio should be equal to one.

$$F = \frac{\text{Between mean square}}{\text{Within mean square}} = \frac{\dfrac{\sum\limits_{j=1}^{m} \sum\limits_{i=1}^{n_j} (\overline{Y}_j - \overline{Y})^2}{m - 1}}{\dfrac{\sum\limits_{j=1}^{m} \sum\limits_{i=1}^{n_j} (Y_{ij} - \overline{Y}_j)^2}{\sum\limits_{j=1}^{m} (n_j - 1)}} \tag{10.12}$$

In addition to testing the omnibus null hypothesis, it is often of interest to make pairwise comparisons of means of the dependent variable. To do this, we use a posterior test designed to keep the experimentwise α error rate equal to a specific value (usually 0.05) regardless of how many pairwise comparisons are made. The best procedure to make all possible pairwise comparisons among the means is the Student-Newman-Keuls procedure. The test statistic for this procedure is similar to a Student's t statistic in that it is equal to the difference between two means minus the hypothesized difference divided by the standard error for the difference.

$$q = \frac{(\overline{Y}_1 - \overline{Y}_2) - (\mu_1 - \mu_2)}{SE_{\overline{Y}_1 - \overline{Y}_2}} \tag{10.14}$$

It is also similar to a Student's t statistic in that the standard error for the difference between two means includes a pooled estimate of the variance of data represented by the dependent variable. In analysis of variance, the pooled estimate of the variance of data is the within mean square.

$$\text{SE}_{\bar{Y}_1 - \bar{Y}_2} = \sqrt{\frac{s_p^2}{2} \cdot \left(\frac{1}{n_1} + \frac{1}{n_2} \right)} \tag{10.13}$$

The important difference between the Student's t procedure and the Student-Newman-Keuls procedure is that the latter requires a specific order in which pairwise comparisons are made. The first comparison must be between the largest and the smallest means. If and only if we can reject the null hypothesis that those two means are equal in the population can we compare less extreme means.

If all the nominal independent variables identify different categories of a single characteristic or factor (e.g., different races), we say that we have a one-way analysis of variance. If, on the other hand, some of the nominal independent variables specify categories of one factor (e.g., race), and other nominal independent variables specify categories of another factor (e.g., gender), we say that we have a factorial analysis of variance.

Factorial analysis of variance involves estimation of total, within, and between variation of data represented by the dependent variable just like one-way analysis of variance. The difference between factorial and one-way analyses of variance is that, in factorial analysis of variance, we consider components of the between variation. Some of these components estimate the variation among the means of the dependent variable corresponding to categories of that particular factor and are called main effects. Another component reflects the consistency of the relationship among categories of one factor for different categories of another factor. This source of variation is called the interaction. Only if there does not seem to be a statistically significant interaction can the main effects be interpreted easily.

It is very common that a data set contains both continuous and nominal independent variables. The procedure we use to analyze such a data set is called analysis of covariance. An analysis of covariance can be thought of as a multiple regression in which the nominal independent variable(s) is represented numerically, often with the values zero and one. The numeric representation of a nominal independent variable is called an indicator variable. An additional independent variable is created by multiplying an indicator variable by another independent variable. This is called an interaction.

$$Y = \alpha + (\beta_1 \cdot X) + (\beta_2 \cdot I) + (\beta_3 \cdot X \cdot I) \tag{10.19}$$

where

X = continuous independent variable
I = indicator variable created from a nominal independent variable

In its simplest form, analysis of covariance can be thought of as a method to compare regression equations for the categories specified by values of the nominal independent variable(s). In that interpretation, the regression coefficient for the indicator variable gives the difference between the intercepts of the regression equations, and the regression coefficient for the interaction gives the difference between the slopes for those regression equations.

Another way to think about analysis of covariance is that it is a method to compare group means while controlling for the confounding effects of a continuous independent variable. This is not really different than the regression interpretation. In fact, all the procedures we have examined for continuous dependent variables in *Statistical First Aid* can be thought of as regression analyses.

|| PRACTICE PROBLEMS

10.1 Imagine that we conduct a clinical trial of a drug that is designed to lower serum cholesterol levels compared to a placebo. In the analysis of the resulting observations we wish to control for the potential confounding effects of age and gender. What is the regression equation that describes the relationship in which we are interested? How would the regression coefficients of that equation be interpreted?

10.2 Suppose we collect data on systolic blood pressure (in mm Hg) in a geriatric population, with the intent to examine the relationship between that dependent variable and independent variables representing gender and age (in years). We analyze those data using a computer program for multiple regression. For that analysis, we create an indicator of gender (SEX = 1 for males and SEX = 0 for females) and an interaction variable for age and gender (A · S). Suppose we observe the following results.

SOURCE	DF	SUM OF SQS	MEAN SQ
REGRESSION	3	970.735	323.578
RESIDUAL	50	3,247.665	64.953

VARIABLE	B	SE B	F	P
AGE	1.001	0.287	12.190	0.001
SEX	10.100	3.184	10.061	0.002
A · S	0.094	0.046	4.101	0.050
(CONSTANT)	74.389	21.476	11.997	0.001

What do the results of that analysis suggest about the relationships between age and systolic blood pressure and between gender and systolic blood pressure?

10.3 Using the results of the analysis in Problem 10.2, answer the following questions.
   a) What was the sample size in this study?
   b) What proportion of the variation in systolic blood pressure measurements is associated with the combination of age and gender?
   c) How do these data relate to the hypothesis that there is no relationship between systolic blood pressure and the combination of age and gender?

10.4 In a particular disease known to be associated with damage to the liver, we recognize four stages in the progression of the disease. To evaluate the amount of liver damage at each stage, we measure serum glutamic transaminase (AST) in ten patients at each stage. Suppose we observe the following AST measurements (units/ml).

Stage I	Stage II	Stage III	Stage IV
38	23	57	30
22	36	42	26
41	44	36	42
12	33	39	23
37	42	42	21
29	48	43	43
32	19	29	39
18	28	52	32
25	34	65	39
31	40	51	31

Test the null hypothesis that the mean AST values are the same for all stages of this disease, allowing a 5% chance of making a Type I error.

10.5 For the observations in Problem 10.4, make all pairwise comparisons of mean AST values to test the null hypothesis that each difference between two means is equal to zero in the population from which the sample was drawn. As an alternative, hypothesize that the difference between the means is not equal to zero. Allow a 5% chance of making a Type I error.

10.6 Suppose that we are interested in examining a new treatment for the disease described in Problem 10.4 that is designed to reduce liver damage. We perform a clinical trial of that treatment (TX) versus a placebo (PL) and observe the following results.

Stage I		Stage II		Stage III		Stage IV	
TX	PL	TX	PL	TX	PL	TX	PL
29	38	36	23	41	57	26	30
23	22	30	36	55	42	34	26
25	41	25	44	43	36	28	42
29	12	14	33	20	39	29	23
27	37	42	42	34	42	38	21
26	29	37	48	34	43	17	43
13	32	30	19	27	29	18	39
38	18	35	28	28	52	38	32
19	25	32	34	34	65	21	39
34	31	19	40	45	51	26	31

Using a computer program for factorial analysis of variance, we obtain the following computer output:

Source of Variation	Degrees of Freedom	Sum of Squares	Mean Square
Total	79	8,435.87	106.78
Within	72	5,686.90	78.98
Between	7	2,748.97	392.71
Stage	3	2,033.02	677.67
Treatment	1	577.79	577.79
Interaction	3	137.48	45.83

Test the following null hypotheses, allowing a 5% chance of making a Type I error.
a) All eight means are equal in the population.
b) The means for the four stages of disease are equal in the population.
c) The means for the two treatments are equal in the population.
d) The relationship between the treatments is the same for all stages of the disease in the population.

CHAPTER 11

Ordinal Dependent Variables

Like we discussed for univariable and bivariable data sets, multivariable analysis of an ordinal dependent variable can be performed on data that occur naturally on an ordinal scale or on continuous data converted to an ordinal scale. That conversion from a continuous scale to an ordinal scale allows us to circumvent some of the assumptions of the statistical methods that are designed to analyze continuous dependent variables. In either case, observations are converted to a scale of ranks for all of the statistical procedures that we will discuss in this chapter. That conversion to a scale of ranks follows the same procedure that we have used in the past.

CONTINUOUS INDEPENDENT VARIABLES

If we have an ordinal dependent variable and more than one continuous independent variable, the continuous data represented by the independent variables are most often converted to an ordinal scale for analysis. There are no commonly used statistical procedures that permit us to take advantage of the continuous nature of independent variables when the dependent variable is ordinal.

ORDINAL INDEPENDENT VARIABLES

In Chapter 10, two types of analyses were discussed for a continuous dependent variable and more than one continuous independent variable. Those were multiple correlation analysis and multiple regression analysis. When the dependent and independent variables are ordinal rather than continuous, we can use statistical procedures that are similar to multiple correlation analysis. As we can see in Flowchart 9, there are no commonly used procedures for ordinal variables that are parallel to multiple regression analysis.

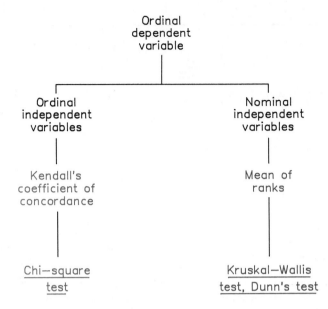

FLOWCHART 9 Multivariable analysis of an ordinal dependent variable. Point estimates are indicated in red. Statistical procedures are indicated in red and underlined.

Recall from our discussion of multiple correlation analysis that the multiple coefficient of determination (the square of the multiple correlation coefficient) reflects the proportion of variation in data represented by the dependent variable that is associated with the entire collection of independent variables. For instance, we found a multiple coefficient of determination of 0.78 for weight as a function of height and age in Example 10.2. That implies that 78% of the variation in weight can be explained by knowing a person's height and age.

With a simple (bivariable) correlation coefficient, we would obtain the same value regardless of which of the two continuous variables is considered to be the dependent variable. This is true of Pearson's correlation coefficient for continuous variables and for Spearman's correlation coefficient for ordinal variables. This is not true, however, of the correlation coefficient calculated from a multivariable set of continuous variables. The value of a multiple correlation coefficient (and, thus, of a multiple coefficient of determination) is influenced by which of a collection of continuous variables is considered to be the dependent variable. For example, if we considered age to be represented by the dependent variable and weight and height to be represented by independent variables in the data set from Example 10.2, the multiple coefficient of determination would be 0.59 instead of 0.78. That difference is due to the fact that we are asking how the combination of weight and height are associated with age instead of how the combination of height and age are associated with weight.

When we have an ordinal dependent variable and more than one ordinal independent variable, the measure of association that is most often used to examine those variables is called **Kendall's coefficient of concordance.** Equation 11.1 shows how that coefficient is calculated.[1]

$$W = \frac{\Sigma R_j^2 - \frac{(\Sigma R_j)^2}{n}}{\frac{[k^2 \cdot (n^3 - n)] - (k \cdot \Sigma T)}{12}} \tag{11.1}$$

where

W = Kendall's coefficient of concordance

R_j = sum of the ranks for all the variables for the jth observation

k = number of variables (dependent and independent)

ΣT = correction for ties where t_i is the number of tied ranks in the ith group of ties and $\Sigma T = \Sigma(t_i^3 - t_i)$

Kendall's coefficient of concordance is like the multiple correlation coefficient in that it is a measure of association among several variables. Kendall's coefficient of concordance, however, has an interpretation that is very different from the interpretation of the multiple correlation coefficient. Rather than measuring the strength of the association between the dependent variable and the entire collection of independent variables (like a multiple correlation coefficient), Kendall's coefficient of concordance is approximately equal to the mean value of the Spearman's correlation coefficients that would be obtained if we calculated a bivariable Spearman's correlation coefficients for each possible pair of variables (see Example 11.1). In other words, Kendall's coefficient of concordance can be interpreted to reflect the average strength with which all the variables are associated if those variables were considered two at a time. Thus, Kendall's coefficient of concordance, unlike many other procedures for ordinal variables, cannot be thought of as exactly parallel to any procedure for continuous variables. Rather, Kendall's coefficient of concordance has its own unique interpretation.

Kendall's coefficient of concordance is a combination of all possible pairs of variables without distinction between dependent and independent variables in a data set. Therefore, unlike the multiple correlation coefficient (but like a bivariable correlation coefficient), Kendall's coefficient of concordance will have the same value regardless of which variable is considered to be the dependent variable.

The maximum value possible for Kendall's coefficient of concordance is $+1$. A value of positive one indicates that all the variables, when examined two at a time, have perfect (on an ordinal scale) positive associations. We might expect that, like a correlation coefficient, the minimum value for Kendall's coefficient of concordance might be equal to -1. This, however, is *not* the case. The minimum value for Kendall's coefficient of concordance is *zero*. To understand why this is true, remember that Kendall's coefficient of concordance is approximately equal to the mean of all the possible bivariable (Spearman's) correlation coefficients. For Kendall's coefficient of concordance to be equal to -1, all the bivariable correlation coefficients would have to

[1]Actually, there are several methods that can be used to calculate Kendall's coefficient of concordance. The one shown in Equation 11.1 is the simplest of those methods.

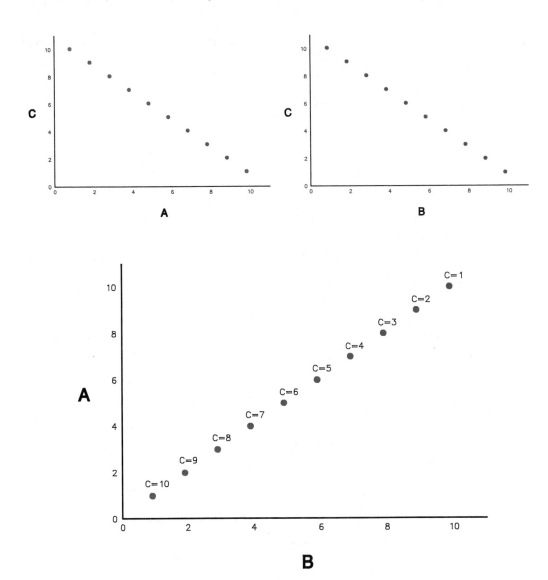

FIGURE 11.1 Illustration of the inability of three variables to have perfect negative associations. Here, variables *A* and *B* have perfect negative associations with variable *C*. Under that condition, variable *A* must have a perfect *positive* association with variable *B*.

be equal to −1. This cannot happen since it is impossible for all variables to be negatively related to one another.[2] If, for example, we have three variables called *A*, *B*, and *C*, *A* and *B* might be negatively correlated with *C*, but then *A* and *B* *must be* positively correlated with each other. This is illustrated in Figure 11.1.

[2]In addition, the correlation coefficients for each variable associated with itself is included in the mean of correlation coefficients. By definition, the correlation of a variable with itself must be equal to +1.

Now that we understand how Kendall's coefficient of concordance is calculated and interpreted, let us take a look at an example.

Example 11.1 Estimate Kendall's coefficient of concordance for the observations of weight, height, and age among twelve nutritionally deficient children presented in Example 10.2.

First, we need to convert those observations to ranks. Then, we calculate the sum of the ranks of all three variables for each observation and the square of that sum of ranks. The procedures are summarized in the following table:

Weight	Rank	Height	Rank	Age	Rank	R_j	R_j^2
64	7	57	8.5	8	4.5	20.0	400.00
71	10	59	10	10	9	29.0	841.00
53	2	49	4	6	1.5	7.5	56.25
67	8	62	12	11	11	31.0	961.00
55	3	51	6	8	4.5	13.5	182.25
58	6	50	5	7	3	14.0	196.00
77	12	55	7	10	9	28.0	784.00
57	5	48	3	9	6.5	14.5	210.25
56	4	42	1.5	10	9	14.5	210.25
51	1	42	1.5	6	1.5	4.0	16.00
76	11	61	11	12	12	34.0	1,156.00
68	9	57	8.5	9	6.5	24.0	576.00
						234.0	5,589.00

There are six groups of tied ranks in this data set. Two of those groups are ranks of height (1.5 and 8.5). Each of those groups includes two members. The other four groups of ties are ranks of age (1.5, 4.5, 6.5, and 9). Three of those four groups include two members, and one of those groups (9) includes three members. Thus, the correction for tied ranks is:

$$\Sigma T = \Sigma(t_i^3 - t_i) = [5 \cdot (2^3 - 2)] + (3^3 - 3) = 54$$

Finally, we use Equation 11.1 to estimate Kendall's coefficient of concordance:

$$W = \frac{\Sigma R_j^2 - \dfrac{(\Sigma R_j)^2}{n}}{\dfrac{[k^2 \cdot (n^3 - n)] - (k \cdot \Sigma T)}{12}} = \frac{5,589.00 - \dfrac{234.0^2}{12}}{\dfrac{[3^2 \cdot (12^3 - 12)] - (3 \cdot 54)}{12}} = 0.806$$

To demonstrate that Kendall's coefficient of concordance is related to the mean of all possible

Spearman's correlation coefficients, let us take a look at the following matrix of all possible Spearman's correlation coefficients for this data set:

	Weight	Height	Age
Weight	1.000	0.761	0.747
Height	0.761	1.000	0.616
Age	0.747	0.616	1.000

The mean of those nine Spearman's correlation coefficients is equal to

$$\bar{r}_s = \frac{1.000 + 0.761 + 0.747 + \cdots + 0.616 + 1.000}{9} = 0.805$$

which is very close to the value obtained for Kendall's coefficient of concordance (0.806).   ▭

In statistical inference for Kendall's coefficient of concordance, the most common null hypothesis tested is that the coefficient of concordance in the population from which the sample was drawn is equal to zero. To test that null hypothesis, we can convert the coefficient to a standard scale (a chi-square statistic with $n - 1$ degrees of freedom) as shown in Equation 11.2.

$$\chi^2 = k \cdot (n - 1) \cdot W \qquad (11.2)$$

where k = number of variables.

This conversion to a chi-square value is a good approach as long as the sample's size is equal to five or more. For smaller samples a special table of Kendall's coefficients of concordance should be used to evaluate the test statistic.

Example 11.2   Test the null hypothesis that Kendall's coefficient of concordance in the population from which the sample in Example 11.1 was drawn is equal to zero versus the alternative hypothesis that it is not equal to zero. Allow a 5% chance of making a Type I error.

Using Equation 11.2, we calculate the following chi-square value:

$$\chi^2 = k \cdot (n - 1) \cdot W = 3 \cdot (12 - 1) \cdot 0.803 = 26.499$$

From Table B.7, we find that a chi-square value corresponding to $12 - 1 = 11$ degrees of freedom and an α of 0.05 is equal to 19.675. Since our calculated chi-square value (26.499) is greater than 19.675, we reject the null hypothesis and accept, by elimination, the alternative hypothesis that the coefficient of concordance is not equal to zero in the population.   ▭

NOMINAL INDEPENDENT VARIABLES

In Chapter 10, we learned that a collection of nominal independent variables divides values of a continuous dependent variable into groups. Testing of the null hypothesis that the means of all of those groups in the population are equal (the omnibus null hypothesis) was accomplished with an analysis of variance. In that chapter, we looked at two different types of analyses of variance. A one-way analysis of variance was used to examine more than two categories of one factor (such as the four different drugs in Example 10.3). A factorial analysis of variance was used to examine categories of more than one factor (such as the three clinics and two treatments in Example 10.6). When the dependent variable is ordinal instead of continuous, we have a similar interest in comparing the several groups of ordinal dependent variable values specified by values of the nominal independent variables. The procedures that we use are parallel to those used in Chapter 10, but they circumvent assumptions about the distribution of dependent variable values required by an analysis of variance.[3]

The procedure that we use for values of an ordinal dependent variable divided into more than two categories of a single factor is called the **Kruskal-Wallis test.** Like the other procedures that we have discussed for ordinal dependent variables, the Kruskal-Wallis test is based on values of a dependent variable converted to a scale of ranks. That conversion follows the same rules that we have used in those other procedures. The Kruskal-Wallis test statistic (H) is calculated from the sums of the ranks for each of the categories of dependent variable values, as shown in Equation 11.3.

$$H = \left[\frac{12}{n_T \cdot (n_T + 1)} \cdot \sum \frac{R_j^2}{n_j} \right] - [3 \cdot (n_T + 1)] \qquad (11.3)$$

where

n_T = total number of observations
R_j = sum of the ranks for the jth category
n_j = number of observations in the jth category

Equation 11.3 is applicable to data sets in which the ranks of the dependent variable values are not tied. When tied ranks exist, a corrected Kruskal-Wallis test statistic (H_c) can be calculated, as shown in Equation 11.4.

$$H_c = \frac{H}{1 - \dfrac{\sum (t_i^3 - t_i)}{n_T^3 - n_T}} \qquad (11.4)$$

where t_i = number of ties in the ith groups of ties.

The null hypothesis that is tested with the Kruskal-Wallis test statistic is that the values of the dependent variable are the same in all of the categories in the population from which the sample was drawn. This is parallel to the omnibus null hypothesis

---

[3]Two of the most commonly violated assumptions in analysis of variance are that the means of the dependent variable come from a Gaussian distribution and that the variance of data represented by the dependent variable is the same within each group.

tested with the F ratio in a one-way analysis of variance. To evaluate a calculated Kruskal-Wallis test statistic, its value is compared with a value from a table of critical values (such as Table B.9). For samples larger than those in Table B.9, the Kruskal-Wallis test statistic can be considered a chi-square value with $m - 1$ (m = number of groups) degrees of freedom and can be compared to chi-square values in Table B.7.

Example 11.3   Let us consider the observations of minimum effective doses of a particular drug from four different manufacturers to treat migraine headache presented in Example 10.3. Suppose that we have some reason to believe that the assumptions required by analysis of variance are not satisfied in this data set. Therefore, we want to test the null hypothesis that the minimum effective doses (dependent variable) are the same for all four groups (independent variables) in the population from which the sample was drawn without making assumptions about the distribution of minimum effective doses. We will allow a 5% chance of making a Type I error.

First, we need to convert the observations in Example 10.3 to ranks. Then, in preparation for calculating the Kruskal-Wallis test statistic, we need to sum those ranks for each of the drug groups. Those operations are illustrated in the following table.

Drug 1	Rank	Drug 2	Rank	Drug 3	Rank	Drug 4	Rank
17	5	29	39.5	17	5	18	8.5
16	1.5	28	37	25	30	20	16
21	20	23	23.5	24	26	25	30
22	22	26	34	19	11.5	24	26
23	23.5	26	34	28	37	16	1.5
18	8.5	19	11.5	21	20	20	16
20	16	25	30	20	16	20	16
17	5	29	39.5	25	30	17	5
25	30	26	34	19	11.5	19	11.5
21	20	28	37	24	26	17	5
	151.5		320.0		213.0		135.5

Then, we use Equation 11.3 to calculate the Kruskal-Wallis test statistic.

$$H = \left[\frac{12}{n_T \cdot (n_T + 1)} \cdot \sum \frac{R_j^2}{n_j} \right] - [3 \cdot (n_T + 1)]$$

$$= \left[\frac{12}{40 \cdot (40 + 1)} \cdot \left(\frac{151.5^2}{10} + \frac{320.0^2}{10} + \frac{213.0^2}{10} + \frac{135.5^2}{10} \right) \right]$$

$$- [3 \cdot (40 + 1)] = 15.352$$

This data set contains tied ranks, so we need to use Equation 11.4 to correct the Kruskal-Wallis test statistic for those ties. There are four groups of two tied ranks (1.5, 8.5, 23.5, and 39.5), four groups of three tied ranks (20, 26, 34, and 37), one group of four tied ranks (11.5), and three groups of five tied ranks (5, 16, and 30). Thus, the corrected Kruskal-Wallis test statistic is as follows:

$$H_c = \cfrac{H}{1 - \cfrac{\Sigma(t_i^3 - t_i)}{n_T^3 - n_T}}$$

$$= \cfrac{15.352}{1 - \cfrac{[4 \cdot (2^3 - 2)] + [4 \cdot (3^3 - 3)] + (4^3 - 4) + [3 \cdot (5^3 - 5)]}{40^3 - 40}} = 15.483$$

Since Kruskal-Wallis test statistics corresponding to four groups with 10 observations in each group do not appear in Table B.9, we compare our calculated Kruskal-Wallis test statistic to a chi-square value from Table B.7 with $4 - 1 = 3$ degrees of freedom. From that table, we find a value of 7.815 associated with an α of 0.05. Since 15.483 is greater than 7.815, we reject the omnibus null hypothesis and accept, by elimination, the alternative hypothesis that not all the drugs are associated with the same minimum effective doses in the population.

    The Kruskal-Wallis procedure tests the omnibus null hypothesis which states that values of the dependent variable (e.g., minimum effective dose) in all of the categories corresponding to values of the independent variables (e.g., different manufacturers) are the same in the population from which the sample was drawn. If we are able to reject that omnibus null hypothesis, we conclude that values of the dependent variable differ in the population for at least some of the categories (e.g., that the means of minimum effective dose from some of the manufacturers are different from one another). We cannot determine from the test of the omnibus null hypothesis, however, which of those categories of dependent variable values are different from one another. In Chapter 10, we made pairwise comparisons of the means of categories with a statistical test called the Student-Newman-Keuls procedure. When we have an ordinal dependent variable, we can use a parallel procedure. To our knowledge, this posterior test for ordinal dependent variables has not been given a special name. We will refer to this test as **Dunn's procedure** in acknowledgment of the statistician who first proposed it.[4]

    There are three differences between the Student-Newman-Keuls procedure and Dunn's procedure. First, Dunn's procedure compares the mean of the ranks of the dependent variable values, rather than the mean of the dependent variable values themselves. The mean of the ranks for a particular category is found by dividing the sum of the ranks for all of the observations for that category by the number of observations in the category. Thus, the mean of the ranks is just like the mean of the data except that the ranks, rather than the data, are summed. This is the only difference between Dunn's procedure and the Student-Newman-Keuls procedure that affects interpretation.

---

[4]Like the Student-Newman-Keuls procedure, we refer to Dunn's procedure as a posterior test even though it is not necessary to test the omnibus null hypothesis before making pairwise comparisons.

The second difference is that a special formula is used to calculate the standard error for the difference between two means of ranks. That standard error, shown in Equation 11.5, can compare categories with different numbers of observations and allows correction for tied ranks.

$$SE_{\overline{R}_1 - \overline{R}_2} = \sqrt{\left[\frac{n_T \cdot (n_T + 1)}{12} - \frac{\Sigma(t_i^3 - t_i)}{12 \cdot (n_T - 1)}\right] \cdot \left(\frac{1}{n_1} + \frac{1}{n_2}\right)} \tag{11.5}$$

where

n_T = total number of observations

n_j = number of observations in group j (j is equal to 1 or 2)

t_i = number of tied ranks in the ith group of ties

The third difference between Dunn's procedure and the Student-Newman-Keuls procedure is that the test statistic resulting from Dunn's procedure (symbolized by Q) is compared to different values than are test statistics resulting from the Student-Newman-Keuls procedure (symbolized by q). Critical values of Q statistics are found in Table B.10. Q is calculated for each pair of categories, as shown in Equation 11.6.

$$Q = \frac{\overline{R}_1 - \overline{R}_2}{SE_{\overline{R}_1 - \overline{R}_2}} \tag{11.6}$$

where $\overline{R}_j$ = mean of the ranks for the jth group.

Everything else about these two procedures is the same, including the general method of arranging the means of the ranks in order of their magnitudes and testing first the null hypothesis that the highest and lowest means of the ranks in the sample are equal in the population from which the sample was drawn. If and only if we are able to reject that null hypothesis can we compare the lowest mean of the ranks to the second highest mean of the ranks and also the highest mean rank to the second lowest mean of the ranks. That is to say, we must be able to reject the null hypothesis that two more extreme means of the ranks are equal before we can compare two less extreme means of the ranks.

Example 11.4 Examine the data in Example 11.3 to determine which categories are different in the population which was sampled. Allow a 5% chance of making a Type I error.

First, we calculate the means of the ranks for each drug category by dividing the sum of the ranks in that category by the number of observations.

$$\overline{R}_{Drug1} = \frac{151.5}{10} = 15.15 \qquad \overline{R}_{Drug2} = \frac{320.0}{10} = 32.00$$

$$\overline{R}_{Drug3} = \frac{213.0}{10} = 21.30 \qquad \overline{R}_{Drug4} = \frac{135.5}{10} = 13.55$$

Next, we arrange those means of the ranks in ascending order of magnitude.

Drug 4	Drug 1	Drug 3	Drug 2
13.55	15.15	21.30	32.00

Since all four groups have the same number of observations (10), the standard errors for all the comparisons will be equal to the same value. Equation 11.5 is used to calculate that value.

$$SE_{\bar{R}_1-\bar{R}_2} = \sqrt{\left(\frac{n_T \cdot (n_T + 1)}{12} - \frac{\Sigma(t_i^3 - t_i)}{12 \cdot (n_T - 1)}\right) \cdot \left(\frac{1}{n_1} + \frac{1}{n_2}\right)}$$

$$= \sqrt{\left(\frac{40 \cdot (40 + 1)}{12} - \frac{[4 \cdot (2^3 - 2)] + [4 \cdot (3^3 - 3)] + (4^3 - 4) + [3 \cdot (5^3 - 5)]}{12 \cdot (40 - 1)}\right) \cdot \left(\frac{1}{10} + \frac{1}{10}\right)}$$

$$= 5.206$$

Now, we can make our pairwise comparisons. That process is summarized in the following table. The critical values of Q are from Table B.10.

Compare Drugs	Difference	SE	Q	k	$Q_{0.05,k}$	Reject H_0?
4 and 2	18.45	5.206	3.544	4	2.639	Yes
4 and 3	7.75	5.206	1.489	3	2.394	No
1 and 2	16.85	5.206	3.237	3	2.394	Yes
4 and 1	This comparison is not examined (Drug 4 vs. Drug 3 not rejected).					
1 and 3	This comparison is not examined (Drug 4 vs. Drug 3 not rejected).					
3 and 2	10.7	5.206	2.055	2	1.960	Yes

In Chapter 10, we learned that, when a collection of nominal independent variables represents more than one characteristic or factor, we use a factorial analysis of variance rather than a one-way analysis of variance for a continuous dependent variable. A factorial analysis of variance permits us to compare the categories within each factor separately. For example, suppose that we were interested in diastolic blood pressure and its relationship to gender and race. Then, diastolic blood pressure would be the dependent variable and nominal independent variables would define the genders (one variable distinguishing males and females) and the races (two variables distinguishing blacks, whites, and others). Gender and race are the factors, and male, female, black, white, and other are the categories within those factors. Factorial analysis of variance allows us to test separately the null hypotheses that: (1) there is no difference between the genders, (2) there are no differences among the races, and (3) there is no interaction between gender and race.

When we have more than one factor and an ordinal dependent variable, we are also interested in a statistical procedure that will allow us to compare categories within the factors separately. In other words, we are interested in a procedure that is parallel to a factorial analysis of variance. The Kruskal-Wallis test that we used to examine categories within a single factor can be expanded to examine more than one factor. Before we look at the details of how this is done, however, let us take a closer look at the Kruskal-Wallis test as it is applied to a single factor.

Actually, the Kruskal-Wallis procedure is more closely related to the analysis of variance procedure for continuous dependent variables than it seems from examination of Equations 11.3 and 11.4. The Kruskal-Wallis test statistic (or the corrected statistic if there are tied ranks) is equal to the between sum of squares divided by the total mean square calculated from the ranks of dependent variable values (Equation 11.7). This is not very different from the F ratio calculated in analysis of variance which is equal to the between mean square divided by the within mean square. This is demonstrated in Example 11.5.

$$H \text{ or } H_c = \frac{\text{Between sum of squares}}{\text{Total mean square}} = \frac{\sum_{j=1}^{m} n_j (\overline{R}_j - \overline{R})^2}{\dfrac{\sum_{j=1}^{m} \sum_{i=1}^{n_j} (R_{ij} - \overline{R})^2}{\left(\sum_{j=1}^{m} n_j\right) - 1}} \tag{11.7}$$

where

  m = number of categories
  n_j = number of observations in the jth category
  $\overline{R}_j$ = mean of the ranks in the jth category
  $\overline{R}$ = overall mean of the ranks
  R_{ij} = rank of the ith dependent variable value in the jth category

Example 11.5   Calculate the Kruskal-Wallis test statistic as the ratio of the between sum of squares and the total mean square for the ranks of the data in Example 11.3.

First, let us calculate the overall mean of the ranks for all n_T dependent variable values.

$$\overline{R} = \frac{\sum_{j=1}^{m} R_{ij}}{n_T} = \frac{5 + 1.5 + 20 + \cdots + 5 + 11.5 + 5}{40} = 20.5$$

Next, we calculate the between sum of squares (the numerator of Equation 11.7).

$$\text{Between sum of squares} = \sum_{j=1}^{m} n_j (\overline{R}_j - \overline{R})^2$$

$$= [(10 \cdot (15.15 - 20.5)^2] + [10 \cdot (32.00 - 20.5)^2]$$
$$+ [10 \cdot (21.30 - 20.5)^2] + [10 \cdot (13.55 - 20.5)^2] = 2{,}098.15$$

Then, we calculate the total mean square (the denominator of Equation 11.7).

$$\text{Total mean square} = \frac{\sum_{j=1}^{m} \sum_{i=1}^{n_j} (R_{ij} - \overline{R})^2}{\left(\sum_{j=1}^{m} n_j\right) - 1}$$

$$= \frac{(5 - 20.5)^2 + (1.5 - 20.5)^2 + \cdots + (11.5 - 20.5)^2 + (5 - 20.5)^2}{10 + 10 + 10 + 10 - 1} = 135.51$$

Finally, we calculate the Kruskal-Wallis test statistic.

$$H_c = \frac{\text{Between sum of squares}}{\text{Total mean square}} = \frac{2{,}098.15}{135.51} = 15.483$$

This is the same value for the Kruskal-Wallis test statistic that we obtained in Example 11.5 when we used Equations 11.3 and 11.4.

When we expand the Kruskal-Wallis procedure to allow analysis of more than one factor, we take advantage of the fact that the Kruskal-Wallis test statistic can be calculated by dividing the between sum of squares or any of its components by the total mean square. Then, a procedure parallel to factorial analysis of variance can be performed by calculating the sums of squares for the main effects and the interaction just as they are calculated for a continuous dependent variable, but here they are calculated from the ranks of the dependent variable values.

One null hypothesis for factorial analysis of variance for an ordinal dependent variable states that, within a particular factor, values of the dependent variable are the same among categories within that factor in the population from which the sample was drawn. This null hypothesis is tested by dividing the corresponding factor sum of squares by the total mean square to produce a Kruskal-Wallis test statistic. The null hypothesis that there is no interaction between the factors is tested by dividing the interaction sum of squares by the total mean square. The resulting Kruskal-Wallis values are evaluated by comparing them with a chi-square value with the number of degrees of freedom that would be associated with the numerator sum of squares if we were performing a factorial analysis of variance for a continuous dependent variable (Chapter 10). To see how this works, let us take a look at an example.

Example 11.6   In Example 10.6, we examined data from a clinical trial of a treatment for herpes labialis. In that trial, 12 patients at each of three clinics were randomized to receive either the treatment (TX) or a placebo (PL). The dependent variable in that data set was the number of days until the lesion disappeared. Now, let us examine those data using an extension of the Kruskal-Wallis procedure, allowing a 5% chance of making a Type I error.

To begin, we need to convert the continuous observations in Example 10.6 to a scale of ranks.

Clinic A				Clinic B				Clinic C			
PL	Rank	TX	Rank	PL	Rank	TX	Rank	PL	Rank	TX	Rank
13	12.5	10	4.5	13	12.5	7	1	17	27	19	33
20	34.5	14	16	10	4.5	8	2	23	36	12	10
18	30.5	17	27	18	30.5	15	20.5	17	27	11	7
15	20.5	9	3	15	20.5	12	10	20	34.5	15	20.5
12	10	14	16	11	7	14	16	14	16	16	24
16	24	16	24	14	16	11	7	18	30.5	18	30.5
	132.0		90.5		91.0		56.5		171.0		125.0

Now, we need to use a computer program to analyze these data. Using a factorial analysis of variance program to analyze the ranks of the days until cure, we would observe the following results:

Source of Variation	Degrees of Freedom	Sum of Squares	Mean Square
Total	35	3,854.000	110.157
Within	30	2,516.083	83.869
Between	5	1,337.917	267.583
Clinics	2	918.875	459.438
Treatments	1	413.444	413.444
Interaction	2	5.597	2.798

Now, we can calculate a Kruskal-Wallis test statistic to test the omnibus null hypothesis by dividing the between mean square by the total sum of squares, as shown in Equation 11.7.

$$H_c = \frac{\text{Between sum of squares}}{\text{Total mean square}} = \frac{1,337.917}{110.157} = 12.146$$

Then, to test the null hypothesis that there are no differences in the population among the six groups of dependent variable values, we compare the calculated Kruskal-Wallis test statistic to a chi-square value from Table B.7 that corresponds to $m - 1 = 5$ degrees of freedom and an α of 0.05. That chi-square value is equal to 11.070. Since 12.146 is greater than 11.070, we reject the null hypothesis and accept, by elimination, the alternative hypothesis that there are at least some differences among the six groups of dependent variable values in the population.

To test the null hypothesis that the dependent variable values for the three clinics are the same in the population, we calculate a Kruskal-Wallis statistic from the clinic sum of squares and the total mean square.

$$H_c = \frac{\text{Clinic sum of squares}}{\text{Total mean square}} = \frac{918.875}{110.157} = 8.341$$

That calculated value is compared to a chi-square value from Table B.7 corresponding to $3 - 1 = 2$ degrees of freedom and an α of 0.05. That chi-square value is equal to 5.991. Since 8.341 is greater than 5.991, we reject the null hypothesis and accept, by elimination, the alternative hypothesis that there are at least some differences among the three clinics in the population.

To test the null hypothesis that values of the dependent variable for the two treatments are the same in the population, we calculate a Kruskal-Wallis statistic from the treatment sum of squares and the total mean square.

$$H_c = \frac{\text{Treatment sum of squares}}{\text{Total mean square}} = \frac{413.444}{110.157} = 3.753$$

That calculated value is compared to a chi-square value from Table B.7 corresponding to $2 - 1 = 1$ degrees of freedom and an α of 0.05. That chi-square value is equal to 3.841. Since 3.753 is less than 3.841, we do not reject the null hypothesis.

The final portion of the between sum of squares reflects the variation in dependent variable values associated with the interaction between clinics and treatment. We can test the null hypothesis that there is no interaction in the population which was sampled by calculating a Kruskal-Wallis test statistic as follows:

$$H_c = \frac{\text{Interaction sum of squares}}{\text{Total mean square}} = \frac{5.597}{110.157} = 0.051$$

Then, we compare that calculated value to a chi-square value from Table B.7 corresponding to $5 - (2 + 1) = 2$ degrees of freedom and an α of 0.05. That chi-square value is equal to 5.991. Since 0.051 is less than 5.991, we do not reject the null hypothesis. We take this result to imply that we can interpret the tests for main effects making the assumption that there is no interaction among those factors in the population.

MIXED INDEPENDENT VARIABLES

In Chapter 10, we learned that we can examine a continuous dependent variable and a combination of continuous and nominal independent variables by using regression analysis. When the dependent variable is ordinal or the data it represents are converted to an ordinal scale to circumvent assumptions of the methods for continuous dependent variables, there is no commonly used procedure that is parallel to regression analysis. Thus, continuous (or ordinal) independent variables must be converted to a nominal scale for analysis with an ordinal dependent variable and nominal independent variables. As we learned in previous chapters, such a conversion of scale results in a loss of information and, thus, a loss of statistical power.

||| SUMMARY

When we have an ordinal dependent variable, we can examine that variable relative to more than one ordinal independent variable or more than one nominal independent variable. When the independent variables are all ordinal, we can calculate Kendall's coefficient of concordance (Equation 11.1).

$$W = \frac{\sum R_j^2 - \frac{(\sum R_j)^2}{n}}{\frac{[k^2 \cdot (n^3 - n)] - (k \cdot \sum T)}{12}} \tag{11.1}$$

Kendall's coefficient of concordance is different from the multiple correlation coefficient or its square, the coefficient of multiple determination, that are used to examine a continuous dependent variable and more than one continuous independent variable. Those estimates evaluate the relationship between the dependent variable and the entire collection of independent variables. Kendall's coefficient of concordance, on the other hand, is approximately equal to the average of all possible bivariable (Spearman's) correlation coefficients among the variables taken two at a time. Thus, Kendall's coefficient of concordance, unlike many procedures for ordinal variables, cannot be thought of as exactly parallel to any procedure for continuous variables. Rather, Kendall's coefficient of concordance has its own unique interpretation.

Kendall's coefficient of concordance does not distinguish between the dependent variable and the independent variables. Thus, for a particular collection of ordinal variables, we would get the same value for Kendall's coefficient of concordance regardless of which variable we considered to be the dependent variable.

The maximum value of Kendall's coefficient of concordance is $+1$, indicating that all the variables share perfect positive associations. The minimum value of that coefficient is zero, indicating that, on the average there is no association among the variables. The null hypothesis that Kendall's coefficient of concordance is equal to zero in the population from which the sample was drawn can be tested by converting the coefficient to a chi-square value with $n - 1$ degrees of freedom (Equation 11.2).

$$\chi^2 = k \cdot (n - 1) \cdot W \tag{11.2}$$

Kendall's coefficient of concordance is parallel to multivariable techniques for continuous dependent and independent variables only in the sense that it can be calculated from a multivariable data set. Statistical procedures for an ordinal dependent variable and more than one nominal independent variable, on the other hand, are quite similar in operation and interpretation to procedures for continuous variables. A parallel procedure to a one-way analysis of variance is the Kruskal-Wallis test. The test statistic for the Kruskal-Wallis test (H) is calculated from the sum of the ranks of the dependent variable values in each group specified by values of the nominal independent variables (Equation 11.3).

$$H = \left[\frac{12}{n_T \cdot (n_T + 1)} \cdot \sum \frac{R_j^2}{n_j} \right] - [3 \cdot (n_T + 1)] \tag{11.3}$$

If there are tied ranks, a corrected test statistic should be calculated (Equation 11.4).

$$H_c = \frac{H}{1 - \dfrac{\Sigma(t_i^3 - t_i)}{n_T^3 - n_T}} \tag{11.4}$$

Kruskal-Wallis test statistics calculated from a sample's observations can be compared to values in Table B.9 to test the omnibus null hypothesis. This is parallel to the F ratio test in analysis of variance. If the numbers of observations in each group are greater than the values in Table B.9, the Kruskal-Wallis test statistic can be considered to be a chi-square value with degrees of freedom equal to the number of groups minus one and compared to values in Table B.7.

When the dependent variable is continuous, we usually use a procedure such as the Student-Newman-Keuls procedure to compare two groups of values of the dependent variable. When the dependent variable is ordinal, we use a parallel procedure that we call Dunn's procedure. Dunn's procedure is very much like the Student-Newman-Keuls procedure except that the means of the ranks of the dependent variable values are compared rather than the means of the values of the dependent variable themselves. The standard error for the difference between two means of ranks is given in Equation 11.5.

$$SE_{\bar{R}_1 - \bar{R}_2} = \sqrt{\left(\frac{n_T \cdot (n_T + 1)}{12} - \frac{\Sigma(t_i^3 - t_i)}{12 \cdot (n_T - 1)} \right) \cdot \left(\frac{1}{n_1} + \frac{1}{n_2} \right)} \tag{11.5}$$

The test statistic in Dunn's procedure (Equation 11.6) is compared to values in Table B.10 to test the null hypothesis that the difference is equal to zero in the population from which the sample was drawn.

$$Q = \frac{\bar{R}_1 - \bar{R}_2}{SE_{\bar{R}_1 - \bar{R}_2}} \tag{11.6}$$

To perform an analysis that is parallel to factorial analysis of variance for continuous dependent variables on ordinal dependent variables, we take advantage of the fact that the Kruskal-Wallis test statistic can be calculated by dividing the between sum of squares for the ranks of values of the dependent variable by the total mean square for those ranks (Equation 11.7).

$$H \text{ or } H_c = \frac{\text{Between sum of squares}}{\text{Total mean square}} = \frac{\sum_{j=1}^{m} n_j (\overline{R}_j - \overline{R})^2}{\dfrac{\sum_{j=1}^{m} \sum_{i=1}^{n_j} (R_{ij} - \overline{R})^2}{\left(\sum_{j=1}^{m} n_j\right) - 1}} \qquad (11.7)$$

When we have more than one factor among the independent variables, we can partition the between sum of squares for the ranks in the same way that we partitioned the between sum of squares in factorial analysis of variance. Null hypotheses that the means of the ranks of the categories within each factor are equal or that there is no interaction between factors in the population can be tested by dividing the appropriate partition of the between sum of squares by the total mean square and comparing the resulting test statistic to the values in Table B.9.

||| **PRACTICE PROBLEMS**

11.1 Suppose that we are interested in the relationship among age, systolic blood pressure (SBP), and diastolic blood pressure (DBP) among persons in a particular population. To investigate this relationship, we measure blood pressure and record the ages for 15 individuals and observe the following results:

Age	DBP	SBP
41	85	123
56	90	137
51	87	132
62	90	139
48	90	124
55	89	125
46	86	127
59	87	130
43	91	128
60	93	130
51	89	136
54	87	130
47	84	133
44	84	127
48	87	126

Estimate Kendall's coefficient of concordance for those observations. Test the null hypothesis that Kendall's coefficient of concordance is equal to zero in the population that was sampled versus the alternative that it is not equal to zero. Allow a 5% chance of making a Type I error.

11.2 In Problem 10.4, we examined serum glutamic transaminase (AST) measurements among ten persons at each of four stages of a particular disease. The following data were observed:

Stage I	Stage II	Stage III	Stage IV
38	23	57	30
22	36	42	26
41	44	36	42
12	33	39	23
37	42	42	21
29	48	43	43
32	19	29	39
18	28	52	32
25	34	65	39
31	40	51	31

Test the null hypothesis that the AST measurements at all four stages of this disease are the same versus the alternative hypothesis that they are not the same. Do not make any assumptions about the distribution of AST measurements. Allow a 5% chance of making a Type I error.

11.3 For the observations in Problem 11.2, make all possible pairwise comparisons of AST measurements to test the null hypothesis that the AST measurements are the same in the population from which the sample was drawn. As an alternative, hypothesize that the AST measurements are not the same. Do not make any assumptions about the distribution of AST values. Allow a 5% chance of making a Type I error.

11.4 Compare the answers to Problems 11.2 and 11.3 to the answers you got for Problems 10.4 and 10.5 and explain any differences.

11.5 In Problem 10.6, we examined data from a clinical trial of a treatment designed to reduce liver damage compared to a placebo. In that trial, we recognized four stages of liver damage, and we used factorial analysis of variance to examine the influence of stage of disease and treatment on AST measurements. Now, suppose that we convert AST measurements to ranks and use factorial analysis of variance on those ranks. Imagine that we obtain the following computer output:

Source of Variation	Degrees of Freedom	Sum of Squares	Mean Square
Total	79	42,527.28	538.32
Within	72	30,272.94	420.46
Between	7	12,254.34	1,750.62
Stage	3	9,007.26	3,002.42
Treatments	1	2,928.20	2,928.20
Interaction	3	318.86	106.29

Without making any assumptions about the distribution of AST values, test the following null hypotheses allowing a 5% chance of making a Type I error.
a)   All eight groups are the same in the population.
b)   The AST values for the four stages of disease are the same in the population.
c)   The AST values for the two treatments are the same in the population.
d)   The relationship between the treatments is the same for all stages of the disease in the population.

CHAPTER 12

Nominal Dependent Variables

Two facts place multivariable analyses of nominal dependent variables among the most useful of the statistical methods discussed in *Statistical First Aid*. First, the complexity of health and disease and, thus, the number of characteristics that must be considered make multivariable analyses the appropriate approach to most of the research data we encounter. Second, most of the variables of primary interest in health research are nominal, such as diseased/not diseased, cured/not cured, or dead/alive. Thus, the procedures discussed in this chapter are ones we will often encounter in reading the health research literature and use in analyzing data.

CONTINUOUS INDEPENDENT VARIABLES

When we have a nominal dependent variable and more than one continuous independent variable, the statistical methods that we use for estimation and inference are much like multiple regression analysis that we discussed in Chapter 10 for continuous dependent variables. There are some differences in the regression methods we most often use for nominal dependent variables, however.

The most important difference between regression methods for continuous dependent variables and methods for nominal dependent variables is in the basic way in which regression coefficients are estimated. Recall that multiple regression for continuous dependent variables uses the method of least squares, in which we find coefficient estimates that minimize the sum of the squared differences between observed and estimated values of the dependent variable. In regression methods for nominal dependent variables, we most often use the **maximum likelihood** method to estimate those coefficients.

In the maximum likelihood method, the regression coefficients are estimated so that the probability of getting the values of the dependent variable in the sample is as high as possible if the population regression coefficients were equal to their estimated values. If we applied the method of maximum likelihood to estimating the regression

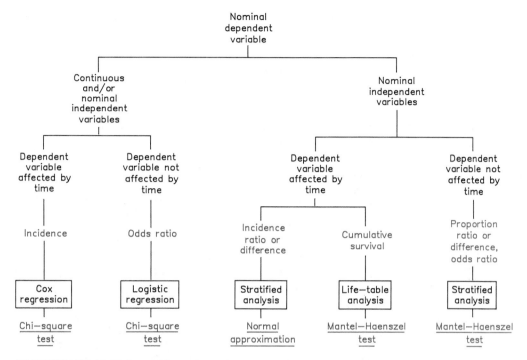

FLOWCHART 10 Multivariable analysis of a nominal dependent variable. Point estimates are indicated in red. Statistical procedures are indicated in red and underlined. Common names for a general class of statistical procedures appear in boxes.

coefficients for a continuous dependent variable and one or more independent variables, we would obtain estimates of those coefficients that would be identical to the ones obtained using the method of least squares. We use the method of least squares for continuous dependent variables because it is easier to compute.[1] For a nominal dependent variable, the method of maximum likelihood does not result in regression coefficient estimates that are identical to those that would result from the least squares approach. When the dependent variable is nominal, coefficient estimates are more likely to be close to the population's values if the maximum likelihood method is used than if the least squares method were used. Thus, we most often use maximum likelihood, rather than least squares, for regression analysis of nominal dependent variables.

Hypotheses are tested in regression analysis of a nominal dependent variable using **likelihood ratios.** A likelihood ratio is the probability of obtaining the observed values of the dependent variable if the null hypothesis were true, divided by the probability of

[1] The maximum likelihood method involves iterative computations that virtually require a computer to perform.

obtaining those values of the dependent variable if the sample's estimates accurately reflect the population's parameters (Equation 12.1).

$$\text{LR} = \frac{L_0}{L} \qquad (12.1)$$

where

LR = likelihood ratio

L_0 = likelihood (probability) of obtaining the observed data if the null hypothesis were true

L = likelihood (probability) of obtaining the observed data if the population's coefficients were equal to the estimates derived from the sample

Let us take a moment to examine the likelihood ratio. The way that the likelihood ratio is used in regression analysis for a nominal dependent variable is similar to the way that the F ratio is used in multiple regression. Recall from Chapter 10 that an F ratio can be used to test the omnibus null hypothesis that the entire collection of independent variables does not help us to estimate values of the dependent variable. An F ratio (specifically, the partial F ratio) also can be used to test the null hypothesis that a particular coefficient is equal to zero in the population from which the sample was drawn. We learned in Chapter 10 that a partial F ratio is calculated by comparing the full model (with all the independent variables included) to a reduced model. If we are interested in examining a single coefficient, the reduced model contains all the independent variables except the one of interest. Although we did not make this explicit in Chapter 10, the F ratio testing the omnibus null hypothesis also can be calculated using this comparison of the full model with a reduced model. For the omnibus null hypothesis, the reduced model contains none of the independent variables (it contains only the intercept).

The likelihood ratio can be used to test the omnibus null hypothesis or a null hypothesis that a particular coefficient is equal to zero in the population by comparing the full model with a reduced model. In either of those types of null hypotheses, what we are really saying in the null hypothesis is that the full and reduced models are equally good at estimating values of the dependent variable. If the null hypothesis is true, the denominator of the likelihood ratio will be (on the average) equal to the numerator. Thus, the likelihood ratio will tend to be equal to one when the null hypothesis is true. One is the maximum value that we can obtain for a likelihood ratio. When the null hypothesis is not true, the denominator will be greater than the numerator. This is because the likelihood based on the null hypothesis always uses less information for estimating values of the dependent variable than is contained in the sample (i.e., null hypotheses assume that independent variables do nothing to improve estimation of values of the dependent variable). Thus, the likelihood ratio will be less than one when the null hypothesis is not true. Since both the numerator and denominator are probabilities that must have values between zero and one, the smallest value possible for a likelihood ratio is zero.[2]

---

[2] Note that this is the opposite of what we expect with an F ratio, which will (on the average) be greater than one when the null hypothesis is not true. Thus, F ratios range (on the average) between one and infinity, while likelihood ratios range between one and zero.

Thus, we expect likelihood ratios to be close to one when the null hypothesis (either the omnibus null hypothesis or the null hypothesis that a particular coefficient is equal to zero) is true and to be less than one when the null hypothesis is not true. To determine if a particular likelihood ratio is sufficiently far from a value of one so that we suspect that the null hypothesis is not true, we need to convert the likelihood ratio to a standard scale. The standard scale that we use for likelihood ratios is the chi-square distribution. Mathematical examination of the likelihood ratio has led to the discovery that the natural logarithm of a likelihood ratio multiplied by -2 is equal to a chi-square value. By taking the natural logarithm of the likelihood ratio, we obtain a value of zero when the ratio is equal to one and values of increasingly large negative numbers as the ratio becomes increasingly small (i.e., as we get values that differ more from those expected under the null hypothesis). Multiplying that negative number by -2 converts it to a positive number that can be shown mathematically to be approximately equal to a chi-square value (Equation 12.2). The number of degrees of freedom of that chi-square value is equal to the difference between the number of independent variables specified in the null hypothesis (i.e., in the reduced model) and the total number of independent variables.[3]

$$\chi^2_{kdf} = -2 \cdot \ln \text{LR} \qquad (12.2)$$

As we pointed out earlier, we can examine the relationship between a nominal dependent variable and the entire collection of independent variables or we can examine each of the independent variables individually. Looking at the entire collection of independent variables tests the omnibus null hypothesis, which says that all the independent variables taken together do not improve estimation of values of the dependent variable. The likelihood ratio used to test the omnibus null hypothesis has in its numerator the probability of obtaining the observed values of the dependent variable if all the independent variables were ignored (L_0). In other words, in calculating that probability, we are using a reduced model that assumes that all the regression coefficients are equal to zero in the population and that the dependent variable is equal to the intercept.[4] In the denominator of the likelihood ratio testing the omnibus null hypothesis, we have the probability of obtaining the observed values of the dependent variable if the regression coefficients in the population were equal to the regression coefficients estimated from the sample's observations (L).

To actually test the omnibus null hypothesis (versus the alternative hypothesis that some of the independent variables help estimate values of the dependent variable), we convert that likelihood ratio to a chi-square value (Equation 12.2) and compare it to a chi-square value from Table B.7 corresponding to an area of α and with degrees of freedom equal to the number of independent variables.[5]

[3] This is the same as the numerator degrees of freedom in an F ratio test.

[4] When all of the regression coefficients are equal to zero, the intercept is equal to the mean of the dependent variable.

[5] Here, we are interested in only one tail of the chi-square distribution. Recall from Chapter 9 that a one-tailed chi-square corresponds to the square of a two-tailed standard normal deviate. When we square, for example, either $+1.96$ or -1.96, we obtain $+3.841$. Thus, both tails of the standard normal distribution are represented by the upper tail of the chi-square distribution. This leads to a potentially confusing situation in which we are testing a two-tailed alternative to the omnibus null hypothesis, but we use a one-tailed chi-square value to do so. This also was true of the F test discussed in Chapter 10 since an F ratio is the square of a Student's t value.

Rather than (or in addition to) testing the omnibus null hypothesis, which compares the dependent variable to the entire collection of independent variables, we can examine the relationships between the dependent variable and each of the independent variables individually (while taking the other independent variables into account). In multiple regression analysis, we test the null hypothesis that a particular regression coefficient is equal to zero in the population by calculating a partial F ratio (Equation 10.5). With a nominal dependent variable, we test that same null hypothesis that a particular coefficient is equal to zero in the population by computing another type of likelihood ratio. Since this likelihood ratio is parallel to the partial F ratio, we will call it the **partial likelihood ratio.**

The partial likelihood ratio used to test null hypotheses about individual coefficients is the same as Equation 12.1, but the numerator is based on a different model than the one used in testing the omnibus null hypothesis. The numerator of any likelihood ratio must reflect the particular null hypothesis that we are testing. Here, we are testing the null hypothesis that a particular coefficient is equal to zero. Thus, this partial likelihood ratio has in its numerator the probability of obtaining the observed values of the dependent variable if the particular regression coefficient were equal to zero in the population and the regression coefficients for all the other independent variables were equal to the values estimated from the sample's observations (i.e., the reduced model, which excludes only the independent variable of interest). The denominator of this partial likelihood ratio is the same as the denominator of the likelihood ratio used to test the omnibus null hypothesis. Thus, the denominator of the partial likelihood ratio contains the probability of obtaining the observed values of the dependent variable values if all the regression coefficients in the population were equal to the estimates derived from the sample (i.e., the full model). Since the null hypothesis in this case considers one fewer than the total number of independent variables, the difference between the number of independent variables in the full and reduced models is equal to one, and the corresponding chi-square value has one degree of freedom.

Thus, a likelihood ratio, like the F ratio in regression analysis of a continuous dependent variable, compares a reduced model with a full model to test either the omnibus null hypothesis or null hypotheses about particular regression coefficients. An important consequence of our discovery that the likelihood ratio compares a reduced model with the full model is the realization that multicollinearity in multivariable analysis of nominal dependent variables works the same way that it does in analysis of continuous dependent variables. To reject the null hypothesis that a particular regression coefficient is equal to zero in the population by looking at the partial likelihood ratio, the numerator of the partial likelihood ratio must be smaller than its denominator. In other words, the probability of observing the values of the dependent variable estimated by the reduced model must be lower than the probability of observing the values of the dependent variable estimated by the full model. The greater the degree of multicollinearity, the less the distinction we will observe between the reduced and full models and the closer the partial likelihood ratio will be to one (the null value for a likelihood ratio). As we discovered in Chapter 10, the same thing happens with the partial F ratio in multiple regression analysis (except an F ratio becomes larger than one and a likelihood ratio becomes less than one as the null hypothesis becomes less consistent with the data).

There are two different types of multivariable regression analyses for nominal dependent variables that are commonly used in health research. The first of these that we will examine is **logistic regression.** Logistic regression is used for probabilities. Next, we will discuss **Cox regression.** Cox regression, which is also known as proportional hazards regression, is used for rates.

LOGISTIC REGRESSION   For the most part, logistic regression looks like any multiple regression equation. That is to say, logistic regression includes an intercept and a series of independent variables multiplied by regression coefficients. The elements of this series are added together as they are in multiple regression for continuous dependent variables. The dependent variable in logistic regression, however, is not used in its natural form (i.e., as a probability). Rather, dependent variables are mathematically altered or **transformed** (the reason for this transformation will be discussed a little later). The particular transformation used in logistic regression is called a **logit transformation** (thus, the name "logistic" regression). In the logit transformation, we take the natural logarithm of the probability of an event divided by the probability of the complement of that event (Equation 12.3).

$$\text{logit} = \ln \frac{p}{(1 - p)} \tag{12.3}$$

Logistic regression analysis uses the method of maximum likelihood to estimate the coefficients of the following regression equation. Notice that the dependent variable of that equation is the logit transformation of the (population's) probability of the nominal dependent variable event:

$$\ln \left(\frac{\theta}{1 - \theta} \right) = \alpha + \beta_1 X_1 + \beta_2 X_2 + \ldots + \beta_k X_k \tag{12.4}$$

Algebraically solving for the dependent variable expressed as the probability of the event, Equation 12.4 becomes:

$$\theta = \frac{1}{1 + e^{-(\alpha + \beta_1 X_1 + \beta_2 X_2 + \ldots + \beta_k X_k)}} \tag{12.5}$$

where e = base of the natural log scale = 2.718.

So, the consequence of the logit transformation in regression analysis of a nominal dependent variable is a rather complicated-looking regression equation. It might seem strange that we use such a complicated regression equation in logistic regression since the solutions that statisticians pose to statistical problems are usually the simplest ones possible. As you might expect, there are good reasons for using the logit transformation. One reason is to avoid the possibility of the regression equation estimating probabilities that are less than zero or greater than one (which we know are impossible values for probabilities). If we plot the probabilities estimated from a logistic regression for values of any independent variable, we get an S-shaped or **sigmoid** curve (Figure 12.1). That curve can never reach values less than zero or greater than one.

Another reason that the logit transformation is used is that the ratio of the probabilities of an event and its complement has a number of statistical advantages over a probability itself. Actually, we have mentioned these advantages in Chapter 9. The context of that previous discussion might be clearer if we multiply the numerator and denominator of this ratio by the sample's size (n).

$$\frac{n}{n} \cdot \frac{p}{(1-p)} = \frac{\text{Number of observations with event}}{\text{Number of observations without event}} \tag{12.6}$$

Compare the right side of Equation 12.6 with Equation 9.9. We can see by that comparison that the ratio of the probabilities of an event and its complement is the same as the odds of the event. Thus, the dependent variable in logistic regression is the natural logarithm of the odds of the nominal dependent variable. We call the natural logarithm of the odds the **log odds** of the nominal dependent variable. This is a very important discovery, for it implies that we can summarize the results of logistic regression analysis using *odds ratios*. To calculate an odds ratio for two values of a specific independent variable, we use Equation 12.7.

$$OR = \frac{e^{\beta X}}{e^{\beta X'}} = e^{\beta(X-X')} \tag{12.7}$$

where
X = one value of the independent variable
X' = another value of the independent variable

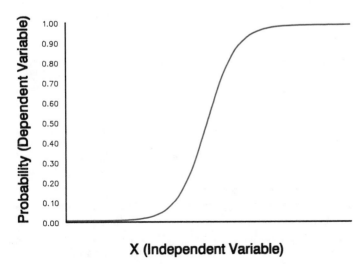

FIGURE 12.1 The relationship between estimated values of a nominal dependent variable and values of a continuous independent variable when the logit transformation has been used.

We can see from Equation 12.7 that an odds ratio between any two values of an independent variable is also the odds ratio between any other two values of that independent variable that differ by the same amount $(X - X')$. Now, let us take a look at an example of a computer output for logistic regression analysis and how to interpret the results.

Example 12.1 Suppose that we conducted a clinical trial of a beta blocker to prevent post–myocardial infarction (MI) mortality among high-risk patients. In this trial, we are interested in the relationship between dose and the probability of surviving five years post-MI. We randomize 100 patients to receive either 5, 10, 15, 20, or 25 mg of the experimental drug (20 to each dose) and follow them all for five years. We are concerned about age as a potential confounder. To analyze the resulting data, we use a statistical program for logistic regression with survival (yes/no) represented by the dependent variable and dose and age represented by continuous independent variables. Suppose that we obtained the following computer output:

LIKELIHOOD RATIO = 1.36917E−09

VARIABLE	B	CHISQ
DOSE	0.2076	23.814
AGE	−0.1349	7.900
(CONSTANT)	3.6805	2.513

Interpret the results of that computer analysis.

Parts of this output are familiar to us from our study of multiple regression in Chapter 10. Other parts are not so familiar. Let us first interpret parts that are most similar to multiple regression output. The table in this output gives us estimates of regression coefficients in the column labeled B just as multiple regression programs do. From this information, we know that our sample's estimate of the logistic regression equation is:

$$\ln \left[\frac{p\,(\text{survival})}{1 - p\,(\text{survival})} \right] = 3.6805 + (0.2076 \cdot \text{DOSE}) + (-0.1349 \cdot \text{AGE})$$

This tells us that the log odds of survival increase as dose increases and decrease as age increases. To interpret the logistic regression equation more fully, we can either estimate the probability of survival (i.e., the complement of the five-year risk of death) for various combinations of dose and age, or we can compare the odds (i.e., estimate odds ratios) for different values of age and dose.

First, let us use Equation 12.5 to estimate the probabilities of survival for each of the five doses and ages of 50 and 60 years. For a dose of 5 mg and an age of 50 years, that probability is:

$$p = \frac{1}{1 + e^{-[3.6805 + (0.2076 \cdot 5) + (-0.1349 \cdot 50)]}} = 0.116$$

Using that same procedure, we find the following probabilities of surviving five years for all five doses and ages of 50 and 60 years:

	Dose	p (Survival)
Age = 50 years	5	0.116
	10	0.271
	15	0.512
	20	0.748
	25	0.893
Age = 60 years	5	0.033
	10	0.088
	15	0.214
	20	0.435
	25	0.685

That method of interpreting the results of logistic regression analysis is most useful when we are interested in estimating the probability that patients of a certain age will survive for five years if they receive a given dose of the drug under investigation. It is not very easy, however, to appreciate the relationship between dose and survival or between age and survival from those probability estimates. That is easier to do from estimates of odds ratios. Since the independent variables are continuous,[6] we need to choose specific values of those variables to compare in an odds ratio. For example, we might calculate an odds ratio to compare the odds of surviving with a dose of 10 mg to the odds of surviving with a dose of 5 mg. We make that calculation using Equation 12.7.

$$OR = e^{0.2076(10-5)} = 2.824$$

Thus, the odds of surviving with a dose of 10 mg are 2.824 times as great as the odds of surviving with a dose of 5 mg. More generally, the odds ratio for any 5-mg increment in dose (within the 5- to 25-mg range) is also estimated to be equal to 2.824 (since we use the difference between the independent variable values in Equation 12.7). That is to say, the odds of surviving are 2.824 times as great with a dose of 15 mg compared to a dose of 10 mg and they are 2.824 times as great with a dose of 20 mg compared to a dose of 15 mg.

Now, let us estimate an odds ratio for age comparing 50- and 60-year-old patients. Remember that the same odds ratio is applicable to any ten-year age range.

$$OR = e^{-0.1349(50-60)} = 3.854$$

That implies that the odds of survival are 3.854 times greater for patients compared to other patients who are 10 years older.

Those odds ratios give us a better idea about the relationships between the independent

---

[6]The fact that a limited number of doses (five) have been considered in this study is a reflection of purposive sampling, not an indication that dose has a limited number of potential values. Since dose exists in the population as continuous data, it is represented by a continuous variable.

variables and survival. We need to be a little careful here, however. We must remember that we have chosen particular ranges of independent variable values to calculate those odds ratio estimates. We cannot compare the odds ratio of 2.824 for dose with the odds ratio of 3.854 for age and conclude that age is a more important predictor of (i.e., more strongly associated with) survival than is dose. The reason we cannot make that comparison is because we cannot say that a 5-mg increment in dose is equivalent to a 10-year increment in age (or any other increment in age).

In addition to interpreting the estimates of the regression coefficients from logistic regression analysis, we also can perform statistical inference. As in multivariable analysis of continuous dependent variables, we can test the omnibus null hypothesis that the entire collection of independent variables does not help us to estimate dependent variable values, and/or we can test hypotheses that the individual regression coefficients are equal to zero in the population from which the sample was drawn (i.e., that they do not help estimate dependent variable values).

The likelihood ratio at the top of the computer output compares the full model with a reduced model containing none of the independent variables. In other words, we are provided with a likelihood ratio that can be used to examine the omnibus null hypothesis. (Notice that the computer gives us $1.36917E-09$ for that likelihood ratio. That is the same as 1.36917 times 10^{-9} or 0.00000000136917.) To test the omnibus null hypothesis, we use Equation 12.2 and that likelihood ratio from the computer output.

$$\chi^2_{kdf} = -2 \cdot \ln LR = -2 \cdot \ln(1.36917 \cdot 10^{-9}) = 40.818$$

Since there are two independent variables, that chi-square value has two degrees of freedom. From Table B.7, we find that a chi-square value of 5.991 corresponds to two degrees of freedom and an α of 0.05. Since 40.818 is larger than 5.991, we reject the omnibus null hypothesis that the combination of age and dose does not help us estimate the probability of survival and accept, by elimination, that those independent variables do help estimate the probability of survival.

Testing null hypotheses about individual coefficients being equal to zero in the population is easier than testing the omnibus null hypothesis since this computer program provides us with the chi-square values rather than likelihood ratios. Thus, we do not need to use Equation 12.2 to convert likelihood ratios to chi-square values. Rather, we need only to compare the chi-square values provided to those in Table B.7.

Each of the chi-square values testing the null hypothesis that a particular coefficient is equal to zero in the population has one degree of freedom since they compare the full model (including both dose and age) with a reduced model in which the particular independent variable being tested has been removed. From Table B.7, we find that a chi-square value of 3.841 corresponds to one degree of freedom and an α of 0.05. Comparing the chi-square values from the computer output to 3.841, we find that we can reject the null hypothesis that the regression coefficient for dose is equal to zero ($23.814 > 3.841$), and we can reject the null hypothesis that the regression coefficient for age is equal to zero ($7.900 > 3.841$) in the population that was sampled. Thus, we can accept, by elimination, the alternative hypotheses that the coefficients for those variables are not equal to zero in the population from which the sample was drawn. We cannot, however, reject the null hypothesis that the intercept (CON-STANT) is equal to zero in the population ($2.513 < 3.841$).

The test of the null hypothesis that the intercept is equal to zero may or may not be interesting. Here, it is not very interesting since our inability to reject that null hypothesis implies that we are unable to say that the log odds of survival for a dose of zero and an age of zero is equal to a value different from zero (i.e., different from an odds ratio of one). An age of zero is not relevant to this study.

COX REGRESSION   Logistic regression can be used for proportions or probabilities, but it should not be used for rates. Recall from Chapter 6 that rates are used to summarize nominal dependent variables that are affected by time. That is to say, whether or not we observe a particular event is influenced by how long we look for it. For example, if a nominal dependent variable represented mortality, we would expect a greater number of deaths the longer we followed a group of persons. This is not a problem if everyone in a study was followed for the same period of time (such as in Example 12.1). In that case, we can simply count the number of events and use logistic regression to analyze our observations. If, on the other hand, persons in a study were followed for various periods of time (as is often the case in controlled clinical trials), we need to take the period that each person was followed into account. Logistic regression does not take time into account and, therefore, should not be used to analyze nominal dependent variables that are affected by time. Rather, Cox regression should be used if persons in a study have various periods of follow-up.

The regression equation for Cox regression is less complicated to interpret than the equation for logistic regression since the dependent variable is the natural logarithm of the rate (Equation 12.8). It is more complicated to calculate, however, since the intercept is a function of time. That should not bother us since the job of calculation is left to the computer.

$$\ln(\text{rate}) = \alpha_t + \beta_1 X_1 + \beta_2 X_2 + \ldots + \beta_k X_k \tag{12.8}$$

where α_t = the intercept expressed as a function of time.

The usual way to interpret the coefficients in Cox regression is to calculate a rate ratio (the rate for one condition divided by the rate for another condition).[7] Equation 12.9 shows us how to calculate a rate ratio (RR[8]) for two values of one independent variable. Notice that we do not include the intercept in that calculation.

$$\text{RR} = \frac{e^{\beta X}}{e^{\beta X'}} = e^{\beta(X - X')} \tag{12.9}$$

Other than this difference in interpretation, we can think of Cox regression as being much like logistic regression. That is to say, Cox regression uses the same basic principles as logistic regression to estimate regression coefficients and to test null hypotheses. This is illustrated in the next example.

Example 12.2   In Example 12.1, we examined data from a clinical trial of survival post-MI using a logistic regression analysis. To do that, we had to assume that all 100 subjects in the study were followed for five years or until they died. Since subjects are usually recruited into a study over a period of time (perhaps over several years), this study would have taken a long time to complete. A common design for a study like this is to recruit subjects into the study over a

---

[7] We also can interpret the results of a Cox regression by taking the antilog of an estimated dependent variable value to get the rate, but this is complicated by the intercept being a function of time.

[8] We have used RR to stand for relative risk (the ratio of two risks) in previous chapters. We use it here to indicate the rate ratio. We are comfortable doing this since a rate ratio is algebraically the same as the relative risk.

period of time and to end follow-up of the subjects on a specified date. That design implies that some subjects will be followed for less than five years even though they are alive on the date that follow-up ends.

Thus, in a more realistic study design, many of the persons in the study will not have been followed for the entire study period. Since we do not know if those subjects would have survived the entire study period (in this case, five years) or if they would have died, we cannot use these data in a logistic regression. If we calculate survival rates instead of probabilities of survival, however, we can use all these data to estimate survival rates.

Let us now assume that the clinical trial in Example 12.1 had this more usual design and analyze the resulting data with Cox regression. Suppose that we observed the following computer output:

$$\text{LIKELIHOOD RATIO} = 9.8841\text{E} - 05$$

VARIABLE	B	CHISQ
DOSE	0.082	13.191
AGE	−0.048	3.115

Interpret the results of that computer analysis.

Computer output from Cox regression analysis usually looks very much like computer output from logistic regression analysis. The only difference we see here from the output in Example 12.1 is the absence of an estimate for the intercept. The reason for this omission is that the intercept in Cox regression is not a simple constant, but rather a function of time. For the usual interpretation of the results of Cox regression analysis, it is not necessary to know the form of this function for the intercept.

To interpret the sample's estimates of the regression coefficients for the independent variables, we use Equation 12.9 to estimate rate ratios. As we did for odds ratios in logistic regression analysis, we need to specify a range of values for continuous independent variables to calculate a rate ratio. Let us first estimate the rate ratio for a 5-mg difference in dose (e.g., 5 mg to 10 mg) of the drug under investigation.

$$\text{RR} = e^{0.082(10-5)} = 1.507$$

Thus, we estimate that the rate of survival is 1.507 times higher for each 5-mg increase in dose. Now, let us estimate the rate ratio for a 10-year difference in age (e.g., 50 years to 60 years).

$$\text{RR} = e^{-0.048(50-60)} = 1.616$$

This tells us that our best estimate is that the rate of survival in the population is 1.616 times higher for each decade that age is reduced.

Next, let us consider statistical inference for this Cox regression. The omnibus null hypothesis, that the combination of dose and age do not contribute to the estimation of the rate of survival in the population that was sampled, is tested using Equation 12.2 as it was in logistic regression analysis.

$$\chi^2_{kdf} = -2 \cdot \ln \text{LR} = -2 \cdot \ln(9.8841 \cdot 10^{-5}) = 18.444$$

This chi-square value has two degrees of freedom, representing the difference in the number of independent variables between the full model (that includes both independent variables) and the reduced model for the omnibus null hypothesis (that includes neither of the independent variables). From Table B.7, we find that a chi-square value of 5.991 corresponds to an α of 0.05 and two degrees of freedom. Since 18.444 is larger than 5.991, we reject the omnibus null hypothesis and accept, by elimination, the alternative hypothesis that the combination of dose and age helps estimate the rate of survival in the population.

The chi-square values associated with each of the individual regression coefficients have one degree of freedom (since the full model includes both independent variables and the reduced model contains one independent variable). Therefore, we compare them to 3.841, the value from Table B.7 that corresponds to an α of 0.05 and one degree of freedom. The chi-square value calculated to test the null hypothesis that the regression coefficient for dose is equal to zero in the population (13.191) is larger than 3.841, allowing us to reject that null hypothesis and conclude, by default, that the coefficient for dose is equal to some value other than zero in the population. The corresponding value for age (3.115), however, is smaller than 3.841. Thus, we cannot reject the null hypothesis that this regression coefficient is equal to zero in the population. That implies that we are unable to say that the rate of survival differs for persons of different ages in the population.   ▤

ORDINAL INDEPENDENT VARIABLES

There are no statistical procedures for analyzing more than one ordinal independent variable and a nominal dependent variable that are frequently used in health statistics. The usual practice is to convert ordinal independent variables into a series of nominal independent variables (one fewer than the number of ordinal categories) and, then, to use one of the procedures that we will discuss in the next two sections of this chapter.

NOMINAL INDEPENDENT VARIABLES

We learned in Chapter 9 that observations for a nominal dependent variable and a nominal independent variable are most often organized in a 2 × 2 table. What we do when we have more than one nominal independent variable depends on whether those nominal independent variables represent one or more than one factor or characteristic. For example, if we are interested in looking at levels of serum cholesterol for different races and we record race as white, black, Asian, or other, then the three nominal variables we would use to represent those four race categories are all representative of the same factor or characteristic (namely, race). If, on the other hand, we were interested in looking at serum cholesterol levels by treatment type (drug versus placebo) and gender, the two nominal independent variables (one to designate treatment type and one to designate gender) that we would use in analysis would be representative of two separate factors (namely, treatment and gender).

If the collection of nominal independent variables in a data set all represent various categories of a single characteristic or factor, the usual approach to inference (we will look at estimation in a moment) is an expansion of the chi-square procedure discussed in Chapter 9 for 2×2 tables. As mentioned in that chapter, the most important advantage of the chi-square test is its ability to analyze $R \times C$ tables. When we have one nominal dependent variable and more than one nominal independent variable and those nominal independent variables designate categories of a single factor (i.e., a $2 \times C$ table), we calculate a chi-square value (Equation 9.20) by summing all the squared differences between observed and expected values divided by their respective expected values. The number of degrees of freedom for that chi-square is equal to the number of independent variables.[9]

When the nominal independent variables designate more than one factor (such as exposure and gender), we cannot organize the data in a single table. Rather, the data must be organized into a series of tables. Generally, one of the independent variables is selected to specify two groups (such as an exposed and an unexposed group) between which we wish to compare values of the dependent variable. We refer to this independent variable as the independent variable of main interest. The remaining independent variable(s) are included in the analysis to control for confounding. These independent variables are often called **confounding variables.** Then we organize our observations in a series of 2×2 tables with the dependent variable and the independent variable of main interest specifying the rows and columns of each table and the independent variables that are likely to be confounders (i.e., the confounding variable) specifying the individual tables themselves. This procedure of constructing a series of 2×2 tables is called **stratification** and is illustrated in the following example.

Example 12.3 Suppose that we were interested in the probability of developing cataracts (dependent variable) among persons on long-term hormonal therapy (independent variable of main interest). To investigate the probability of developing cataracts, we identify 100 persons on this therapy and 100 control patients with the same age distribution. Further suppose that we are concerned about the potential confounding effect of gender. Imagine that we make the following observations:

	Independent Variable of Main Interest			
	Hormonal Therapy		No Hormonal Therapy	
Confounding Variable	*Dependent Variable*		*Dependent Variable*	
	Cataracts	No Cataracts	Cataracts	No Cataracts
Females	21	49	13	37
Males	7	23	9	41

Organize these observations in 2×2 tables.

[9] Recall that the number of degrees of freedom for an $R \times C$ table is $(R - 1) \cdot (C - 1)$. For a $2 \times C$ table, that is equal to $(C - 1)$ because $(R - 1)$ is equal to 1. Since k independent variables specify $k + 1$ categories, the number of independent variables equals $C - 1$.

We are primarily interested in the probability of developing cataracts. Therefore, the dependent variable in this study is the nominal variable that represents the presence or absence of a cataract, and the independent variables include one that represents the two genders and one that represents exposure and nonexposure to hormonal therapy. Our main interest is to compare the probabilities of developing cataracts for the two hormonal therapy groups. Thus, we will construct two 2 × 2 tables: one for females and one for males (the two values of the confounding variable). Each of those 2 × 2 tables will have the rows representing the two values of the dependent variable (presence or absence of cataracts) and columns representing the independent variable of main interest (exposure or nonexposure to hormonal therapy).

For females:

	Therapy	No Therapy
Cataracts	21	13
No Cataracts	49	37

For males:

	Therapy	No Therapy
Cataracts	7	9
No Cataracts	23	41

We refer to the general class of statistical procedures that we perform on data divided into a series of 2 × 2 tables as **stratified analysis.** The purpose of stratified analysis is to allow estimation and inference on the nominal dependent variable and one of the nominal independent variables (the independent variable of main interest), while controlling for the confounding effects of the other nominal independent variables (the confounding variables). First, let us consider how we can use stratified analysis techniques in estimation.

ESTIMATION   We have the choice of two strategies for making estimates in stratified analysis. The first strategy is to estimate the nature of the relationship between the dependent variable and the independent variable of main interest for each of the strata (i.e., each of the 2 × 2 tables). These estimates are called **strata-specific estimates.** The other strategy is to combine the information from all the strata to make a single estimate (called a **summary estimate**) of the nature of the relationship between the independent variable of main interest and the dependent variable. In both cases, we can estimate that relationship by using ratios or differences of probabilities or rates or by using ratios of odds. Making a single summary estimate provides us with a simpler task in interpretation (we only need to interpret one estimate), but it only makes sense if we think that the relationship is the same in each of the strata. Suppose, for example, that we thought that the lenses of females, but not the lenses of males, were sensitive to hormonal therapy. If we then combined the information for males and females, we would underestimate the relationship between hormonal therapy and cataracts for females and overestimate that relationship for males by making a single estimate for both genders.

If we think that the relationship is the same in each of the strata, it is to our advantage to combine the information from the strata to produce a single estimate. The method we choose to combine that information must do two things. First, it must give us the best possible guess at the nature of the relationship in the population. Second, it must take into account (or control for) the confounding effects of the other independent variable(s). The way that we can take confounding into account is to combine the estimates obtained from each of the strata (i.e., the strata-specific estimates) instead of initially combining the data from those strata. In other words, we want to maintain the separate 2×2 tables instead of creating a single 2×2 table. If we were to combine all the observations in a single 2×2 table, that would be tantamount to ignoring the independent variable(s) that represent confounders. If those variables are ignored, confounding will influence the results of our analysis. On the other hand, confounding does not influence strata-specific estimates[10] since all the observations in a single 2×2 table share the same confounding characteristic (for instance, in the first 2×2 table in Example 12.3, everyone is female).

Now, we have to decide the best way to combine the strata-specific estimates so that we obtain our best possible estimate of the population's value. One possibility would be to take the mean of the strata-specific estimates (i.e., add up the estimates and divide by the number of estimates). A problem with this approach is that each strata-specific estimate contributes equally to the mean even though we might be more confident of the estimates from some strata than we are of the estimates from other strata (perhaps because the strata contain different numbers of observations).

To solve this problem, we do the same thing we have done many times before: we take a weighted average of the strata-specific estimates. As weights, we use the inverse of the variances of the strata-specific estimates. The larger the variance of an estimate, the less confident we are in it. Larger variances have smaller inverses. Thus, using the inverse of the variance of the strata-specific estimates as weights will give more weight to the more precise estimates. This procedure will give us our best estimate of the population's value.

When our observations are proportions or probabilities, the strata-specific estimates of the relationship between the nominal dependent variable and the independent variable of main interest can be expressed as a probability difference, a probability ratio, or an odds ratio. We discussed the choice among these estimates for a bivariable

[10]This is true for a confounder that is truly nominal (such as gender). If, as is commonly done, strata are constructed to represent categories of continuous data (such as age) converted to a nominal scale (i.e., age groups), there is likely to be some residual confounding of strata-specific estimates. This residual confounding is assumed to be small. That assumption may or may not be justified.

data set in Chapter 9. There, we said that it made little difference whether we chose a difference or a ratio of probabilities. In multivariable analysis, it does make a difference. To understand the reason for this, we need to remember that in making a summary estimate we are assuming that the parameter we are estimating is the same in each stratum. If differences between probabilities are the same for all the strata, it is virtually impossible for the strata-specific ratios of probabilities also to be the same over the strata. For instance, look at the strata in Example 12.3. The probability differences in the two strata are very similar (0.04 and 0.05), but the probability ratios are not so similar (1.15 and 1.28).[11]

The reasons for choosing the odds ratio have additional aspects, two of which we discussed in Chapter 9. The odds ratio is the only estimate that makes sense for case-control studies. In addition, the odds ratio is insensitive to certain kinds of bias.[12]

The method that we use to calculate a weighted average of the strata-specific estimates depends on whether those estimates are probability differences, probability ratios, or odds ratios. First, let us consider probability differences. The probability difference mathematically describing the relationship between the dependent variable and the independent variable of main interest estimated by combining information from all the strata is a weighted average of the strata-specific probability differences (Equation 12.10).

$$\text{PD} = \frac{\Sigma\,(w_i \cdot \text{PD}_i)}{\Sigma\,w_i} \tag{12.10}$$

where

PD = probability difference for all strata combined
PD_i = strata-specific probability difference for the ith stratum
w_i = weight for the ith stratum

Equation 12.11 shows the weights that are used to combine strata-specific probability differences. These weights are (approximations of) the inverse of the variance of strata-specific estimates of the probability difference. Equation 12.11 uses the 2×2 table notation introduced in Chapter 9 (see Table 9.1).

$$w_i = \frac{(a_i + c_i) \cdot (b_i + d_i) \cdot n_i}{(a_i + b_i) \cdot (c_i + d_i)} \tag{12.11}$$

Example 12.4   Combine the data presented in Example 12.3 to calculate the best possible summary estimate of the difference in probabilities of developing cataracts for persons receiving hormonal therapy compared to persons not receiving hormonal therapy.

First, we need to calculate strata-specific estimates of the probability difference and the weights that will be used to combine those estimates. Those weights are calculated using Equation 12.11

---

[11]The discrepancy between differences and ratios among strata can be much more marked than in this example.

[12]A third reason for selecting the odds ratio will be presented when we discuss inference.

For females:

	Therapy	No Therapy
Cataracts	21	13
No Cataracts	49	37

The estimate of the probability difference for females is:

$$PD_f = \frac{21}{21 + 49} - \frac{13}{13 + 37} = 0.30 - 0.26 = 0.04$$

The weight for that estimate is:

$$w_f = \frac{(a_f + c_f) \cdot (b_f + d_f) \cdot n_f}{(a_f + b_f) \cdot (c_f + d_f)}$$

$$= \frac{(21 + 49) \cdot (13 + 37) \cdot (21 + 13 + 49 + 37)}{(21 + 13) \cdot (49 + 37)} = 143.6$$

For males:

	Therapy	No Therapy
Cataracts	7	9
No Cataracts	23	41

The estimate of the probability difference for males is:

$$PD_m = \frac{7}{7 + 23} - \frac{9}{9 + 41} = 0.23 - 0.18 = 0.05$$

The weight for that estimate is:

$$w_m = \frac{(a_m + c_m) \cdot (b_m + d_m) \cdot n_m}{(a_m + b_m) \cdot (c_m + d_m)}$$

$$= \frac{(7 + 23) \cdot (9 + 41) \cdot (7 + 9 + 23 + 41)}{(7 + 9) \cdot (23 + 41)} = 117.2$$

Before we combine the strata-specific estimates, let us take a look at those estimates and their weights. First, we notice that the two estimates of the probability difference are very close. Therefore, it makes sense to combine them in a single estimate. Second, we see that the weight for the estimate in females is larger than the weight for the estimate in males. This implies that we are more confident of the estimate calculated in the female stratum than we are of the one calculated in the male stratum. This makes sense since the study contains more females than it does males.

Now, let us use Equation 12.10 to calculate a weighted average for the probability difference.

$$PD = \frac{\Sigma (w_i \cdot PD_i)}{\Sigma w_i} = \frac{(143.6 + 0.04) + (117.2 \cdot 0.05)}{143.6 + 117.2} = 0.044$$

Thus, 0.044 is our best estimate of the population's value of the difference in the probabilities of developing cataracts for persons on hormonal therapy compared to persons not on hormonal therapy.   ▤

Next, let us see how to combine strata-specific estimates of probability ratios. This is a little different from the procedure for probability differences since we combine the natural logarithms of the ratios rather than the ratios themselves.[13] After we calculate a weighted average of the logarithms of the ratios, we convert back to a probability ratio by taking the antilog of the weighted average. Equation 12.12 shows both of those operations combined.

$$PR = e^{\Sigma(w_i \cdot \ln PR_i)/\Sigma w_i} \tag{12.12}$$

where
PR = probability ratio for all strata combined
PR_i = strata-specific probability ratio for the ith stratum

Equation 12.13 shows the weights that are used to combine the natural logarithms of the strata-specific probability ratios. Those weights are the inverse of (an approximation of) the variance of the strata-specific estimates of the probability ratio.

$$w_i = \frac{(a_i + c_i) \cdot (b_i + d_i) \cdot (a_i + b_i)}{(c_i + d_i) \cdot n_i} \tag{12.13}$$

Example 12.5   Combine the data presented in Example 12.3 to estimate the ratio of probabilities of developing cataracts for persons receiving hormonal therapy compared to persons not receiving hormonal therapy.

As we did for probability differences in Example 12.4, we first need to calculate strata-specific estimates of the probability ratio and the weights that will be used to combine those estimates. Those weights are calculated using Equation 12.13.

For females:

	Therapy	No Therapy
Cataracts	21	13
No Cataracts	49	37

---

[13] When we use the inverse of the variance of an estimate as an indicator of the precision of that estimate, we are assuming that the strata-specific estimates have a Gaussian distribution. This is not a bad assumption for differences, but ratios tend to have a **log normal** distribution rather than a Gaussian distribution. The logarithm of a ratio, however, can be assumed to have a Gaussian distribution. To see why this might be so, recall that division on a log scale is performed by finding a difference.

The estimate of the probability ratio for females is:

$$PR_f = \frac{\dfrac{21}{21 + 49}}{\dfrac{13}{13 + 37}} = \frac{0.30}{0.26} = 1.15$$

The weight for that estimate is:

$$w_f = \frac{(a_f + c_f) \cdot (b_f + d_f) \cdot (a_f + b_f)}{(c_f + d_f) \cdot n_f} = \frac{(21 + 49) \cdot (13 + 37) \cdot (21 + 13)}{(49 + 37) \cdot (21 + 13 + 49 + 37)} = 11.53$$

For males:

	Therapy	No Therapy
Cataracts	7	9
No Cataracts	23	41

The estimate of the probability ratio for males is:

$$PR_m = \frac{\dfrac{7}{7 + 23}}{\dfrac{9}{9 + 41}} = \frac{0.23}{0.18} = 1.28$$

The weight for that estimate is:

$$w_m = \frac{(a_m + c_m) \cdot (b_m + d_m) \cdot (a_m + b_m)}{(c_m + d_m) \cdot n_m} = \frac{(7 + 23) \cdot (9 + 41) \cdot (7 + 9)}{(23 + 41) \cdot (7 + 9 + 23 + 41)} = 4.69$$

When we examine the strata-specific probability ratios, we find that they are not as close to each other as were the strata-specific estimates of the probability difference. Still, they are close enough that we might be interested in an overall (summary) estimate. Therefore, we use Equation 12.12 to calculate a weighted average for the probability ratio.

$$PR = e^{\Sigma(w_i \cdot \ln PR_i)/\Sigma w_i} = e^{(11.53 \cdot \ln 1.15) + (4.69 \cdot \ln 1.28)/11.53 + 4.69} = e^{0.1707} = 1.186$$

Thus, 1.186 is our best estimate of the population's value of the ratio of the probabilities of developing cataracts for persons on hormonal therapy compared to persons not on hormonal therapy if we are willing to assume that the ratios are equal for the two genders in the population. If we are not willing to make that assumption, we should use the strata-specific estimates rather than calculate a summary estimate. ▭

The procedure for combining strata-specific information to estimate the odds ratio appears to be quite different from the procedures for the probability difference or the probability ratio although it is based on the same principle of calculating a weighted average of strata-specific estimates. Due to algebraic simplification, however, the procedure for the odds ratio is also considerably easier to calculate. Equation 12.14 shows that calculation.

$$OR = \frac{\sum \frac{(a_i \cdot d_i)}{n_i}}{\sum \frac{(b_i \cdot c_i)}{n_i}} \tag{12.14}$$

Example 12.6 Combine the data presented in Example 12.3 to estimate the odds ratio for developing cataracts, comparing persons receiving hormonal therapy to persons not receiving hormonal therapy.

As we did for probability differences and probability ratios, we should first calculate strata-specific estimates of the odds ratio.

For females:

	Therapy	No Therapy
Cataracts	21	13
No Cataracts	49	37

The estimate of the odds ratio for females is:

$$OR_f = \frac{21 \cdot 37}{13 \cdot 49} = 1.22$$

For males:

	Therapy	No Therapy
Cataracts	7	9
No Cataracts	23	41

The estimate of the odds ratio for males is:

$$OR_m = \frac{7 \cdot 41}{9 \cdot 23} = 1.39$$

As we found when we examined the strata-specific probability ratios, the strata-specific odds ratios are not as close to each other as were the strata-specific estimates of the probability difference. Still, those odds ratios are close enough that we might be interested in an overall (summary) estimate. Therefore, we use Equation 12.14 to calculate a weighted average for the odds ratio.

$$OR = \frac{\sum \frac{(a_i \cdot d_i)}{n_i}}{\sum \frac{(b_i \cdot c_i)}{n_i}} = \frac{\dfrac{21 \cdot 37}{21 + 13 + 49 + 37} + \dfrac{7 \cdot 41}{7 + 9 + 23 + 41}}{\dfrac{13 \cdot 49}{21 + 13 + 49 + 37} + \dfrac{9 \cdot 23}{7 + 9 + 23 + 41}} = 1.274$$

Thus, 1.274 is our best estimate of the population's value of the odds ratio if we are willing to assume that the odds ratios are equal for the two genders in the population. If we are not willing to make that assumption, we should use the strata-specific estimates rather than calculate a summary estimate.   ▭

The procedures that we have discussed so far are for probabilities and proportions. If the nominal dependent variable is expressed as a function of time (i.e., as a rate) and we have more than one nominal independent variable, we can also perform a stratified analysis. To combine strata-specific estimates of rates, we use Equation 12.10 for differences between rates and Equation 12.12 for ratios of rates (i.e., the same calculations we used for probability differences and ratios). The weights that we use for rates, however, are slightly different from those that we use for probabilities. For differences between rates, the weights are as shown in Equation 12.15. Those weights are the inverse of the variance of the strata-specific rate difference estimates.

$$w_i = \frac{py_{1_i} \cdot py_{2_i}}{a_i + b_i} \qquad (12.15)$$

where

py_{1_i} = number of person-years of follow-up in group 1 in the ith stratum
py_{2_i} = number of person-years of follow-up in group 2 in the ith stratum
   a_i = number of events in group 1 in the ith stratum
   b_i = number of events in group 2 in the ith stratum

Equation 12.16 shows how the weights are calculated for rate ratios. These weights are (an approximation of) the inverse of the variance of the strata-specific estimates of the rate ratio.

$$w_i = \frac{py_{2_i} \cdot (a_i + b_i)}{(py_{1_i} + py_{2_i})^2} \qquad (12.16)$$

Example 12.7 Suppose that the study described in Example 12.3 involved following persons receiving hormonal therapy and persons not receiving hormonal therapy (the independent variable of main interest) for various periods of time (up to five years) or until they developed a cataract (the dependent variable). Then, our interest would be in comparing the rate (incidence) at which cataracts developed in these two groups. Further suppose that we are still concerned about gender as a possible confounding factor. Imagine that we made the following observations:

	Independent Variable of Main Interest			
	Hormonal Therapy		No Hormonal Therapy	
Confounding Variable	*Dependent Variable*		*Dependent Variable*	
	Number with Cataracts	Follow-up Time (py)	Number with Cataracts	Follow-up Time (py)
Females	21	324	13	241
Males	7	145	9	238

Estimate the rate difference and the rate ratio for the population from which this sample was derived.

First, we need to calculate the strata-specific estimates of the rate difference and rate ratio as well as the weights that we will use to combine those estimates.

For females:

	No	
	Therapy	Therapy
Number with Cataracts	21	13
Follow-up Time (py)	324	241

The estimate of the rate difference for females is:

$$RD_f = \frac{21}{324} - \frac{13}{241} = 0.011 \text{ cataracts per person-year}$$

The weight for the rate difference for females is (using Equation 12.15):

$$w_f = \frac{py_{1_f} \cdot py_{2_f}}{a_f + b_f} = \frac{324 \cdot 241}{21 + 13} = 2{,}296.59$$

The estimate of the rate ratio for females is:

$$RR_f = \frac{\dfrac{21}{324}}{\dfrac{13}{241}} = 1.20$$

The weight for the rate ratio for females (using Equation 12.16) is:

$$w_f = \frac{py_{2_f} \cdot (a_f + b_f)}{(py_{1_f} + py_{2_f})^2} = \frac{241 \cdot (21 + 13)}{(324 + 241)^2} = 0.0257$$

For males:

	No	
	Therapy	Therapy
Number with Cataracts	7	9
Follow-up Time (py)	145	238

The estimate of the rate difference for males is:

$$RD_m = \frac{7}{145} - \frac{9}{238} = 0.010 \text{ cataracts per person-year}$$

The weight for the rate difference for males (using Equation 12.15) is:

$$w_m = \frac{py_{1_m} \cdot py_{2_m}}{a_m + b_m} = \frac{145 \cdot 238}{7 + 9} = 2{,}156.88$$

The estimate of the rate ratio for males is:

$$RR_m = \frac{\dfrac{7}{145}}{\dfrac{9}{238}} = 1.28$$

The weight for the rate ratio for males (using Equation 12.16) is:

$$w_m = \frac{py_{2_m} \cdot (a_m + b_m)}{(py_{1_m} + py_{2_m})^2} = \frac{238 \cdot (7 + 9)}{(145 + 238)^2} = 0.0260$$

Both the strata-specific rate differences and the strata-specific rate ratios are close enough for the two genders that calculating estimates for the two strata combined makes sense. For the rate difference, we use Equation 12.10.

$$RD = \frac{\Sigma (w_i \cdot RD_i)}{\Sigma w_i} = \frac{(2{,}296.59 \cdot 0.011) + (2{,}156.88 \cdot 0.010)}{2{,}296.59 + 2{,}156.88}$$

$$= 0.0105 \text{ cataracts per person-year}$$

Thus, 0.0105 cataracts per person-year is our best estimate of the difference between the incidences of cataracts among persons on hormonal therapy and persons not on hormonal therapy in the population.

To calculate an estimate of the rate ratio over the two strata, we use Equation 12.12.

$$RR = e^{\Sigma(w_i \cdot \ln RR_i)/\Sigma w_i} = e^{(0.0257 \cdot \ln 1.20) + (0.0260 \cdot \ln 1.28)/(0.0257 + 0.0260)} = 1.240$$

Thus, 1.240 is our best estimate of the ratio of the incidence of cataracts among persons on hormonal therapy and persons not on hormonal therapy in the population.   ▱

Thus, when it is appropriate to calculate a summary estimate of the difference or ratio of a probability or a rate over all strata, we can obtain the best possible estimate by finding a weighted average of the individual strata-specific estimates, using the inverse of the variances as the weights.

LIFE-TABLE ANALYSIS   As in univariable and bivariable analyses, nominal dependent variables that are affected by time can be expressed as rates to allow for variable intervals of follow-up. The use of rates, however, has one important drawback. That drawback is that rates are, for most of us, more difficult to understand than are probabilities. Fortunately, there is another type of stratified analysis that allows us to calculate a probability for an irreversible, once-in-a-lifetime event (such as death) even if persons are followed for different intervals of time. This procedure is called **life-table analysis.**

Life-table analysis treats follow-up time as a confounding variable. As for other confounders, we reduce the influence of variable lengths of follow-up by creating strata within which any differences in length of follow-up are not expected to influence the probability of observing the event represented by the dependent variable.[14] Since time is continuous data and strata are defined by nominal variables, we must convert time to a nominal scale. In other words, each time that stratum represents an interval of time (often one year) in life-table analysis. The way that those strata are organized to aid calculation of point estimates is different from the way stratified data are usually organized. Let us see how those strata are constructed to create a life table in the following example.

Example 12.8   Suppose that we followed a group of 100 persons for up to five years to observe the number who died during that interval of time. Of those 100 persons, 10 died during the first year that they were in the study and 10 other persons were followed for only one year before the study ended (i.e., they entered the study at the beginning of the last year of follow-up). In addition to those 10 persons who died during their first year in the study, 19 other persons died: 8 during the second year, 6 during the third year, 4 during the fourth year, and 1 during the fifth year of follow-up. In addition to the 10 persons who survived the one year that they were in the study, of the remaining 61 persons who survived the interval of follow-up, 13 were followed for five years, 20 were followed for four years, 16 were followed for three years, and 12 were followed for two years.

Construct a life table for these observations, with each year of the study represented by a single stratum.

In a life table, we organize the data into separate columns indicating the length of follow-up time (t), the number of persons in the study at the beginning of that follow-up interval (N_t), the number of persons dying (or experiencing any irreversible event of interest) during that follow-up interval (D_t), and the number of persons who left the study (or "withdrew") during the interval of follow-up without dying (W_t). For the data in this example, the following life table could be constructed:

t	N_t	D_t	W_t
1	100	10	10
2	80	8	12
3	60	6	16
4	38	4	20
5	14	1	13

In life-table analysis, we assume that all the persons who did not die (or have the event of interest) in a time stratum were followed for the same interval of time. The most common assumption is that all those persons were followed for the entire time interval that the stratum represents. This is the same as assuming that those persons who were not followed during the next time interval (i.e., those who withdrew) left

---

[14]Actually, follow-up time is no different than any other confounding factor. It can influence our observations only if it has a different distribution in the groups being compared and it is a determinant of the outcome.

the study at the end of the last time interval during which they were in the study. In Example 12.8, that implies that the persons who withdrew during the first year of the study are assumed to have been followed for the entire first year. Making this assumption, we are using a particular method of analyzing our life table, known as the **Kaplan-Meier** (or **product-limit**) method.[15]

Since we are assuming that all the persons who did not die in a particular time stratum were followed for the same interval of time (the entire interval with the Kaplan-Meier method), we do not need to use a rate to account for follow-up time within each time stratum. Rather we can calculate a probability. One probability we calculate in life-table analysis is the probability of surviving the time interval (or the probability of not having the event of interest). Since this is a probability of something happening during a specified interval of time, the probability of surviving the time interval is a risk. Specifically, it is the risk of surviving (or the complement of the risk of dying) that time interval. Equation 12.17 shows how that probability is calculated, using the information contained in a life table.

$$P_t = 1 - \frac{D_t}{N_t} \tag{12.17}$$

where
   P_t = probability of surviving time interval t
   D_t = number of persons dying during time interval t
   N_t = number of persons alive at the beginning of time interval t

Using Equation 12.17 makes very efficient use of the data collected in a study in which persons are followed for various intervals of time. No matter how long a person remains in the study or what their outcome is, they contribute information to the estimation of probabilities of surviving certain time intervals. Everyone in the study contributes information to the denominator of the probability of surviving the first time interval. This includes persons who were followed for the entire study period and persons who were followed for shorter intervals of time. The probability of surviving the second time interval is estimated using data from all the persons in the study except those who were followed only for the first time interval.

To make such efficient use of information collected in a study in which persons were followed for various intervals of time, we need to make an assumption about that information. Specifically, we need to assume that the survival experience of those followed for shorter intervals of time would have been the same as those who remained in the study for the entire study period. If the reason for persons not being followed for the entire study period is that they entered the study too late to be followed for that long, this assumption is probably justified. If, on the other hand, the reason for persons not being followed for that interval is that they could not be contacted or refused to continue to participate, we need to consider carefully if it is appropriate to

---

[15]Another method of analyzing life-table data, known as the **Cutler-Ederer** (or **actuarial**) method, assumes that withdrawals occur uniformly over the time interval. Although this is probably a more realistic assumption than assuming that withdrawals occur at the end of the time interval, the Kaplan-Meier method is more commonly used in health research.

allow them to contribute information to the time intervals during which they were followed.

Thus, life-table analysis requires the assumption that each time interval of follow-up is the same for all persons in the study during that time interval regardless of how long after that time interval those persons will remain in the study. Although we have not made this assumption explicit for other methods of analyzing data that are affected by time, it is important to realize that it also is a necessary assumption in estimation of rates. Recall from Chapter 6 that we estimate incidence by allowing each person to contribute the number of years they were followed to the denominator of the estimate (Equation 6.3). In that calculation, it is assumed that each year of follow-up is the same as any other year. Cox regression uses a similar principle to estimate rates and, therefore, is subject to the same assumption. Whenever we wish to use all the information available to estimate a nominal dependent variable that is affected by time, we must assume that each unit of follow-up time is comparable among all of the persons in the study. In other words, when some individuals are followed for shorter intervals of time and others are followed for longer intervals of time, the statistical methods most commonly used to estimate probabilities or rates assume that those persons followed for shorter intervals of time would have developed the event at the same rate as those persons followed for longer intervals of time if they had continued to be followed.

There is another probability that we calculate in life-table analysis that takes advantage of a special feature of follow-up time that other confounders do not have. That feature is that follow-up time is sequential. In other words, in order for someone in a study to have the potential of having the event (e.g., death) in the second time stratum, that person must have survived the first time interval without having the event. This feature allows us to summarize survival over all the time strata by calculating the **cumulative probability** of survival. A cumulative probability is the probability of surviving a particular time interval and surviving all the preceding time intervals. In other words, a cumulative probability is the intersection of two events: surviving that particular time interval and surviving all the previous time intervals. We know from Chapter 1 that the probability of the intersection of two events is calculated using the multiplication rule of probability theory. In this case, the probabilities that we multiply together are the probability of surviving the time interval and the cumulative probability from the previous time interval (Equation 12.18).

$$P_T = P_t \cdot P_{T-1} \qquad (12.18)$$

where
P_T = cumulative probability of surviving up to and including time interval t
P_t = probability of surviving time interval t, given that the person survived to the beginning of time interval t
P_{T-1} = cumulative probability of surviving up to and including the time interval prior to time interval t

Example 12.9   For the life table in Example 12.8, calculate the probabilities of surviving each time interval and the cumulative probabilities of survival for each of the time intervals.

To calculate the probability of surviving any particular time interval, we calculate the complement of the probability of dying in that interval, as shown in Equation 12.17. For the first two time intervals, those probabilities are:

$$P_{t=1} = 1 - \frac{D_{t=1}}{N_{t=1}} = \frac{10}{100} = 0.90$$

$$P_{t=2} = 1 - \frac{D_{t=2}}{N_{t=2}} = 1 - \frac{8}{80} = 0.90$$

To calculate the cumulative probability of surviving up to and including any particular time interval, we multiply the probability of surviving that time interval by the probability of surviving up to that time interval (i.e., the cumulative probability for the previous time interval), as shown in Equation 12.18. For the first time interval, the probability of surviving up to that time interval is equal to one. The cumulative probabilities for the first two time intervals are:

$$P_{T=1} = P_{t=1} \cdot P_{T=0} = 0.90 \cdot 1 = 0.90$$

$$P_{T=2} = P_{t=2} \cdot P_{T=1} = 0.90 \cdot 0.90 = 0.81$$

Those probabilities and corresponding probabilities for the remaining time intervals appear in the following life table:

t (Period of Follow-up)	N_t (Number at Beginning)	D_t (Number Dying)	W_t (Number Withdrawing)	P_t (Probability of Survival)	P_T (Cumulative Probability)
1	100	10	10	0.90	0.90
2	80	8	12	0.90	0.81
3	60	6	16	0.90	0.73
4	38	4	20	0.89	0.65
5	14	1	13	0.93	0.61

Thus, the probability of surviving five years for persons in the population from which this sample was drawn is estimated to be 0.61. Or, in other words, the estimated five-year risk of death is equal to the complement of 0.61 or 0.39. This estimate takes into account variable intervals of follow-up under the assumption that everyone who was alive at the beginning of a particular time interval either died during that time interval or was followed for the entire time interval.

To see that we gained something by using the life-table procedure to calculate the five-year risk of death, let us see what we would have estimated to be the five-year risk of death if we had ignored the fact that not everyone who survived was followed for the full five-year period. If we did not take into account variable follow-up times, we would have calculated the five-year risk by dividing the total number of persons who died (29) by the total number of persons in the study (100). Then, we would have estimated the five-year risk of death to be equal to 0.29, which is considerably different from 0.39 obtained from the life-table analysis. Ignoring variable follow-up times will always underestimate the risk of the event since it overestimates the actual time persons were followed and, thus, had an opportunity to have the event.   ▤

So far in our discussion of life-table analysis, the only independent variables that we have considered are those that specify follow-up time intervals. Since follow-up times can be considered a confounding variable, we have not yet considered a parallel to other types of stratified analysis in which we had another independent variable that defined groups between which we are interested in comparing dependent variable values (i.e., an independent variable of main interest). Usually, life-table analysis includes such an independent variable. For example, we might use life-table analysis to analyze the results of a clinical trial in which we wish to compare survival of persons receiving a particular treatment to survival of persons receiving a placebo. In that case, we would have a nominal independent variable that represents the type of treatment a person received. When we have such an independent variable, we construct separate life tables for each of the two groups being compared.

One way to compare the life tables of two groups is to examine cumulative probabilities for any particular time interval as a difference or as a ratio. There is no need to calculate weighted averages of those cumulative probabilities if follow-up time is the only confounding variable being considered. The reason for this is that each group provides one and only one estimate of the cumulative survival for that time interval.[16]

Example 12.10 Let us suppose that the life table in Example 12.8 represents the survival of persons in a clinical trial who received a particular treatment. Let us further suppose that the following life table represents survival of 100 persons in that clinical trial who received a placebo.

t	N_t	D_t	W_t	P_t	P_T
1	100	19	10	0.81	0.81
2	71	13	11	0.82	0.66
3	47	8	13	0.83	0.55
4	26	4	14	0.84	0.46
5	8	1	7	0.88	0.41

Estimate the difference in the three-year risk of death for persons in the two treatment groups in the population.

In Example 12.9, we found that the three-year cumulative probability of survival for persons receiving the treatment was 0.73. The three-year risk of death for persons receiving the

---

[16]If other confounding factors need to be taken into account, life tables can be stratified, and weighted averages of differences or ratios of cumulative probabilities can be calculated.

treatment is the complement of that probability, or 0.27. In the life table for persons receiving the placebo, we see that the three-year cumulative probability of survival is 0.55. Thus, the three-year risk of death among those persons is 0.45, and the difference between the three-year risks of death in the population is estimated to be $0.45 - 0.27 = 0.18$.   ▱

Another way to compare life tables of the two groups is to examine the survival experience over the entire period of follow-up. This is usually accomplished graphically by comparing **survival curves.** A survival curve is a plot of the cumulative probability of survival (on the ordinate) versus the length of follow-up (on the abscissa). Most commonly, survival curves are drawn using "steps" between the estimated cumulative probabilities of survival as shown in Example 12.11.

Example 12.11   Compare the survival experience for persons in the sample presented in Example 12.8 (treated persons) to persons in the sample presented in Example 12.10 (untreated persons) by constructing survival curves.

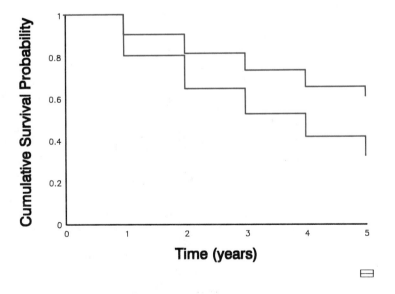

INFERENCE   Statistical inference in stratified analysis is easier than estimation because separate methods are not needed for differences and ratios as they were in estimation. Further, the methods for inference are extensions of methods with which we are familiar. For example, to test the null hypothesis that a probability difference is equal to zero or that a probability ratio or an odds ratio are equal to one in the population that was sampled, we use an extension of the Mantel-Haenszel chi test that we discussed to test those hypotheses in bivariable data sets (see Equation 9.19). To consider more than one stratum of observations, we sum the values in one of the cells of the 2×2 tables and subtract the sum of the values that we would expect if the null hypothesis were true. Then we divide that difference by the square root of the sum of the variances for the expected value. That calculation is shown in Equation 12.19.

$$\chi_{\text{M-H}} = \frac{\sum [a_i] - \sum \left[\frac{(a_i + b_i) \cdot (a_i + c_i)}{n_i} \right]}{\sqrt{\sum \dfrac{(a_i + b_i) \cdot (c_i + d_i) \cdot (a_i + c_i) \cdot (b_i + d_i)}{n_i^2 \cdot (n_i - 1)}}} \qquad (12.19)$$

Example 12.12 Test the null hypothesis that the difference between the probabilities of developing cataracts for persons on hormonal therapy versus persons not on hormonal therapy is equal to zero in the population that was sampled in Example 12.3. As an alternative hypothesis, consider that the probability difference is not equal to zero in the population. Allow a 5% chance of making a Type I error.

Using the stratified data from Example 12.3 and Equation 12.19, we calculate the following chi value.

$$\chi_{\text{M-H}} = \frac{\sum [a_i] - \sum \left[\frac{(a_i + b_i) \cdot (a_i + c_i)}{n_i} \right]}{\sqrt{\sum \dfrac{(a_i + b_i) \cdot (c_i + d_i) \cdot (a_i + c_i) \cdot (b_i + d_i)}{n_i^2 \cdot (n_i - 1)}}}$$

$$= \frac{[21 + 7] - \left[\dfrac{(21 + 13) \cdot (21 + 49)}{120} + \dfrac{(7 + 9) \cdot (7 + 23)}{80} \right]}{\sqrt{\dfrac{(21 + 13) \cdot (49 + 37) \cdot (21 + 49) \cdot (13 + 37)}{120^2 \cdot (120 - 1)} + \dfrac{(7 + 9) \cdot (23 + 41) \cdot (7 + 23) \cdot (9 + 41)}{80^2 \cdot (80 - 1)}}}$$

$$= 1.12$$

As we know from Chapter 9, the Mantel-Haenszel chi is a standard normal deviate. Therefore, we compare 1.12 to a standard normal deviate from Table B.1 with an area of $0.05/2 = 0.025$ in each tail of the distribution. That standard normal deviate is equal to 1.96. Since 1.12 is less than 1.96, we do not reject the null hypothesis.

Note that we have simultaneously tested the null hypothesis that the probability difference is equal to zero, the null hypothesis that the probability ratio is equal to one, and also the null hypothesis that the odds ratio is equal to one in the population from which the sample was drawn (see Chapter 9 to review the reason that this is true). ▱

If the nominal dependent variable is affected by time (i.e., the probability of observing the event is influenced by how long we wait for it, and persons are followed for various intervals of time), we have the choice of estimating the rate of the event or calculating cumulative probabilities using life-table methods. If we choose to estimate the rate of the event, we can test the null hypothesis that the rate difference is equal to zero or that the rate ratio is equal to one in the population. This can be done from stratified data, using an extension of the procedure described in Chapter 9 for comparing two rates (see Equation 9.21). The extension of the method for rates is similar to the extension of the Mantel-Haenszel chi calculation (Equation 12.19) for probabilities. The method for analysis of rates from stratified data is shown in Equation 12.20.

$$\chi = \frac{\sum [a_i] - \sum \left[(a_i + b_i) \cdot \dfrac{py_{1_i}}{py_{total_i}} \right]}{\sqrt{\sum \dfrac{(a_i + b_i) \cdot (py_{1_i}) \cdot (py_{2_i})}{py^2_{total_i}}}} \tag{12.20}$$

Example 12.13   For the observations in Example 12.7, test the null hypothesis that the rate ratio is equal to one in the population from which the sample was drawn versus the alternative hypothesis that it is not equal to one. Allow a 5% chance of making a Type I error.

To test that null hypothesis (or the null hypothesis that the rate difference is equal to zero), we use Equation 12.20.

$$\chi = \frac{\sum [a_i] - \sum \left[(a_i + b_i) \cdot \dfrac{py_{1_i}}{py_{total_i}} \right]}{\sqrt{\sum \dfrac{(a_i + b_i) \cdot (py_{1_i}) \cdot (py_{2_i})}{py^2_{total_i}}}}$$

$$= \frac{[21 + 7] - \left[\left((21 + 13) \cdot \dfrac{324}{324 + 241} \right) + \left((7 + 9) \cdot \dfrac{145}{145 + 238} \right) \right]}{\sqrt{\dfrac{(21 + 13) \cdot 324 \cdot 241}{(324 + 241)^2} + \dfrac{(7 + 9) \cdot 145 \cdot 238}{(145 + 238)^2}}} = 0.56$$

Like the Mantel-Haenszel chi, this is a standard normal deviate. Thus, we compare 0.56 to 1.96 (from Table B.1). Since 0.56 is less than 1.96, we do not reject the null hypothesis.   ▱

If we choose to represent a dependent variable that is affected by time with a cumulative probability rather than a rate, we can perform life-table analysis as described previously. In life-table analysis, we have a choice between two types of null hypotheses that we can test. Most commonly, inference in life-table analysis tests the null hypothesis that the entire survival experiences for two groups are the same.[17] To

---

[17] The other type of null hypothesis is that the cumulative probabilities for two groups are the same for a particular time stratum. In other words, we might test the null hypothesis that the difference between the cumulative probabilities of survival in the three-year interval is equal to zero in the population from which the sample was drawn for the study described in Examples 12.8 and 12.10. Once we have selected a particular time interval, this is really a bivariable test of statistical inference since we have one nominal dependent variable (survival) and one nominal independent variable (treatment group). We will not examine the details of this procedure in *Statistical First Aid*.

test this null hypothesis, we recall that life-table analysis can be thought of as a stratified analysis, with the strata identifying time intervals. Then, the approach to inference can be exactly the same as for any other stratified nominal data that can be summarized with a probability. Specifically, we can use the Mantel-Haenszel chi procedure (Equation 12.19) to compare two life tables.[18] The next example shows how that procedure can be applied to life-table data.

Example 12.14   Test the null hypothesis that the survival experiences in Example 12.11 are the same in the population that was sampled versus the alternative hypothesis that they are not the same. Allow a 5% chance of making a Type I error.

To see how we apply the Mantel-Haenszel procedure to life-table data, it is probably helpful to arrange the life-table data into a series of 2 × 2 tables, each representing a particular time interval. For the data in Examples 12.8 and 12.10, those 2 × 2 tables are as follows:

Year 1:

		Treatment Group		
		Treatment	Placebo	
Survival	Yes	90	81	171
	No	10	19	29
		100	100	200

Year 2:

		Treatment Group		
		Treatment	Placebo	
Survival	Yes	72	58	130
	No	8	13	21
		80	71	151

Year 3:

		Treatment Group		
		Treatment	Placebo	
Survival	Yes	54	39	93
	No	6	8	14
		60	47	107

[18] An alternative name for the Mantel-Haenszel procedure is the **log-rank test.** Curiously, the term "log-rank test" is more often used to refer to calculation of a Mantel-Haenszel chi to compare two life tables than is the term "Mantel-Haenszel procedure." Calculation and interpretation of the Mantel-Haenszel procedure and the log-rank test are identical.

Year 4:

Treatment Group

		Treatment	Placebo	
Survival	Yes	34	22	56
	No	4	4	8
		38	26	64

Year 5:

Treatment Group

		Treatment	Placebo	
Survival	Yes	13	7	20
	No	1	1	2
		14	8	22

Now, we use Equation 12.19 to calculate a Mantel-Haenszel chi statistic for all those 2×2 tables, just as we would for any stratified analysis of probabilities or odds.

$$\chi_{\text{M-H}} = \frac{\sum [a_i] - \sum \left[\frac{(a_i + b_i) \cdot (a_i + c_i)}{n_i} \right]}{\sqrt{\sum \frac{(a_i + b_i) \cdot (c_i + d_i) \cdot (a_i + c_i) \cdot (b_i + d_i)}{n_i^2 \cdot (n_i - 1)}}}$$

$$= \frac{(90 + 72 + 54 + 34 + 13) - \left(\frac{171 \cdot 100}{200} + \frac{130 \cdot 80}{151} + \frac{93 \cdot 60}{107} + \frac{56 \cdot 38}{64} + \frac{20 \cdot 14}{22} \right)}{\sqrt{\frac{171 \cdot 29 \cdot 100 \cdot 100}{200^2 \cdot 199} + \frac{130 \cdot 21 \cdot 80 \cdot 71}{151^2 \cdot 150} + \frac{93 \cdot 14 \cdot 60 \cdot 47}{107^2 \cdot 106} + \frac{56 \cdot 8 \cdot 38 \cdot 26}{64^2 \cdot 63} + \frac{20 \cdot 2 \cdot 14 \cdot 8}{22^2 \cdot 21}}}$$

$$= 2.63$$

Since the Mantel-Haenszel chi statistic is a standard normal deviate, we compare our calculated value to the value in Table B.1 that corresponds to 0.05 split between the two tails of the standard normal distribution. That value is 1.96. Since 2.63 is greater than 1.96, we reject the null hypothesis and accept, by elimination, the alternative hypothesis that the survival experiences are not the same for the two treatment groups in the population.

So, we have seen that testing the null hypothesis that two survival curves are the same in the population from which the sample was drawn is just like testing a null hypothesis that the ratio of two probabilities is equal to one (or, equivalently, that their difference is equal to zero) when we have stratified the data to diminish the influence of some confounder. In both cases, we use the Mantel-Haenszel chi procedure. That procedure combines information from all the strata in such a way that we can examine probabilities within strata without relationships between strata influencing our conclusion. That is not to say, however, that each stratum has equal impact on the Mantel-Haenszel chi calculation.

In general, strata that contain more observations contribute more to the Mantel-Haenszel chi value than do strata with fewer observations. In life-table analysis, this is an important feature to keep in mind, for the number of observations in life-table analysis is always greatest for the first time interval and becomes smaller for each subsequent time interval. Thus, our ability to demonstrate statistical significance for true differences between survival curves (i.e., the statistical power) is greatest when those survival curves differ in the early intervals of follow-up and is least when the survival curves differ only in the later intervals of follow-up. Another way to express this relationship among time intervals is to say that the precision of estimates of the interval-specific risks is greatest for the early time intervals and least for the later time intervals. If we were to calculate confidence intervals for those risks, we would find that the most narrow confidence intervals would correspond to the beginning of follow-up and that the confidence intervals would become quite wide for the final time interval.

MIXED INDEPENDENT VARIABLES

In Chapter 10, we discussed how a mixture of nominal and continuous independent variables can be analyzed using multiple regression techniques. With that approach, nominal independent variables are converted into indicator variables, and indicator variables are multiplied by other independent variables to create interaction terms in the regression model. We do the same thing for nominal dependent variables when we have a mixture of nominal and continuous independent variables. In this case, logistic regression is used for probabilities and odds, and Cox regression is used for rates.

Over the past few years, we have seen logistic regression being used with increasing frequency in the health research literature in situations in which stratified analyses of probabilities or odds used to be the analysis of choice. Also, we have seen Cox regression replacing stratified analysis of rates or life-table analysis of nominal dependent variables that are affected by time.[19] There are several reasons for this decrease in popularity of stratified analysis procedures and the corresponding increase in the use of regression techniques for nominal dependent variables. One of these reasons is the fact that health research data most often include a mixture of nominal and continuous independent variables.

We can use stratified analysis procedures on sets of data that include a mixture of nominal and continuous independent variables, but to do that, the continuous independent variables must be converted to nominal independent variables. For example, if we wish to control for age in a stratified analysis, that continuous variable must be converted into a series of nominal variables specifying age groups. As we know from previous discussions, conversion of continuous data to a nominal scale

---

[19]The results of Cox regression also can be used to construct survival curves which can be interpreted in the same way that survival curves in life-table analysis are interpreted.

results in a loss of information. Loss of information for the independent variable of primary interest results in a loss of statistical power, making it more difficult to reject a false null hypothesis. Loss of information for independent variables that represent confounders results in poor control of confounding. For instance, it is possible (or even likely) that age differences within age strata will influence our conclusions about the dependent variable and the independent variable of primary interest to some degree. In life-table analysis, this is a common problem since time is continuous and life-table techniques force us to convert time to a nominal scale by dividing follow-up time into a series of time intervals.[20]

Therefore, when we have a mixture of continuous and nominal independent variables, it is better, from a statistical point of view, to use logistic or Cox regression procedures rather than employ a stratified approach. Even if all the independent variables are nominal, we might choose to use logistic or Cox regression rather than stratified analysis. The reason for that choice is that those regression techniques allow us to obtain a deeper understanding about the relationships between the nominal dependent variable and the independent variables (when the data set includes independent variables in addition to time and the independent variable of primary interest) than does stratified analysis.

In stratified analysis, we only can examine the relationship between the dependent variable and one of the nominal independent variables. Although we can take confounders into account, we cannot estimate the degree to which those confounders are associated with the dependent variable or test hypotheses about whether those variables are associated with the dependent variable in the population from which the sample was drawn. In a regression approach, however, coefficients for confounding variables allow us to perform such estimation and inference.[21] Stratified analysis also does not allow us to investigate formally how the relationship between the dependent variable and the independent variable of primary interest differs for different values of the other independent variables. This differing of the relationship between one independent variable and the dependent variable for different values of another independent variable can be examined by including interaction terms in the regression model (see Chapter 10).

Thus, logistic or Cox regression procedures are often a better choice than stratified analysis when we have a mixture of nominal and continuous independent variables or even when all the independent variables are nominal. Why then do we learn about stratified analysis techniques? There are three reasons. First, it is still not uncommon to encounter these techniques in the health research literature. We must, therefore, understand how to interpret the results of stratified analysis.

---

[20] The best techniques for life-table analysis place each event in a separate stratum. If this is done, there is no residual effect of time.

[21] Estimation of the relationship between a confounding variable and the dependent variable is accomplished in logistic or Cox regression by estimation of the regression coefficient associated with the independent variable representing the confounder. We can test the null hypothesis that the coefficient associated with that independent variable is equal to zero in the population by examining the partial likelihood ratio associated with its coefficient.

Second, many researchers believe that stratified analysis is easier to understand than logistic or Cox regression. Interpretability of a statistical technique is a desirable feature that must be balanced with the ability of the technique to provide reasonable statistical power and ability to control confounding. If stratified analysis is more easily interpreted and it does not result in a substantial loss of power nor endanger our conclusions by allowing the confounder to be poorly controlled, it may well be the analysis of choice.

The third reason for our consideration of stratified analysis as a useful method for analyzing a multivariable data set with a nominal dependent variable is that stratified analyses require less stringent assumptions than do regression analyses. In regression analyses, we have a very particular model that we are trying to fit to our data. For instance, in logistic regression, we force a linear combination of independent variables to be related to the log odds of the dependent variable. For a continuous independent variable such as age, we assume that each unit increase in that independent variable is related to a unit increase in the log odds. This may or may not be a good reflection of the true relationship among the independent variables and the dependent variable. Deviations between the true relationship and the one dictated by the regression model will result in a loss of statistical power and poor control of confounding. In that case, stratified analysis would be the better choice.

||| SUMMARY

We have two choices for our basic approach to multivariable analysis of a nominal dependent variable. One approach that is applicable to continuous and/or nominal independent variables is comparable to multiple regression analysis for a continuous dependent variable. The other approach is stratified analysis, which can be performed only with nominal independent variables or independent variables converted to a nominal scale.

In the regression approach to the analysis of nominal dependent variables, there are two techniques that we encounter most often in health research. When the nominal dependent variable is expressed as a probability or as odds, we use logistic regression. Logistic regression uses a transformation of the nominal dependent variable known as the logit. The logit is equal to the natural logarithm of the ratio of the probabilities of an event and its complement. This is the same as the natural logarithm of the odds of the dependent variable (known as the log odds).

$$\text{logit} = \ln \frac{p}{(1 - p)} \tag{12.3}$$

To estimate values of the logit transformed dependent variable, logistic regression analysis uses a linear combination of the independent variables that is the same as in multiple regression analysis of continuous dependent variables.

$$\ln\left(\frac{\theta}{1 - \theta}\right) = \alpha + \beta_1 X_1 + \beta_2 X_2 + \ldots + \beta_k X_k \tag{12.4}$$

There are two ways in which the estimated values of the dependent variable in logistic regression can be expressed. One way is by estimating probabilities for specific values of all the independent variables.

$$\theta = \frac{1}{1 + e^{-(\alpha + \beta_1 X_1 + \beta_2 X_2 + \ldots + \beta_k X_k)}} \tag{12.5}$$

The other way to interpret estimated values of the dependent variable in logistic regression is by estimating odds ratios for specific values of the independent variables, one at a time (Equation 12.7).

$$OR = \frac{e^{\beta X}}{e^{\beta X'}} = e^{\beta(X - X')} \tag{12.7}$$

Cox regression is the regression approach that is most often used when the nominal dependent variable is affected by time and expressed as a rate. The dependent variable in the Cox regression equation is the natural logarithm of the rate.

$$\ln(\text{rate}) = \alpha_t + \beta_1 X_1 + \beta_2 X_2 + \ldots + \beta_k X_k \tag{12.8}$$

It is possible to interpret the estimated values of the dependent variable in Cox regression as the rate corresponding to specific values for all the independent variables, but this is a little complicated since the intercept is a function of time. More often, dependent variable values are interpreted as a rate ratio corresponding to an increment in a specific independent variable.

$$RR = \frac{e^{\beta X}}{e^{\beta X'}} = e^{\beta(X - X')} \tag{12.9}$$

Both logistic regression and Cox regression rely on the maximum likelihood method for estimating values of regression coefficients and testing hypotheses. In the maximum likelihood method, values for the coefficients are chosen so that the probability of obtaining the sample's observations from a population with those coefficients is as high as possible. Inference in logistic and Cox regression uses a likelihood ratio. That likelihood ratio contains the probability of obtaining the sample's observations if the null hypothesis were true (L_0) in the numerator and the probability of obtaining those observations if the population's coefficients were equal to the sample's estimates of those coefficients (L) in the denominator.

$$LR = \frac{L_0}{L} \tag{12.1}$$

The likelihood ratio can be used to test the omnibus null hypothesis that all the coefficients are equal to zero, or a partial likelihood ratio can be used to test the null hypothesis that a particular coefficient is equal to zero. These likelihood ratios differ in the likelihood used in their numerators. The likelihood ratio for the omnibus null hypothesis has in its numerator the likelihood of obtaining the observed data if all the coefficients were equal to zero. The partial likelihood ratio has in its numerator the likelihood of obtaining the observed data if a particular coefficient were equal to zero and all the other coefficients were equal to the values estimated from the sample's observations.

Regardless of which null hypothesis is being tested, evaluation of whether or not the likelihood ratio is unusual enough to allow rejection of the null hypothesis involves conversion of the likelihood ratio to a chi-square statistic. That chi-square value has degrees of freedom equal to the difference between the number of coefficients considered in the null hypothesis and the total number of coefficients in the regression equation.

$$\chi^2_{kdf} = -2 \cdot \ln \mathrm{LR} \tag{12.2}$$

When all the independent variables are nominal, we can still use logistic or Cox regression techniques to analyze them. An alternative to the regression approach for nominal independent variables, however, is the stratified analysis approach. In stratified analysis, we differentiate between one nominal independent variable that is of main interest and other independent variables that represent potential confounders. We then create a series of 2 × 2 tables, one for each value of the independent variable(s) representing the confounder(s). These 2 × 2 tables are constructed so that values of the independent variable of main interest specify the columns, and values of the dependent variable specify the rows.

With data that have been stratified, we have a choice of examining the relationship between the dependent variable and the independent variable of main interest within each of the strata separately or over all the strata combined. The choice between these two approaches depends on whether or not the relationship appears to be consistent over all the strata. When the relationship does not appear to be consistent over the strata, we choose to examine that relationship within each of the strata separately, using the techniques for bivariable analysis of a nominal dependent variable described in Chapter 9.

If the relationship between the dependent variable and the main independent variable appears to be the same for all the strata, we can facilitate interpretation of that relationship by making one summary estimate combining the estimates for each of the strata. That is done by taking a weighted average of the strata-specific estimates. The weights that we use are (approximations of) the inverse of the variance of the estimate in each of the strata. This method gives the greatest weight to those strata-specific estimates that are associated with the greatest degree of precision. The weights for differences between probabilities are calculated as follows:

$$w_i = \frac{(a_i + c_i) \cdot (b_i + d_i) \cdot n_i}{(a_i + b_i) \cdot (c_i + d_i)} \tag{12.11}$$

The weighted average of strata-specific probability differences is calculated like other weighted averages we have discussed.

$$\mathrm{PD} = \frac{\Sigma (w_i \cdot \mathrm{PD}_i)}{\Sigma w_i} \tag{12.10}$$

We calculate a weighted average for ratios of probabilities by first taking the natural logarithm of the strata-specific probability ratio, finding the weighted average of those natural logarithms, and then converting the weighted average back to its natural scale. That procedure can be done in one step by using Equation 12.12 and the weights in Equation 12.13.

$$\mathrm{PR} = e^{\Sigma (w_i \cdot \ln \mathrm{PR}_i)/\Sigma w_i} \tag{12.12}$$

$$w_i = \frac{(a_i + c_i) \cdot (b_i + d_i) \cdot (a_i + b_i)}{(c_i + d_i) \cdot n_i} \tag{12.13}$$

The method for finding a weighted average of the strata-specific odds ratios is more straightforward since the calculation can be summarized as shown in Equation 12.14.

$$\mathrm{OR} = \frac{\Sigma \dfrac{(a_i \cdot d_i)}{n_i}}{\Sigma \dfrac{(b_i \cdot c_i)}{n_i}} \tag{12.14}$$

The procedure for finding a weighted average of strata-specific estimates of the differences or ratios of rates is similar to the procedure for probabilities. The weights, however, are different. For differences between rates, the weights in Equation 12.15 are used. Equation 12.16 gives the weights for ratios of rates.

$$w_i = \frac{py_{1_i} \cdot py_{2_i}}{a_i + b_i} \tag{12.15}$$

$$w_i = \frac{py_{2_i} \cdot (a_i + b_i)}{(py_{1_i} + py_{2_i})^2} \tag{12.16}$$

When it is more likely that we will observe the nominal dependent variable event the longer we follow individuals and individuals in a study are followed for variable periods of time, we say that the dependent variable is affected by time. In previous chapters, we have examined nominal dependent variables that are affected by time by estimating rates rather than probabilities. In this chapter, we examined an alternative approach to nominal dependent variables that are affected by time with a method called life-table analysis. In life-table analysis, follow-up time is treated like a nominal confounding variable used to create strata. Within each time stratum, the probability of surviving the time interval is calculated (Equation 12.17).

$$P_t = 1 - \frac{D_t}{N_t} \tag{12.17}$$

where

P_t = probability of surviving time interval t

D_t = number of persons dying during time interval t

N_t = number of persons alive at the beginning of time interval t

Of more interest than the probability of surviving a particular time stratum is the cumulative probability of surviving up to and including that time interval. This cumulative probability is calculated using the multiplication rule of probability theory (Equation 12.18).

$$P_T = P_t \cdot P_{T-1} \tag{12.18}$$

where

P_T = cumulative probability of surviving up to and including time interval t

P_t = probability of surviving time interval t given that the person survived to the beginning of time interval t

P_{T-1} = cumulative probability of surviving up to and including the time interval prior to time interval t

It is often of interest to compare the survival experience of two groups. Most commonly, entire life tables are compared graphically by examining survival curves. A survival curve plots time on the abscissa (X-axis) and the cumulative probability of survival on the ordinate (Y-axis).

For both probabilities and rates, methods of estimation differ between differences and ratios. That is not true of inference. The method we use to test the null hypothesis that the probability difference is equal to zero or that the probability or odds ratios are equal to one is an extension of the Mantel-Haenszel procedure first described in Chapter 9.

$$\chi_{\text{M-H}} = \frac{\sum [a_i] - \sum \left[\dfrac{(a_i + b_i) \cdot (a_i + c_i)}{n_i} \right]}{\sqrt{\sum \dfrac{(a_i + b_i) \cdot (c_i + d_i) \cdot (a_i + c_i) \cdot (b_i + d_i)}{n_i^2 \cdot (n_i - 1)}}} \tag{12.19}$$

The Mantel-Haenszel procedure also is used to test the null hypothesis that two life tables are the same in the population from which the sample was drawn. Although the calculations are the same when a Mantel-Haenszel chi is calculated from data stratified by interval of follow-up, there is a feature of inference in life-table analysis that is important to keep in mind. That feature is that the number of observations in each time stratum becomes smaller as we consider strata for later time intervals. Thus, differences in survival early in a study have greater impact on inference than do differences later in a study.

Instead of using life-table analysis to examine a nominal dependent variable that is affected by time, we can estimate rates. In stratified analysis of rates, the method we use to test the null hypothesis that a rate difference is equal to zero or that a rate ratio is equal to one is also an extension of the procedure we used in Chapter 9.

$$\chi = \frac{\sum [a_i] - \sum \left[(a_i + b_i) \cdot \dfrac{py_{1_i}}{py_{\text{total}_i}} \right]}{\sqrt{\sum \dfrac{(a_i + b_i) \cdot (py_{1_i}) \cdot (py_{2_i})}{py_{\text{total}_i}^2}}} \tag{12.20}$$

When a data set contains a nominal dependent variable and a mixture of nominal and continuous independent variables, we can use the regression approaches that were described for continuous independent variables. If the dependent variable is not affected by time (e.g., if all the persons in the study were followed for the same interval of time), we can analyze the data using logistic regression. Otherwise, we can use Cox regression. Those regression techniques can be used even if all the independent variables are nominal. An advantage to using a regression approach rather than stratified analysis is that regression analysis allows us to evaluate the influence of confounders and interactions in a study, not just the independent variable of primary interest.

|| PRACTICE PROBLEMS

12.1 Suppose that we were interested in the relationship between the risk of diabetes (dependent variable) and the presence of high blood pressure (HBP). Further suppose that we were concerned that this relationship might be different for different ages and genders. Imagine that we conduct a study in which all the persons in the study were followed for the same period of time. Then, we could use a logistic regression program to analyze the data we obtain in such a study, using an indicator of hypertension (HYP = 1 for people with hypertension) and an indicator of gender (SEX = 1 for females). Imagine that we observe the following results from a computer program that performs logistic regression:

LIKELIHOOD RATIO = 0.015389

VARIABLE	B	CHISQ
AGE	0.0702	6.95
SEX	0.1519	4.01
HBP	0.3041	7.22
(CONSTANT)	−3.3700	1.43

Test the null hypothesis that the probability of developing diabetes is unrelated to age, gender, and hypertension, allowing a 5% chance of making a Type I error.

12.2 For the observations in Problem 12.1, estimate the probability of developing diabetes for a 50-year-old man with hypertension. For those same observations, estimate the odds ratio for the development of diabetes among persons with hypertension compared to persons without hypertension.

12.3 In a clinical trial of a new treatment for angina, 300 persons with angina were randomly assigned to receive the new treatment, and 300 persons with angina were randomly assigned to receive a standard therapy. After one month, all the subjects in this study were asked if angina pain was reduced. The following table shows the number of subjects in each treatment and age group who either reported a reduction or no reduction in angina pain.

Gender	Age	New Treatment		Standard Therapy	
		Pain Reduced	Pain Not Reduced	Pain Reduced	Pain Not Reduced
Female	50–59	18	42	10	50
	60–69	16	34	7	43
	70–79	13	27	7	33
Male	50–59	22	48	10	60
	60–69	17	43	8	52
	70–79	16	34	9	41

Organize these observations into strata. Determine the best estimate(s) of the odds ratio for pain reduction, comparing the new treatment to the standard therapy. Test the null hypothesis that the odds ratio is equal to one in the population that was sampled versus the alternative that it is not equal to one. Allow a 5% chance of making a Type I error.

12.4 Suppose that we conducted a clinical trial to compare the treatment and placebo from Example 12.10 on a different population of patients. In this clinical trial, we randomly assigned 100 persons to receive the treatment and 100 persons to receive the placebo over a five-year period. Imagine that we obtained the following results:

Time Interval	Placebo		Treatment	
	Deaths	Withdrawals	Deaths	Withdrawals
1	10	8	9	7
2	8	9	8	10
3	7	11	7	13
4	9	11	5	12
5	9	18	3	26

Organize these data as life tables and compare the five-year risks of death between the persons who received the treatment to those persons who received the placebo. How do these risks compare to the risks estimated in Example 12.10?

12.5 Draw survival curves for the data in Problem 12.4. Test the null hypothesis that the entire survival curves are the same in the population from which this sample was drawn versus the alternative hypothesis that those survival curves are not the same. Allow a 5% chance of making a Type I error. Compare this result to the result in Example 12.14 and explain any differences in the conclusions drawn.

APPENDIX A

Answers to Practice Problems

CHAPTER 1

1.1 The observations described in this problem are 50,282 pregnant women participating in the Collaborative Perinatal Project. The events are 3,248 children with congenital malformations born to these women. To calculate the probability that a pregnancy will result in a congenital malformation based on these data, we divide the number of events by the number of observations:

$$p(\text{malformation}) = \frac{\text{Number of malformations}}{\text{Number of pregnancies}} = \frac{3{,}248}{50{,}282} = 0.0646$$

1.2 The answer to this question may be intuitively obvious to you: It is the probability of dying from heart disease (0.05) plus the probability of dying from respiratory disease (0.01) subtracted from 1. In performing what seems like a straightforward calculation, you were actually using some basic principles of probabilities and making some important assumptions. Specifically, you calculated the complement of the union of two events assuming that those events were mutually exclusive. Let us take a closer look at these calculations.

To solve this problem, we need to calculate the union of having heart disease (HD) or respiratory disease (RD) listed as the immediate cause of death on the certificate of death. First, we consider the properties of those events. We can be sure that the events are mutually exclusive, for it is only possible to have one immediate cause of death. That property permits us to use the addition rule of probability theory without including probabilities of intersections (by definition, equal to zero) to determine the union of the events:

$$p(\text{HD or RD}) = p(\text{HD}) + p(\text{RD}) = 0.05 + 0.01 = 0.06$$

Next, we find the probability of the complement of that union:

$$p(\overline{\text{HD}} \text{ and } \overline{\text{RD}}) = 1 - p(\text{HD or RD}) = 1 - 0.06 = 0.94$$

From this approach, we estimate the probability of having neither heart disease nor respiratory disease listed as the immediate cause of death to be equal to 0.94.

There is another, incorrect, approach you might have taken and obtained a probability close to 0.94. That approach is to calculate the intersection of the complements $[p(\overline{\text{HD}}) \cdot p(\overline{\text{RD}})]$. This is an inappropriate approach since those complements are not independent. The probability from this approach happens to be close to the correct answer in this case, but that will not always be true.

1.3 The shaded area in the following diagram corresponds to the probability calculated in Problem 1.2. Note that the areas representing death due to heart disease (HD) and death due to respiratory disease (RD) do not intersect. This implies that those events are mutually exclusive.

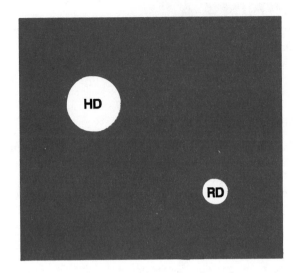

1.4 In this problem, we are asked to determine if two events (smoking and drinking alcohol) are independent. To answer that question, we are provided with four intersections for the two events and their complements:

$$p(S \text{ and } \overline{A}) = 0.05$$

$$p(\overline{S} \text{ and } A) = 0.45$$

$$p(S \text{ and } A) = 0.35$$

$$p(\overline{S} \text{ and } \overline{A}) = 0.15$$

To test for independence, we need to compare unconditional and conditional probabilities for one of the events. Let us calculate those probabilities for smoking.

Those four intersections are collectively exhaustive (everyone must belong to one) and mutually exclusive (everyone can belong to only one). Therefore, we can find the *unconditional* probability of smoking using the addition rule as follows:

$$p(S) = p([S \text{ and } A] \text{ or } [S \text{ and } \overline{A}]) = p(S \text{ and } A) + p(S \text{ and } \overline{A})$$

$$= 0.05 + 0.35 = 0.40$$

The *conditional* probabilities of smoking are calculated using Equation 1.3:

$$p(S|A) = \frac{p(S \text{ and } A)}{p(A)} = \frac{p(S \text{ and } A)}{p(S \text{ and } A) + p(\overline{S} \text{ and } A)} = \frac{0.35}{0.35 + 0.45} = 0.4375$$

$$p(S|\overline{A}) = \frac{p(S \text{ and } \overline{A})}{p(\overline{A})} = \frac{p(S \text{ and } \overline{A})}{p(S \text{ and } \overline{A}) + p(\overline{S} \text{ and } \overline{A})} = \frac{0.05}{0.05 + 0.15} = 0.25$$

Since unconditional and conditional probabilities for smoking are not all equal, we conclude that smoking and drinking alcohol are not independent.

CHAPTER 2

2.1 a) Diagnosis of diabetes as used here is an example of **nominal** data since it consists of information for which only two values are possible (positive or negative for diabetes).

b) Time since diagnosis is an example of **continuous** data since there are a large (theoretically infinite) number of possible evenly spaced values of time.

c) Level of education is best thought of as an example of **ordinal** data since it is likely to be measured in a finite number of categories (e.g., high school, college, etc.) and the distance between those categories is not even (e.g., we probably would not consider the difference between completion of high school and the completion of four years of undergraduate study to be the same as the difference between completion of four years of undergraduate study and four years of graduate study).

d) Place of birth is an example of **nominal** data since it contains information (such as Topeka, Kansas) to which no order can be applied.

e) Visual acuity is probably best thought of as an example of **ordinal** data since the number of categories used are quite limited (usually 11 or fewer categories) and the distance between the categories is not constant.

f) Family income might be considered an example of **continuous** data since there are a large number of evenly spaced values, but information on family income is usually collected by using a few intervals of income, making it more reasonable to consider these data to be **ordinal** rather than continuous.

2.2

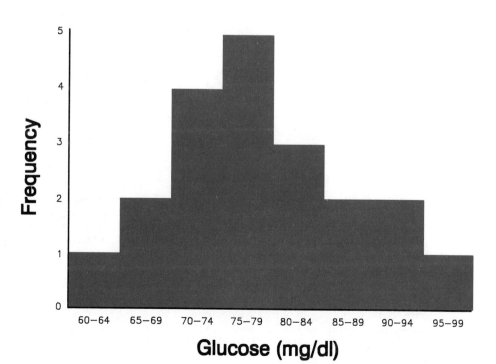

2.3 To calculate the mean, we first sum all the values of fasting blood glucose in Problem 2.2. That sum is 1,573.8 mg/dl. Next, we use Equation 2.1:

$$\mu = \frac{\Sigma Y_i}{N} = \frac{1,573.8}{20} = 78.69 \text{ mg/dl}$$

To determine the median, we begin by listing the data in numeric order. The following table represents the fasting blood glucose values arranged in ascending order.

Patient	Glucose (mg/dl)
TI	63.3
FG	65.4
RP	68.4
EL	70.2
GT	72.7
NS	73.5
CE	73.6
LD	75.3
SH	76.6
MA	76.9
WM	78.8
DV	78.9
BW	80.7
AH	82.0
HR	82.9
KC	86.3
PB	87.7
ON	92.1
JF	92.7
YJ	95.8
Total	1,573.8

Next, we find the value for which half of the data are greater and half are smaller. Since we have 20 patients, the median is between the values for the tenth (patient MA) and eleventh (patient WM) largest fasting blood glucose values. Thus, the median is halfway between 76.9 and 78.8 mg/dl or 77.85 mg/dl.

To determine the mode for continuous data, we must examine a histogram or frequency polygon. The actual value of the mode is influenced by the intervals of data we have decided to use to create the histogram or frequency polygon. If we use the histogram in Problem 2.2, we can see that the most frequent data range is 75–79 mg/dl (representing values from 75.0 up to, but not including, 80.0). Thus, we define the mode as being in the center of this range, which is 77.5 mg/dl.

The first thing we must do in calculating the variance and/or the standard deviation is to determine the sum of the squared deviations of each data value from the mean (the sum of squares). Those squared deviations are presented in the following table, and their sum is found to be equal to 1,539.958 (mg/dl)^2.

Patient	Glucose (mg/dl)	$\Sigma\,(\Upsilon_i - \mu)$	$\Sigma\,(\Upsilon_i - \mu)^2$
WM	78.8	0.11	0.0121
EL	70.2	−8.49	72.0801
RP	68.4	−10.29	105.8841
TI	63.3	−15.39	236.8521
YJ	95.8	17.11	292.7521
ON	92.1	13.41	179.8281
PB	87.7	9.01	81.1801
AH	82.0	3.31	10.9561
SH	76.6	−2.09	4.3681
DV	78.9	0.21	0.0441
FG	65.4	−13.29	176.6241
GT	72.7	−5.99	35.8801
HR	82.9	4.21	17.7241
JF	92.7	14.01	196.2801
KC	86.3	7.61	57.9121
LD	75.3	−3.39	11.4921
CE	73.6	−5.09	25.9081
BW	80.7	2.01	4.0401
NS	73.5	−5.19	26.9361
MA	76.9	−1.79	3.2041
Total	1,573.8	0.00	1,539.9580

Next, we use Equation 2.4 to calculate the variance of data in the population.

$$\sigma^2 = \frac{\Sigma(\Upsilon_i - \mu)^2}{N} = \frac{1,539.958}{20} = 76.9979 \ (mg/dl)^2$$

The standard deviation of the data is the square root of the variance of the data. Thus,

$$\sigma = \sqrt{\sigma^2} = \sqrt{76.9979} = 8.7748 \ mg/dl$$

2.4 To solve this problem, we need to convert 145 µg/dl to a standard normal deviate so that we can use Table B.1 to determine the probability of getting a level of blood iron equal to or higher than this value. Conversion to a standard normal deviate involves subtraction of the population's mean and division by the standard deviation of the data as shown in Equation 2.5.

$$z = \frac{\Upsilon_i - \mu}{\sigma} = \frac{145 - 95}{\sqrt{625}} = 2.00$$

Thus, on the standard normal scale, 145 µg/dl from a population with a mean of 95 µg/dl and a variance of the data of 625 (µg/dl)² is equal to 2.00.

Next, we use Table B.1 to find the area in one tail of the standard normal distribution that is associated with a standard normal deviate of 2.00 or more. That area is 0.0228. Thus, the probability of getting a standard normal deviate equal to or greater than 2.00 or a level of blood iron equal to or greater than 145 µg/dl is 0.0228.

CHAPTER 3

3.1 In Problem 2.3, we calculated the variance and standard deviation as follows:

$$\sigma^2 = \frac{\Sigma(Y_i - \mu)^2}{N} = \frac{1{,}539.958}{20} = 76.9979 \ (\text{mg/dl})^2$$

$$\sigma = \sqrt{\sigma^2} = \sqrt{76.9979} = 8.7748 \ \text{mg/dl}$$

Assuming that the 20 patients are a random sample from a much larger population, we estimate the variance of data in the population using Equation 3.2:

$$s^2 = \frac{\Sigma(Y_i - \overline{Y})^2}{n-1} = \frac{1{,}539.958}{19} = 81.0504 \ (\text{mg/dl})^2$$

$$s = \sqrt{s^2} = \sqrt{81.0504} = 9.0028 \ \text{mg/dl}$$

Thus, the sample's estimates of the variance and standard deviation of data in the population are higher values than are the values we calculated as if the 20 patients had been the entire population. Recall that the reason for the higher value of the sample's estimates of the variance and standard deviation of data in the population is that samples are unlikely to include extreme values from the population.

3.2 In this problem, we are given the following information:

$$\sigma^2 = 1.21 \ \text{mg\%}^2 \qquad \overline{Y} = 4.2 \ \text{mg\%} \qquad n = 16$$

Using this information, we are asked to calculate a 95% confidence interval for the population's mean. The population's distribution of interest to us, therefore, is the distribution of means from all possible samples. To use that distribution, we must know (or estimate) its parameters. The parameters of the population's distribution of means from all possible samples are the population's mean and standard error (the standard deviation of means from all possible samples). The goal of our analysis is to estimate the population's mean. The standard error can be calculated from the variance of the data in the population and the sample's size by taking the square root of the variance of means calculated in Equation 3.4.

$$SE = \sqrt{\sigma_{\overline{Y}}^2} = \sqrt{\frac{\sigma^2}{n}} = \sqrt{\frac{1.21}{16}} = 0.275 \ \text{mg\%}$$

Since we have no reason to believe that the sample's mean deviates in a specific direction from the population's mean, we should calculate a two-tailed interval. From Table B.1, we find that a standard normal deviate with an area of $0.05/2 = 0.025$ in each tail is equal to 1.96. Then, using Equation 3.7:

$$\mu = \overline{Y} \pm (z_{\alpha/2} \cdot SE) = 4.2 \pm (1.96 \cdot 0.275) = 3.66, \ 4.74 \ \text{mg\%}$$

3.3 As in any test of statistical inference, it is the null hypothesis that is appropriate to test. The null hypothesis makes the specific statement that the population's mean is equal to 4.8 mg%. Keeping that in mind, we use Equation 3.5 to convert the sample's mean to a standard normal deviate.

$$z = \frac{\overline{Y} - \mu_{\overline{Y}}}{SE} = \frac{4.2 - 4.8}{0.275} = -2.182$$

Since we have a two-tailed alternative hypothesis and an α of 0.05, we compare our calculated standard normal deviate to the value from Table B.1 that corresponds to an area of $0.05/2 = 0.025$ in each tail of the standard normal distribution. That value is 1.96. Since the absolute value of our calculated value (2.182) is greater than 1.96 (the value from Table B.1), we reject the null hypothesis and accept, by elimination, the alternative hypothesis.

3.4 To solve this problem, we must first calculate the differences between levels of serum cholesterol before and after the intervention.

Patient	Before	After	Difference
1	281	269	12
2	259	245	14
3	272	271	1
4	264	248	16
5	253	229	24
6	297	276	21
7	312	289	23
8	275	260	15
Total			126

Thus, the point estimate for the mean of the differences between levels of cholesterol in the population is (from Equation 3.1):

$$\overline{Y} = \frac{\Sigma Y_i}{n} = \frac{126}{8} = 15.75 \text{ mg/dl}$$

To test the null hypothesis that the population's mean of the differences is equal to zero, we must first estimate the standard error of the mean. To begin, we must calculate the sum of the squared deviations between each difference and the mean of the differences in our sample. The following table shows that calculation.

Patient	Before	After	Difference (Y_i)	$(Y_i - \overline{Y})$	$(Y_i - \overline{Y})^2$
1	281	269	12	-3.75	14.0625
2	259	245	14	-1.75	3.0625
3	272	271	1	-14.75	217.5625
4	264	248	16	0.25	0.0625

Patient	Before	After	Difference (Y_i)	$(Y_i - \overline{Y})$	$(Y_i - \overline{Y})^2$
5	253	229	24	8.25	68.0625
6	297	276	21	5.25	27.5625
7	312	289	23	7.25	52.5625
8	275	260	15	−0.75	0.5625
Total			126	0	383.5000

Next, we can estimate the variance of the data in the population, using Equation 3.2.

$$s^2 = \frac{\Sigma(Y_i - \overline{Y})^2}{n - 1} = \frac{383.5}{7} = 54.7857 \ (\text{mg/dl})^2$$

Then, we use this estimate of the variance of data in the population to calculate the standard error (i.e., the estimate of the standard deviation of the distribution of all possible means of the differences).

$$SE = \sqrt{\frac{s^2}{n}} = \sqrt{\frac{54.7857}{8}} = 2.6169 \ \text{mg/dl}$$

There are two somewhat unusual features to the test of the null hypothesis that we are conducting in this problem. First, we are willing to take only a 1% chance (in contrast to the more usual 5% chance) of making a Type I error. Second, the alternative hypothesis is one-tailed (since we consider an increase in serum cholesterol levels after intervention to be impossible). Thus, the standard normal deviate to which we will compare our sample's value is the value in Table B.1 that corresponds to an area of 0.01 in one tail of the standard normal distribution. That value is 2.33 (or 2.327 if you wish to interpolate a value between 2.32 and 2.33).

With this in mind, we convert our sample's mean of the differences to a standard normal deviate using Equation 3.5. Since inference is performed assuming that the null hypothesis is true, we assume that the mean in the population is equal to zero in that calculation.

$$z = \frac{\overline{Y} - \mu_{\overline{Y}}}{SE} = \frac{15.75 - 0}{2.6169} = 6.02$$

Since our calculated standard normal deviate (6.02) is greater than the value from Table B.1, we reject the null hypothesis and accept, by elimination, the alternative hypothesis that the mean of the differences in the population is greater than zero.

CHAPTER 4

4.1 The first thing we have to do to solve this problem is to estimate the standard error of means from all possible samples.

$$SE = \frac{s}{\sqrt{n}} = \frac{25.1}{\sqrt{18}} = 5.916 \ \text{mm Hg}$$

Next, we use Equation 4.6 to calculate the interval estimate. In that calculation, we use a

Student's t value from Table B.2 that corresponds to $18 - 1 = 17$ degrees of freedom and a two-tailed α equal to 0.05. That Student's t value is equal to 2.110.

$$\mu = \overline{Y} \pm (t_{\alpha/2, df=17} \cdot SE) = 87.5 \pm (2.110 \cdot 5.916) = 75.02, 99.98 \text{ mm Hg}$$

4.2 There are two somewhat unusual features to this problem that we should recognize at the onset. First, the alternative hypothesis is one-tailed rather than two-tailed. Second, the α is equal to 0.01 rather than 0.05. With those features in mind and using the standard error calculated in Problem 4.1, we can use Equation 4.7 to calculate a Student's t value. Since the null hypothesis states that the mean in the population is equal to 60 mm Hg, we use that value in our calculation.

$$t = \frac{\overline{Y} - \mu_0}{SE} = \frac{87.5 - 60}{5.916} = 4.648$$

We compare that Student's t value to a value from Table B.2 corresponding to $18 - 1 = 17$ degrees of freedom and a one-tailed α equal to 0.01. That Student's t value is equal to 2.567. Since our calculated value (4.648) is greater than 2.567, we reject the null hypothesis and accept, by elimination, the alternative hypothesis that the mean is greater than 60 mm Hg in the population.

4.3 The first step in solving this problem is to calculate the differences between body mass index measurements on each individual. Next, we calculate the mean of those differences and the squared deviations between each difference and the mean of the differences. Those steps are summarized in the following table.

Experimental	Standard	Difference	$Y_i - \overline{Y}$	$(Y_i - \overline{Y})^2$
23.4	28.2	−4.8	−2.69	7.2361
27.2	29.3	−2.1	0.01	0.0001
30.3	27.9	2.4	4.51	20.3401
22.7	27.6	−4.9	−2.79	7.7841
28.5	24.8	3.7	5.81	33.7561
33.8	33.3	−0.5	1.61	2.5921
29.3	33.1	−3.8	−1.69	2.8561
26.1	30.0	−3.9	−1.79	3.2041
23.0	27.7	−4.7	−2.59	6.7081
31.9	34.4	−2.5	−0.39	0.1521
		−21.1	0	84.6290

The mean of the differences in body mass indices is equal to $-21.1/10 = -2.11 \text{ kg/m}^2$. The standard error of that mean is estimated from the estimate of the variance of data in the population as follows:

$$s^2 = \frac{\Sigma(Y_i - \overline{Y})^2}{n - 1} = \frac{84.6290}{10 - 1} = 9.4032 \text{ (kg/m}^2)^2$$

$$SE = \sqrt{\frac{s^2}{n}} = \sqrt{\frac{9.4032}{10}} = 0.9697 \text{ kg/m}^2$$

Then we convert our sample's estimate to a Student's t value, using Equation 4.7.

$$t = \frac{\overline{Y} - \mu_0}{SE} = \frac{-2.11 - 0}{0.9697} = -2.176$$

That Student's t value is compared to a value from Table B.2 corresponding to $10 - 1 = 9$ degrees of freedom and a two-tailed α equal to 0.05. Since the absolute value of our calculated Student's t value (2.176) is less than the value from the table (2.262), we do not reject the null hypothesis. (Note that, if we ignored the role of chance in estimating the variance of the data in the population and used the table of standard normal deviates in this problem, we would have compared 2.176 to 1.96 from Table B.1 and incorrectly rejected the null hypothesis.)

4.4 To answer this problem, we use the mean of the differences (-2.11 kg/m^2) and the standard error (0.9697 kg/m^2) estimated in Problem 4.3. The method of calculating this interval estimate is shown in Equation 4.6. The Student's t value that we use in this calculation is the value in Table B.2 that corresponds to $10 - 1 = 9$ degrees of freedom and a two-tailed α equal to 0.01. That Student's t value is 3.250.

$$\mu = \overline{Y} \pm (t_{\alpha/2, df=9} \cdot SE) = -2.11 \pm (3.250 \cdot 0.9697) = -5.26, 1.04 \ \text{kg/m}^2$$

CHAPTER 5

5.1 Conversion to an ordinal scale can be accomplished by ranking. Since we are given no special criterion for this conversion, we can simply rank the differences from lowest to highest.

Experimental	Standard	Difference	Rank
23.4	28.2	−4.8	2
27.2	29.3	−2.1	7
30.3	27.9	2.4	9
22.7	27.6	−4.9	1
28.5	24.8	3.7	10
33.8	33.3	−0.5	8
29.3	33.1	−3.8	5
26.1	30.0	−3.9	4
23.0	27.7	−4.7	3
31.9	34.4	−2.5	6

5.2 In this problem, we are told that we will perform statistical inference on the differences converted to an ordinal scale. We must, therefore, perform that conversion according to the rules of the statistical test we will use. That test is the Wilcoxon signed-rank test. In the Wilcoxon signed-rank test, we rank the observed differences ignoring their signs and then attach the sign of the difference to the rank.

Experimental	Standard	Difference	Rank	Signed Rank
23.4	28.2	−4.8	9	−9
27.2	29.3	−2.1	2	−2
30.3	27.9	2.4	3	3
22.7	27.6	−4.9	10	−10
28.5	24.8	3.7	5	5
33.8	33.3	−0.5	1	−1
29.3	33.1	−3.8	6	−6
26.1	30.0	−3.9	7	−7
23.0	27.7	−4.7	8	−8
31.9	34.4	−2.5	4	−4

The test statistic in the Wilcoxon signed-rank test is the smaller of the sign-specific sums of ranks. In this case, the sum of the ranks for the positive values (T_+ = 8) is smaller than the sum of the ranks for the negative values (T_- = 47). Thus, we compare T_+ = 8 with the value in Table B.3. In Table B.3, we find that a Wilcoxon signed-rank test statistic of 8 is associated with a two-tailed α of 0.05 and a sample size of 10. Normally, we would reject the null hypothesis if our calculated test statistic were less than the value in Table B.3 (remember that this is just the opposite of other test statistics) and fail to reject the null hypothesis if our calculated value were greater than the value in that table. Here, those two values are equal to each other. The usual practice in this situation is to reject the null hypothesis.

5.3 In Problem 4.3, we found a Student's t statistic of −2.176 associated with the null hypothesis that the mean of the differences is equal to zero. That Student's t statistic was less than the corresponding value from Table B.2 (2.262), and we failed to reject the null hypothesis. In Problem 5.2, we were able to reject the null hypothesis. If the assumptions of the Student's t test had been met, we would expect the Student's t test to have more statistical power (i.e., be more able to reject a false null hypothesis) than the Wilcoxon signed-rank test. Since we found the opposite situation here, we suspect that the assumptions of the Student's t test were not met and that the Wilcoxon signed-rank test is more appropriate.

CHAPTER 6

6.1 To estimate a population's risk, we use Equation 6.2.

$$\text{Risk}_{3\text{-yr}} = \frac{\text{Number developing disease from time 0 to time } t}{\text{Total number without disease at time 0}} = \frac{18}{300} = 0.06$$

Since the point estimate of this probability is between 0.05 and 0.95, the normal approximation to the binomial is an appropriate approach to calculate an interval estimate. The standard error for the normal approximation to the binomial is given in Equation 6.5.

$$SE_p = \sqrt{\frac{p \cdot (1 - p)}{n}} = \sqrt{\frac{0.06 \cdot 0.94}{300}} = 0.0137$$

Then, we use Equation 6.7 to calculate the two-tailed confidence interval. From Table B.1, we find that a standard normal deviate corresponding to an area of 0.025 in each tail is equal to 1.96. Thus, we can be 95% confident that the three-year risk of peripheral neuropathy in the population that was sampled lies within the following interval:

$$\theta = p \pm (z_{\alpha/2} \cdot SE_p) = 0.06 \pm (1.96 \cdot 0.0137) = 0.033, 0.087$$

6.2 The first thing we need to do to estimate incidence is to calculate the total person-years of observation during which cases of neuropathy might have developed. Two separate contributions to the total number of person-years of observation time need to be calculated. The first is for those persons who developed neuropathy; we assume that, on the average, they developed neuropathy in the middle of the three-year study period. Once neuropathy developed, observation time for those individuals stopped. Thus, the 18 persons who developed neuropathy contributed $18 \cdot 1.5 = 27$ person-years. The second contribution is for those persons who remained disease-free during the three-year study period. Each of those individuals contribute 3 person-years, or $282 \cdot 3 = 846$ person-years collectively.

Now, we use Equation 6.3 to estimate the incidence (I) of peripheral neuropathy in the population from which the sample was drawn.

$$I = \frac{\text{Number developing disease}}{\text{Number of person-years}} = \frac{18}{27 + 846} = 0.021 \text{ per year}$$

We assume that incidence has a Poisson distribution regardless of the value of the point estimate. Therefore, we use the normal approximation to the Poisson to calculate an interval estimate to solve this problem. Since we want a 95%, two-tailed estimate, we use the standard normal deviate from Table B.1 that corresponds to an area of 0.025 in each tail of the standard normal distribution. That standard normal deviate is equal to 1.96. Then, using Equation 6.12, we calculate the interval estimate for the incidence of peripheral neuropathy in the population.

$$I = \frac{\left[\sqrt{a} \pm \left(z_{\alpha/2} \cdot \frac{1}{2}\right)\right]^2}{\text{person-years}} = \frac{\left[\sqrt{18} \pm \left(1.96 \cdot \frac{1}{2}\right)\right]^2}{873} = 0.012, 0.031 \text{ per year}$$

6.3 To calculate the point estimate for the prevalence of cataracts in the population that was sampled, we use Equation 6.1.

$$\text{Prevalence} = \frac{\text{Number with disease at time } t}{\text{Total number at time } t} = \frac{1,200}{2,000} = 0.60$$

Since the prevalence of cataracts in the population is estimated to be 0.60 and that prevalence is between 0.05 and 0.95, we assume that the prevalence of cataracts in the population has a binomial distribution. Thus, we use Equation 6.7, the normal approximation to the binomial distribution.

First, we need to estimate the standard error of our prevalence estimate from Equation 6.5.

$$SE_p = \sqrt{\frac{p \cdot (1 - p)}{n}} = \sqrt{\frac{0.60 \cdot (1 - 0.60)}{2000}} = 0.011$$

Then, we use Equation 6.7 to calculate the interval estimate. In that calculation, we use the standard normal deviate from Table B.1 associated with an area of 0.025 in one tail ($z = 1.96$).

$$\theta = p \pm (z_{\alpha/2} \cdot SE_p) = 0.60 \pm (1.96 \cdot 0.011) = 0.579, 0.621$$

6.4 Here, again, we use the normal approximation to the binomial. To convert our observed prevalence to the standard normal scale, we use Equation 6.4. The standard error we use in that calculation is not the same as the standard error estimated in Problem 6.3. The reason for using a different standard error is that, in inference, we assume that the null hypothesis is correct. Thus, the standard error is calculated using 0.45 instead of 0.60. That standard error, however, is very close in value to the standard error calculated in Problem 6.3.

$$z = \frac{p - \theta}{\sqrt{\dfrac{\theta \cdot (1 - \theta)}{n}}} = \frac{0.60 - 0.45}{0.011} = 13.48$$

We are told in this problem to allow for a probability of making a Type I error equal to 0.05 and that we should consider a two-tailed alternative hypothesis. Thus, we compare our calculated standard normal deviate to the value from Table B.1 corresponding to an area of 0.025 in each tail of the standard normal distribution. Since 13.48 is greater than the value from Table B.1 (1.96), we reject the null hypothesis and accept, by elimination, the alternative hypothesis.

CHAPTER 7

7.1 To calculate the sample's estimate of the correlation coefficient, we need to calculate the sums of squares and the sum of cross products. Those calculations are illustrated in the following table.

Diastolic Blood Pressure	Systolic Blood Pressure	$X_i - \overline{X}$	$Y_i - \overline{Y}$	$(X_i - \overline{X})^2$	$(Y_i - \overline{Y})^2$	$(Y_i - \overline{Y}) \cdot (X_i - \overline{X})$
70	116	−3.7	−7.2	13.69	51.84	26.64
73	122	−0.7	−1.2	0.49	1.44	0.84
65	119	−8.7	−4.2	75.69	17.64	36.54
77	133	3.3	9.8	10.89	96.04	32.34
81	128	7.3	4.8	53.29	23.04	35.04
68	115	−5.7	−8.2	32.49	67.24	46.74
74	120	0.3	−3.2	0.09	10.24	−0.96
71	124	−2.7	0.8	7.29	0.64	−2.16
82	130	8.3	6.8	68.89	46.24	56.44
76	125	2.3	1.8	5.29	3.24	4.14
737	1,232	0	0	268.10	317.60	235.60

Then, we use Equation 7.3 to calculate the sample's estimate of the population's correlation coefficient.

$$r = \frac{\Sigma(Y_i - \overline{Y})(X_i - \overline{X})}{\sqrt{\Sigma(Y_i - \overline{Y})^2 \cdot \Sigma(X_i - \overline{X})^2}} = \frac{235.60}{\sqrt{317.60 \cdot 268.10}} = 0.807$$

The coefficient of determination is the square of the correlation coefficient (Equation 7.4). The square of 0.807 is 0.652. That implies that 65.2% of the variation in systolic blood pressure is associated with variation in diastolic blood pressure.

To test the null hypothesis that the population's correlation coefficient is equal to zero, we first need to calculate the sample's estimate of the standard error. This is done by using Equation 7.5.

$$SE_r = \sqrt{\frac{1 - r^2}{n - 2}} = \sqrt{\frac{1 - 0.807^2}{10 - 2}} = 0.209$$

Next, we use Equation 7.6 to convert our sample's correlation coefficient to a Student's t value.

$$t = \frac{r - \rho_0}{SE_r} = \frac{0.807 - 0}{0.209} = 3.87$$

Finally, we compare that calculated Student's t value to the value from Table B.2 that corresponds to a two-tailed α of 0.05 and $10 - 2 = 8$ degrees of freedom. Since our calculated value (3.87) is greater than the value from Table B.2 (2.306), we reject the null hypothesis that the correlation coefficient is equal to zero in the population and accept, by elimination, the alternative hypothesis that the correlation coefficient is not equal to zero.

7.2 Here we have a nominal independent variable (training/no training) that divides values of the continuous dependent variable (grade point average) into two groups. To compare values of the dependent variable between those groups, we examine the difference between the means of the dependent variable values. In the following table, we have calculated the sums of the dependent variable values in the two groups, as well as the sums of squares for those values (in preparation for estimation of the variance of data in the population).

Training	$Y_{T_i} - \overline{Y}_T$	$(Y_{T_i} - \overline{Y}_T)^2$	No Training	$Y_{NT_i} - \overline{Y}_{NT}$	$(Y_{NT_i} - \overline{Y}_{NT})^2$
98	9.00	81.00	81	−5.62	31.64
85	−4.00	16.00	86	−0.62	0.39
79	−10.00	100.00	99	12.38	153.14
86	−3.00	9.00	85	−1.62	2.64
93	4.00	16.00	78	−8.62	74.39
94	5.00	25.00	84	−2.62	6.89
88	−1.00	1.00	89	2.38	5.64
			91	4.38	19.14
623	0	248.00	693	0	293.88

First, we calculate an estimate from our sample's observations of the difference between the mean grade point averages in the population from which the sample was drawn.

$$\overline{Y}_T - \overline{Y}_{NT} = \frac{623}{7} - \frac{693}{8} = 2.4$$

Next, in preparation for calculation of the standard error, we estimate the variance of the distribution of data in the population. We begin by calculating separate estimates of that variance for each of the two groups of dependent variable values.

$$s_T^2 = \frac{248.00}{7 - 1} = 41.33$$

$$s_{NT}^2 = \frac{293.88}{8 - 1} = 41.98$$

Then, we combine those variance estimates, using their degrees of freedom as their weights. That pooled estimate is calculated using Equation 7.29.

$$s_p^2 = \frac{[(n_T - 1) \cdot s_T^2] + [(n_{NT} - 1) \cdot s_{NT}^2]}{(n_T - 1) + (n_{NT} - 1)}$$

$$= \frac{[(7 - 1) \cdot 41.33] + [(8 - 1) \cdot 41.98]}{(7 - 1) + (8 - 1)} = 41.68$$

Now, we use Equation 7.30 to calculate the sample's estimate of the standard error of differences between means.

$$SE_{\overline{Y}_T - \overline{Y}_{NT}} = \sqrt{\frac{s_p^2}{n_T} + \frac{s_p^2}{n_{NT}}} = \sqrt{\frac{41.68}{7} + \frac{41.68}{8}} = 3.34$$

To convert our observed difference between mean grade point averages to the Student's t scale, we use Equation 7.31.

$$t = \frac{(\overline{Y}_T - \overline{Y}_{NT}) - (\mu_T - \mu_{NT})}{SE_{\overline{Y}_T - \overline{Y}_{NT}}} = \frac{2.4 - 0}{3.34} = 0.711$$

We compare that calculated Student's t value with a value from Table B.2 that corresponds to a two-tailed α of 0.05 and $15 - 2 = 13$ degrees of freedom ($t = 2.160$). Since our calculated value (0.711) is less than 2.160, we do not reject the null hypothesis.

7.3 To estimate the slope and intercept of the regression line, we need to calculate four estimates from our sample's observations: the mean of the dependent variable, the mean of the independent variable, the sum of squares of the independent variable, and the sum of cross products. The following table shows those calculations.

Dose	Change in Hematocrit	$X_i - \overline{X}$	$(X_i - \overline{X})^2$	$Y_i - \overline{Y}$	$(Y_i - \overline{Y})(X_i - \overline{X})$
0	3	−7.5	56.25	−3.55	26.625
0	−4	−7.5	56.25	−10.55	79.125
0	0	−7.5	56.25	−6.55	49.125
0	1	−7.5	56.25	−5.55	41.625
0	−1	−7.5	56.25	−7.55	56.625
5	2	−2.5	6.25	−4.55	11.375
5	0	−2.5	6.25	−6.55	16.375
5	7	−2.5	6.25	0.45	−1.125
5	−1	−2.5	6.25	−7.55	18.875

Dose	Change in Hematocrit	$X_i - \overline{X}$	$(X_i - \overline{X})^2$	$Y_i - \overline{Y}$	$(Y_i - \overline{Y})(X_i - \overline{X})$
5	5	−2.5	6.25	−1.55	3.875
10	8	2.5	6.25	1.45	3.625
10	4	2.5	6.25	−2.55	−6.375
10	11	2.5	6.25	4.45	11.125
10	16	2.5	6.25	9.45	23.625
10	9	2.5	6.25	2.45	6.125
15	12	7.5	56.25	5.45	40.875
15	17	7.5	56.25	10.45	78.375
15	15	7.5	56.25	8.45	63.375
15	9	7.5	56.25	2.45	18.375
15	18	7.5	56.25	11.45	85.875
150	131	0	625.00	0	627.500

To estimate the slope of the regression line in the population, we use Equation 7.10.

$$b = \frac{\Sigma(Y_i - \overline{Y})(X_i - \overline{X})}{\Sigma(X_i - \overline{X})^2} = \frac{627.500}{625.00} = 1.004$$

To estimate the intercept of the regression line in the population, we use Equation 7.12.

$$a = \overline{Y} - b\overline{X} = \frac{131}{20} - \left(1.004\,\frac{150}{20}\right) = -0.977$$

Thus, the sample's estimate of the population's regression line is:

$$\acute{Y} = -0.977 + 1.004X$$

Next, we want to test the omnibus null hypothesis. In preparation for that test, we need to estimate the three sources of variation for data represented by the dependent variable. The table below shows how we calculate the residual sum of squares $[\Sigma(Y_i - \acute{Y}_i)^2]$ and the total sum of squares $[\Sigma(Y_i - \overline{Y})^2]$.

Dose	Change in Hematocrit	$\acute{Y}_i$	$Y_i - \acute{Y}_i$	$(Y_i - \acute{Y}_i)^2$	$Y_i - \overline{Y}$	$(Y_i - \overline{Y})^2$
0	3	−0.98	3.98	15.816	−3.55	12.60
0	−4	−0.98	−3.02	9.139	−10.55	111.30
0	0	−0.98	0.98	0.954	−6.55	42.90
0	1	−0.98	1.98	3.909	−5.55	30.80
0	−1	−0.98	−0.02	0.001	−7.55	57.00
5	2	4.04	−2.04	4.166	−4.55	20.70
5	0	4.04	−4.04	16.330	−6.55	42.90

Dose	Change in Hematocrit	$\hat{Y}_i$	$Y_i - \hat{Y}_i$	$(Y_i - \hat{Y}_i)^2$	$Y_i - \overline{Y}$	$(Y_i - \overline{Y})^2$
5	7	4.04	2.96	8.756	0.45	0.20
5	−1	4.04	−5.04	25.412	−7.55	57.00
5	5	4.04	0.96	0.920	−1.55	2.40
10	8	9.06	−1.06	1.121	1.45	2.10
10	4	9.06	−5.06	25.593	−2.55	6.50
10	11	9.06	1.94	3.767	4.45	19.80
10	16	9.06	6.94	48.177	9.45	89.30
10	9	9.06	−0.06	0.003	2.45	6.00
15	12	14.08	−2.08	4.314	5.45	29.70
15	17	14.08	2.92	8.544	10.45	109.20
15	15	14.08	0.92	0.852	8.45	71.40
15	9	14.08	−5.08	25.776	2.45	6.00
15	18	14.08	3.92	15.390	11.45	131.10
150	131	131.00	0	218.940	0	848.95

The omnibus null hypothesis is tested by examining the ratio of the regression mean square and the residual mean square. The residual mean square (or the average variation in data represented by the dependent variable remaining after taking into account the relationship with the independent variable) is equal to the residual sum of squares divided by the residual degrees of freedom (Equation 7.15).

$$s_{Y|X}^2 = \frac{\Sigma(Y_i - \hat{Y}_i)^2}{n - 2} = \frac{218.940}{20 - 2} = 12.163$$

The regression mean square (or the average variation in data represented by the dependent variable accounted for by the relationship with the independent variable) is equal to the regression sum of squares divided by the regression degrees of freedom (always equal to one when we have one independent variable). The regression sum of squares is found by subtracting the residual sum of squares from the total sum of squares (Equation 7.16).

$$\Sigma(\hat{Y}_i - \overline{Y})^2 = \Sigma(Y_i - \overline{Y})^2 - \Sigma(Y_i - \hat{Y}_i)^2 = 848.950 - 218.940 = 630.01$$

Thus, the sample's estimate of the regression mean square is equal to the following (from Equation 7.18):

$$s_{reg}^2 = \frac{\Sigma(\hat{Y}_i - \overline{Y})^2}{1} = \frac{630.01}{1} = 630.01$$

To test the omnibus null hypothesis, we divide the regression mean square by the residual mean square. The result is an F ratio (Equation 7.22).

$$F = \frac{s_{reg}^2}{s_{Y|X}^2} = \frac{630.01}{12.163} = 51.796$$

From Table B.4, we find that an F ratio corresponding to an α of 0.05, 1 degree of freedom in the numerator, and $20 - 2 = 18$ degrees of freedom in the denominator is equal to 4.41. Since 51.797 is greater than 4.41, we reject the omnibus null hypothesis and accept, by elimination, the alternative hypothesis that there is a relationship between the dependent and independent variables in the population.

7.4 To estimate the population's correlation coefficient, we need to know the sum of cross products, the sum of squares for the dependent variable, and the sum of squares for the independent variable. All three of those values were calculated in Problem 7.3. Thus, the sample's estimate of the population's correlation coefficient is as follows (from Equation 7.3).

$$r = \frac{\Sigma(Y_i - \overline{Y})(X_i - \overline{X})}{\sqrt{\Sigma(Y_i - \overline{Y})^2 \cdot \Sigma(X_i - \overline{X})^2}} = \frac{627.250}{\sqrt{848.95 \cdot 625.00}} = 0.861$$

In general, a correlation coefficient is interpreted by examining its square (the coefficient of determination). The square of 0.861 is 0.742. That implies that 74.2% of the variation in data represented by the dependent variable is accounted for by the regression with the independent variable. In this particular case, however, the relevance of the correlation coefficient is questionable because the distribution of doses in the sample is not a naturalistic sample from some population of interest. Rather, it is a purposive sample, reflecting the choice of the researcher. Thus, the correlation coefficient has no proper interpretation relative to the population that was sampled to obtain the data in Problem 7.3. If we wish to address the relationship between dose and percentage of fetal hemoglobin in that population, we should estimate the straight line in a regression analysis, such as in Problem 7.3.

CHAPTER 8

8.1 First, we convert values of the dependent and independent variables to ranks. Then, we find the squared differences between the rank of each value of the dependent variable and the rank of its corresponding value of the independent variable. The following table shows those calculations:

Diastolic Blood Pressure (X_i)	Rank X_i	Systolic Blood Pressure (Y_i)	Rank Y_i	d_i	d_i^2
70	3	116	2	1	1
73	5	122	5	0	0
65	1	119	3	−2	4
77	8	133	10	−2	4
81	9	128	8	1	1
68	2	115	1	1	1
74	6	120	4	2	4
71	4	124	6	−2	4
82	10	130	9	1	1
76	7	125	7	0	0
				0	20

To estimate Spearman's correlation coefficient, we use Equation 8.1.

$$r_s = 1 - \frac{6 \cdot \Sigma d_i^2}{n^3 - n} = 1 - \frac{6 \cdot 20}{10^3 - 10} = 0.879$$

In Problem 7.1, we found Pearson's correlation coefficient to be 0.807. The fact that Spearman's correlation coefficient is a little larger than Pearson's correlation coefficient indicates the usual situation in which the ranks of two continuous variables have a relationship that is closer to a perfect linear (straight line) one than is the relationship between those variables when compared on a continuous scale.

8.2 First, we convert values of the dependent and independent variables to ranks. Then, we find the squared differences between the ranks of each value of the dependent variable and the rank of its corresponding value of the independent variable. The following table shows those calculations:

Maternal Age (X_i)	Rank X_i	Birth Weight (Y_i)	Rank Y_i	d_i	d_i^2
31	20.5	3,609	19.5	1.0	1.00
27	15.5	3,831	23	−7.5	56.25
19	4	3,110	9	−5.0	25.00
24	10.5	3,373	15	−4.5	20.25
32	22	4,115	25	−3.0	9.00
37	24	3,740	21.5	2.5	6.25
19	4	2,527	2	2.0	4.00
21	6.5	2,869	6	0.5	0.25
30	18.5	3,392	16	2.5	6.25
28	17	3,319	13	4.0	16.00
18	2	2,532	3	−1.0	1.00
22	8	2,860	5	3.0	9.00
31	20.5	3,452	17	3.5	12.25
17	1	2,484	1	0.0	0.00
39	25	3,507	18	7.0	49.00
26	13.5	3,094	8	5.5	30.25
30	18.5	3,740	21.5	−3.0	9.00
24	10.5	3,368	14	−3.5	12.25
21	6.5	2,842	4	2.5	6.25
19	4	3,010	7	−3.0	9.00
33	23	3,938	24	−1.0	1.00
26	13.5	3,289	12	1.5	2.25
23	9	3,240	11	−2.0	4.00
27	15.5	3,115	10	5.5	30.25
25	12	3,609	19.5	−7.5	56.25
				0.0	376.00

In this set of observations, there are several sets of tied ranks. Thus, we should use Equation 8.2 to estimate the Spearman's correlation coefficient. In preparation for using Equation 8.2, let us first calculate the correction factors for tied ranks. For the independent variable, there are seven groups of ties. One group of ties contains three maternal ages that are the same (19 years). The other six groups of ties each contain two maternal ages that are the same (21, 24, 26, 27, 30, and 31 years). Therefore, the correction factor for tied ranks among values of the independent variable is:

$$\Sigma T_X = \frac{\Sigma(t_X^3 - t_X)}{12} = \frac{(3^3 - 3) + 6(2^3 - 2)}{12} = 5.0$$

For the dependent variable, there are two groups of ties. Both groups contain two birth weights that are the same (3,609 and 3,740 grams). Thus, the correction factor for tied ranks among values of the dependent variable is:

$$\Sigma T_Y = \frac{\Sigma(t_Y^3 - t_Y)}{12} = \frac{2(2^3 - 2)}{12} = 1.0$$

Now, we are ready to use Equation 8.2 to estimate Spearman's correlation coefficient.

$$r_s = \frac{\frac{n^3 - n}{6} - \Sigma d_i^2 - \Sigma T_X - \Sigma T_Y}{\sqrt{\left[\frac{n^3 - n}{6} - (2 \cdot \Sigma T_X)\right] \cdot \left[\frac{n^3 - n}{6} - (2 \cdot \Sigma T_Y)\right]}}$$

$$= \frac{\frac{25^3 - 25}{6} - 376 - 5.0 - 1.0}{\sqrt{\left[\frac{25^3 - 25}{6} - (2 \cdot 5.0)\right] \cdot \left[\frac{25^3 - 25}{6} - (2 \cdot 1.0)\right]}} = 0.855$$

The null hypothesis that Spearman's correlation coefficient is equal to zero in the population is tested in the same way regardless of whether there are tied ranks or not. It is only the point estimate that is calculated differently when the data set includes tied ranks. Thus, we compare our point estimate to a value from Table B.5. From that table, we find that a Spearman's correlation of 0.398 corresponds to a two-tailed α of 0.05 and a sample's size of 25. Since our calculated value (0.855) is greater than 0.398, we reject the null hypothesis and accept, by elimination, that Spearman's correlation coefficient is not equal to zero in the population.

8.3 In this data set, we have a continuous dependent variable (grade point average) and a nominal independent variable (an indicator of assertiveness training). If we wish to avoid the assumption that grade point averages have a Gaussian distribution, we can convert values of that dependent variable to ranks and perform a Mann-Whitney test. Then, we sum the ranks of the dependent variable values separately for each value of the independent variable. Those procedures are illustrated in the following table:

Training	Rank	No Training	Rank
98	14	81	3
85	5.5	86	7.5

Training	Rank	No Training	Rank
79	2	99	15
86	7.5	85	5.5
93	12	78	1
94	13	84	4
88	9	89	10
		91	11
	63.0		57.0

Now, we calculate the Mann-Whitney U statistic taking (arbitrarily) the trained group as group 1. Using Equation 8.3 we find the following:

$$U = (n_1 \cdot n_2) + \frac{n_1 \cdot (n_1 + 1)}{2} - R_1 = (7 \cdot 8) + \frac{7 \cdot (7 + 1)}{2} - 63.0 = 21.0$$

Next, we calculate the Mann-Whitney U statistic taking the untrained group as group 1. Using the shortcut method in Equation 8.4 we get the following value for U':

$$U' = (n_1 \cdot n_2) - U = (7 \cdot 8) - 21.0 = 35.0$$

Finally, we compare the larger of U and U' (since the alternative hypothesis is two-tailed) to a value from Table B.6. In this case, U' is the larger of the two calculated values. From Table B.6, we find that a Mann-Whitney U value of 46 is associated with a two-tailed α of 0.05, 7 observations in one group, and 8 observations in the other group. Since our calculated value (35.0) is less than 46, we do not reject the null hypothesis.

8.4 In this data set, we have an ordinal dependent variable (visual acuity[1]) and a nominal independent variable (treatment). Thus, we are interested in applying the Mann-Whitney procedure to test the null hypothesis that visual acuity is the same in the two treatment groups. Visual acuity is an example of health research data that are considered to occur on a natural ordinal scale. Even with data that are naturally ordinal, we first need to convert those data to a scale of ranks before applying the statistical procedures we have discussed in Chapter 8. The following table shows that conversion and calculation of the sums of the ranks of the dependent variable values for each value of the independent variable. That calculation is easier if we arrange values of the dependent variable into two groups according to values of the independent variable than it is with each variable listed separately (as the data were presented in this problem).

Drug	Rank	Placebo	Rank
20/30	1.5	20/50	7.5
20/50	7.5	20/100	12.5
20/40	3.5	20/40	3.5

[1] As we discussed in Chapter 5, visual acuity is usually considered ordinal data since only a limited number of values are ordinarily possible to observe.

Drug	Rank	Placebo	Rank
20/50	7.5	20/200	15.5
20/50	7.5	20/100	12.5
20/100	12.5	20/50	7.5
20/50	7.5	20/100	12.5
20/30	1.5	20/200	15.5
	49.0		87.0

Now, we calculate the Mann-Whitney U statistic. Since the alternative hypothesis is one-tailed, we must choose group 1 to be the group specified in the alternative hypothesis to have the smaller sum of ranks. In this case, the alternative hypothesis suggests that the visual acuity will be better (i.e., have lower ranks) among persons taking the drug. Thus, the drug group is taken as group 1. Using Equation 8.3 we find the following:

$$U = (n_1 \cdot n_2) + \frac{n_1 \cdot (n_1 + 1)}{2} - R_1 = (8 \cdot 8) + \frac{8 \cdot (8 + 1)}{2} - 49.0 = 51.0$$

With a one-tailed alternative hypothesis, we do not calculate U'. From Table B.6, we find that a Mann-Whitney U value of 49 is associated with a one-tailed α of 0.05 and 8 observations in each group. Since our calculated value (51.0) is greater than the value from Table B.6, we reject the null hypothesis that visual acuity is the same regardless of treatment and accept, by elimination, that the drug improves visual acuity in the population from which the sample was drawn.

CHAPTER 9

9.1 In this problem, we are interested in the trend in a probability (the probability of developing diabetes) relative to the value of a continuous independent variable (time since diagnosis of hypertension). We first need to estimate that probability for each value of the independent variable.

Years Since Diagnosis (X_i)	Number with Hypertension (n_i)	Number with Diabetes	Probability of Diabetes (p_i)
1	306	0	0.0000
2	314	2	0.0064
3	321	2	0.0062
4	264	3	0.0114
5	215	2	0.0093
6	248	4	0.0161
7	179	3	0.0168
8	153	3	0.0196
	2,000	19	

Then, we estimate the mean of the dependent and independent variables.

$$\overline{X} = \frac{\Sigma n_i \cdot X_i}{\Sigma n_i} = \frac{(1 \cdot 306) + (2 \cdot 314) + \cdots + (8 \cdot 153)}{2,000} = 3.9965 \text{ years}$$

$$\overline{p} = \frac{\Sigma \text{ Number with diabetes}}{\Sigma n_i} = \frac{19}{2,000} = 0.0095$$

Next, we calculate the sums of squares and the sum of cross products for the dependent and independent variables.

Years Since Diagnosis (X_i)	Number with Hypertension (n_i)	$n_i(X_i - \overline{X})^2$	Probability of Diabetes (p_i)	$n_i(p_i - \overline{p})^2$	$n_i(X_i - \overline{X}) \cdot (p_i - \overline{p})$
1	306	2,747.6	0.0000	0.02762	8.7108
2	314	1,251.6	0.0064	0.00308	1.9626
3	321	318.8	0.0062	0.00343	1.0458
4	264	0.0	0.0114	0.00092	0.0017
5	215	216.5	0.0093	0.00001	−0.0426
6	248	995.5	0.0161	0.01090	3.2938
7	179	1,614.8	0.0168	0.00943	3.9030
8	153	2,452.3	0.0196	0.01563	6.1914
	2,000	9,597.0		0.07101	25.0665

Now, we are ready to estimate the slope (Equation 9.3) and intercept (Equation 9.4).

$$b = \frac{\Sigma n_i(p_i - \overline{p})(X_i - \overline{X})}{\Sigma n_i(X_i - \overline{X})^2} = \frac{25.0665}{9597.0} = 0.0026 \text{ per year}$$

$$a = \overline{p} - b\overline{X} = 0.0095 - (0.0026 \cdot 3.9965) = -0.0009$$

Thus, the straight line that estimates the probability of having diabetes for various time intervals since diagnosis of hypertension is:

$$\hat{p} = -0.0009 + 0.0026X$$

To prepare to test the omnibus hypothesis that time since diagnosis of hypertension does not help estimate the probability of having diabetes, we calculate the sum of the squared deviations between the estimated values of that probability ($\hat{p}$) and the overall probability ($\overline{p}$).

Years Since Diagnosis (X_i)	Number with Hypertension (n_i)	$\hat{p}_i$	$n_i(\hat{p}_i - \overline{p})^2$
1	306	0.0017	0.01874
2	314	0.0043	0.00854
3	321	0.0069	0.00217

Years Since Diagnosis (X_i)	Number with Hypertension (n_i)	$\hat{p}_i$	$n_i(\hat{p}_i - \bar{p})^2$
4	264	0.0095	0.00000
5	215	0.0121	0.00148
6	248	0.0147	0.00679
7	179	0.0173	0.01102
8	153	0.0200	0.01673
	2,000		0.06547

Finally, we use Equation 9.6 to calculate the chi-square value to test for trend.

$$\chi^2 = \frac{\Sigma n_i(\hat{p}_i - \bar{p})^2}{\bar{p}(1 - \bar{p})} = \frac{0.06547}{0.0095 \cdot 0.9905} = 6.958$$

We compare that chi-square value to the value from Table B.7 corresponding to one degree of freedom and an α of 0.05 (3.841).[2] Since 6.958 is larger than 3.841, we reject the omnibus null hypothesis and accept, by elimination, the alternative hypothesis that there is a relationship between time since diagnosis of hypertension and the probability of developing diabetes in the population from which the sample was drawn.

9.2 Since this is a case-control study, the odds ratio is the best measurement to summarize the association between dementia and reduced cerebral blood flow. Equation 9.10 is used to calculate the point estimate of the odds ratio.

$$OR = \frac{\frac{a}{c}}{\frac{b}{d}} = \frac{ad}{bc} = \frac{51 \cdot 103}{47 \cdot 99} = 1.13$$

9.3 The best way to test this null hypothesis is to use the Mantel-Haenszel chi procedure (Equation 9.19):

$$\chi_{M-H} = \frac{a - \frac{(a+b) \cdot (a+c)}{n}}{\sqrt{\frac{(a+b) \cdot (c+d) \cdot (a+c) \cdot (b+d)}{n^2 \cdot (n-1)}}}$$

$$= \frac{51 - \frac{(51+47) \cdot (51+99)}{300}}{\sqrt{\frac{(51+47) \cdot (99+103) \cdot (51+99) \cdot (47+103)}{300^2 \cdot (300-1)}}} = 0.492$$

[2]Remember that a one-tailed chi-square value with one degree of freedom corresponds to a two-tailed standard normal deviate and, thus, to a two-tailed alternative hypothesis.

We compare this Mantel-Haenszel chi statistic to a standard normal deviate representing an area of $0.05/2 = 0.025$ in each tail (1.96). Since 0.492 is less than 1.96, we do not reject the null hypothesis.

9.4 With paired data, we use a different method to estimate the odds ratio in the population (Equation 9.14):

$$OR = \frac{b}{c} = \frac{21}{17} = 1.24$$

In this case, the odds ratio from the paired data is very close to the odds ratio for the unpaired data (Problem 9.2), but that is not always the case.

Now, we test the null hypothesis that the odds ratio in the population from which the sample was drawn is equal to one using Equation 9.20:

$$\chi^2 = \frac{(b-c)^2}{b+c} = \frac{(21-17)^2}{21+17} = 0.421$$

We compare that chi-square value to the value from Table B.7 corresponding to one degree of freedom and an α of 0.05 (3.841). Since 0.421 is smaller than 3.841, we do not reject the null hypothesis.

9.5 Here, we are interested in the incidences of death in the two groups. The first thing we need to do is determine the number of deaths and the total number of person-years of follow-up time in each group.

Time Period (years)	Number Surviving at End		Number of Deaths		Follow-up Survivors $(p - y)$		Follow-up Deaths $(p - y)$	
	Treated	Not Treated	Treated	Not Treated	Treated	Not Treated	Treated	Not Treated
0–1	91	92	9	8	91	92	4.5	4.0
1–2	82	81	9	11	82	81	4.5	5.5
2–3	74	71	8	10	74	71	4.0	5.0
3–4	67	60	7	11	67	60	3.5	5.5
4–5	60	51	7	9	60	51	3.5	4.5
			40	49	374	355	20.0	24.5

Now, we use Equation 9.21 to test the null hypothesis that the incidences are the same in the two groups.

$$\chi = \dfrac{a - \left[(a + b) \cdot \dfrac{py_1}{py_{total}} \right]}{\sqrt{\dfrac{(a + b) \cdot (py_1) \cdot (py_2)}{py_{total}^2}}}$$

$$= \dfrac{40 - \left[(40 + 49) \cdot \dfrac{374 + 20.0}{374 + 20.0 + 355 + 24.5} \right]}{\sqrt{\dfrac{(40 + 49) \cdot (374 + 20.0) \cdot (355 + 24.5)}{(374 + 20.0 + 355 + 24.5)^2}}} = -1.13$$

We compare -1.13 to 1.96 (the standard normal deviate representing a two-tailed α of 0.05). Since the absolute value of -1.13 is less than 1.96, we do not reject the null hypothesis.

9.6 First, let us organize these data in a 2 × 2 table.

		Gonorrhea Present	Gonorrhea Absent	
Chlamydia	Present	42	33	75
	Absent	8	17	25
		50	50	100

We could use the normal approximation for the difference between two probabilities or Mantel-Haenszel chi to test this null hypothesis, but a chi-square test is most frequently done on data such as these. To use the chi-square test, we need to find the expected values for each cell.

		Gonorrhea Present	Gonorrhea Absent	
Chlamydia	Present	42 {37.5}	33 {37.5}	75
	Absent	8 {12.5}	17 {12.5}	25
		50	50	100

Then, using Equation 9.18:

$$\chi^2 = \Sigma \frac{(O_i - E_i)^2}{E_i} = \frac{(42 - 37.5)^2}{37.5} + \frac{(33 - 37.5)^2}{37.5}$$

$$+ \frac{(8 - 12.5)^2}{12.5} + \frac{(17 - 12.5)^2}{12.5} = 4.32$$

Comparing this to the chi-square value from Table B.7 corresponding to one degree of freedom and an α of 0.05 (3.841), we find that 4.32 is larger than the value from the table. Thus, we reject the null hypothesis and accept, by elimination, the alternative hypothesis that the rates are different in the population that was sampled.

CHAPTER 10

10.1 This data set contains a continuous dependent variable (Y = serum cholesterol), two nominal independent variables (X_1 = treatment and X_2 = gender), and a continuous independent variable (X_3 = age). Before we can mathematically define a regression equation, we need to create indicator variables for the two nominal independent variables. We do that by assigning the value of one to one of the nominal states for each variable and the value of zero to the other nominal state. Our choice of which nominal state will be assigned the value of one is arbitrary. To illustrate, let us choose to let the indicator for treatment (I_1) equal one for the drug and zero for the placebo and the indicator for gender (I_2) equal one for males and zero for females. Then our regression equation, including interaction terms, would be as follows:

$$Y = \alpha + (\beta_1 \cdot I_1) + (\beta_2 \cdot I_2) + (\beta_3 \cdot X_3) + (\beta_4 \cdot I_1 \cdot I_2)$$
$$+ (\beta_5 \cdot I_1 \cdot X_3) + (\beta_6 \cdot I_2 \cdot X_3) + (\beta_7 \cdot I_1 \cdot I_2 \cdot X_3)$$

To determine how each of the coefficients of that equation can be interpreted, let us take a look at the regression equations corresponding to the four groups specified by the two nominal independent variables. (Note that four groups are specified by two nominal variables here because each defines two categories of a separate factor. Specifically, we have two categories of a treatment factor and two categories of a gender factor.)

For males ($I_2 = 1$) receiving the drug ($I_1 = 1$):

$$Y = \alpha + (\beta_1 \cdot 1) + (\beta_2 \cdot 1) + (\beta_3 \cdot X_3) + (\beta_4 \cdot 1 \cdot 1)$$
$$+ (\beta_5 \cdot 1 \cdot X_3) + (\beta_6 \cdot 1 \cdot X_3) + (\beta_7 \cdot 1 \cdot 1 \cdot X_3)$$
$$= [\alpha + \beta_1 + \beta_2 + \beta_4] + ([\beta_3 + \beta_5 + \beta_6 + \beta_7] \cdot X_3)$$

For males ($I_2 = 1$) receiving the placebo ($I_1 = 0$):

$$Y = \alpha + (\beta_1 \cdot 0) + (\beta_2 \cdot 1) + (\beta_3 \cdot X_3) + (\beta_4 \cdot 0 \cdot 1)$$
$$+ (\beta_5 \cdot 0 \cdot X_3) + (\beta_6 \cdot 1 \cdot X_3) + (\beta_7 \cdot 0 \cdot 1 \cdot X_3)$$
$$= [\alpha + \beta_2] + ([\beta_3 + \beta_6] \cdot X_3)$$

For females ($I_2 = 0$) receiving the drug ($I_1 = 1$):

$$Y = \alpha + (\beta_1 \cdot 1) + (\beta_2 \cdot 0) + (\beta_3 \cdot X_3) + (\beta_4 \cdot 1 \cdot 0)$$
$$+ (\beta_5 \cdot 1 \cdot X_3) + (\beta_6 \cdot 0 \cdot X_3) + (\beta_7 \cdot 0 \cdot 0 \cdot X_3)$$
$$= [\alpha + \beta_1] + ([\beta_3 + \beta_5] \cdot X_3)$$

For females ($I_2 = 0$) receiving the placebo ($I_1 = 0$):

$$Y = \alpha + (\beta_1 \cdot 0) + (\beta_2 \cdot 0) + (\beta_3 \cdot X_3) + (\beta_4 \cdot 0 \cdot 0)$$
$$+ (\beta_5 \cdot 0 \cdot X_3) + (\beta_6 \cdot 0 \cdot X_3) + (\beta_7 \cdot 0 \cdot 0 \cdot X_3)$$
$$= \alpha + (\beta_3 \cdot X_3)$$

As we examine those regression equations, we notice several things. First, we see that α and β_3 occur in all four regression equations. Thus, we can think of α and β_3 as being the basic intercept and slope that all the other coefficients will modify for specific states of the nominal variables. More specifically, α estimates the serum cholesterol level when age is equal to zero,[3] and β_3 estimates the change in serum cholesterol for each unit change in age when both indicator variables are equal to zero. Since both indicator variables are equal to zero for females receiving the placebo, all the remaining coefficients will tell us something about how the slope or intercept changes as gender is changed from female to male and/or as treatment is changed from placebo to drug.

Next, we notice that β_1 and β_5 occur in both equations for persons receiving the treatment and they are absent from both equations for persons receiving the placebo. Thus, β_1 estimates the effect of the treatment on the intercept, and β_5 estimates the effect of the treatment on the slope of the relationship between age and cholesterol. We also can see that β_2 and β_6 serve the same sort of functions to compare genders. The difference between the intercepts for males compared to females is estimated by β_2, and the difference between the slopes for males compared to females is estimated by β_3.

All the coefficients discussed so far give us estimates of the main effects of treatment and gender. That is to say, their interpretation depends on the assumption that the treatment effect is the same for both genders and that the differences between the genders is the same regardless of which treatment the subject received. The degree to which that assumption is violated is estimated by β_4 (for the intercept) and β_7 (for the slope). Notice that those regression coefficients are retained (i.e., not multiplied by zero) in only one of the equations (males who received the drug).

10.2 In this problem, we are asked to examine each of the independent variables (age and gender) as they relate to the dependent variable (systolic blood pressure). Therefore, we need to consider the estimates of the regression coefficients and the partial F ratios that test the null hypotheses that the coefficients are equal to zero in the population. First, let us take a look at what the regression coefficients tell us. Using the sample's estimates, we can write the regression equation as follows:

$$SBP = 74.389 + (10.100 \cdot SEX) + (1.001 \cdot AGE) + (0.094 \, M \, AGE \cdot SEX)$$

Another way to express that regression equation is as separate equations for the two genders. For females, SEX is equal to zero. Thus, the estimated regression equation for females is:

$$SBP = 74.389 + (1.001 \cdot AGE)$$

For males, SEX is equal to one, making the estimated equation for males:

$$SBP = [74.389 + 10.100] + ([1.001 + 0.094] \cdot AGE)$$
$$= 84.489 + (1.095 \cdot AGE)$$

Thus, the intercept for males is estimated to differ from the intercept for females by 10.100 mm Hg (the regression coefficient for SEX), and the slope for males is estimated to differ from the slope for females by 0.094 mm Hg per year (the regression coefficient for A $\cdot$ S, the interaction). Those estimated regression lines are shown in the following figure.

---

[3]Since an age of zero is unlikely to be of interest, it is more helpful to think of the intercept as telling us something about the elevation of the regression line in general.

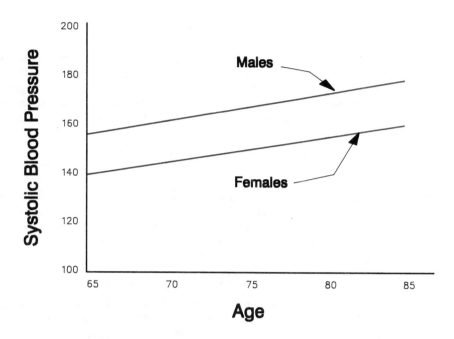

Now, let us take a look at the partial F ratios corresponding to each of the regression coefficient estimates. The partial F ratio for the coefficient of AGE is 12.190, which is associated with an area in the F distribution of 0.001 (the P-value). Since 0.001 is less than the usual α of 0.05, we reject the null hypothesis that the coefficient of AGE is equal to zero in the population. In other words, we conclude that there is an association between age and systolic blood pressure in the population when gender is also taken into account.

The partial F ratio of 10.061 associated with the independent variable SEX tells us that we can reject the null hypothesis that the regression coefficient for this indicator of gender is equal to zero in the population (P-value = 0.002). That implies that we can reject the notion that the intercepts for the two genders are equal in the population. Likewise, we can reject the hypothesis that the slopes of the lines for the two genders are equal in the population since the partial F ratio for the coefficient of the interaction $(A \cdot S)$ is 4.101 (P-value = 0.050).

The final F ratio in this computer output (11.997) tells us that we can reject the null hypothesis that the intercept is equal to zero (P-value = 0.001). In summary, we can conclude from all those tests of inference that the straight line in the population estimating values of systolic blood pressure based on knowledge of age has an intercept and slope not equal to zero for females and that the intercept and slope for males differs from the intercept and slope for females.

10.3 These three questions can be answered by looking at the table of sources of variation for systolic blood pressure in Problem 10.2.
    a)   The sample's size was equal to 54 persons. We know that was the sample's size because the number of regression degrees of freedom is equal to 3 and the number of residual degrees of freedom is equal to 50. Added together, those degrees of freedom give us the total number of degrees of freedom (3 + 50 = 53), which is equal to the sample's size minus

one. Thus, the sample's size is equal to the total degrees of freedom plus one $(53 + 1 = 54)$.

b) The proportion of variation in the data represented by the dependent variable that is associated with the entire collection of independent variables is given by the coefficient of determination. We calculate the coefficient of determination by dividing the regression sum of squares by the total sum of squares (Equation 7.24). Although the total sum of squares is not given, we can calculate it by adding the regression sum of squares and the residual sum of squares.

$$R^2 = \frac{\text{Regression sum of squares}}{\text{Total sum of squares}} = \frac{970.735}{970.735 + 3{,}247.665} = 0.230$$

c) The hypothesis that there is no relationship between the dependent variable and the entire collection of independent variables is the omnibus null hypothesis. To test the omnibus null hypothesis, we calculate an F ratio by dividing the regression mean square by the residual mean square.

$$F = \frac{\text{Regression mean square}}{\text{Residual mean square}} = \frac{323.578}{64.953} = 4.982$$

We evaluate that F ratio by comparing it to a value from Table B.4 corresponding to an α of 0.05, 3 degrees of freedom in the numerator, and 50 degrees of freedom in the denominator. That F ratio is equal to 2.79. Since 4.982 is greater than 2.79, we reject the omnibus null hypothesis and accept, by elimination, the alternative hypothesis that there is a relationship between the dependent variable and the entire collection of independent variables in the population.

10.4 First, we need to calculate the squared deviations between each of the observations and the overall mean of the AST measurements. To prepare for those calculations, we estimate the overall mean to be:

$$\overline{Y} = \frac{\sum_{j=1}^{m} \sum_{i=1}^{n_j} Y_{ij}}{\sum_{j=1}^{m} n_j} = \frac{38 + 22 + 41 + \cdots + 39 + 31}{10 + 10 + 10 + 10} = 35.35 \text{ units/ml}$$

Then, we calculate the squared differences between that mean and each observation. Those calculations are summarized in the following table.

Stage I	$(Y_{i1} - \overline{Y})^2$	Stage II	$(Y_{i2} - \overline{Y})^2$	Stage III	$(Y_{i3} - \overline{Y})^2$	Stage IV	$(Y_{i4} - \overline{Y})^2$
38	7.02	23	152.52	57	468.72	30	28.62
22	178.22	36	0.42	42	44.22	26	87.42
41	31.92	44	74.82	36	0.42	42	44.22
12	545.22	33	5.52	39	13.32	23	152.52
37	2.72	42	44.22	42	44.22	21	205.92
29	40.32	48	160.02	43	58.52	43	58.52

Stage I	$(\Upsilon_{i1} - \overline{\Upsilon})^2$	Stage II	$(\Upsilon_{i2} - \overline{\Upsilon})^2$	Stage III	$(\Upsilon_{i3} - \overline{\Upsilon})^2$	Stage IV	$(\Upsilon_{i4} - \overline{\Upsilon})^2$
32	11.22	19	267.32	29	40.32	39	13.32
18	301.02	28	54.02	52	277.22	32	11.22
25	107.12	34	1.82	65	879.12	39	13.32
31	18.92	40	21.62	51	244.92	31	18.92
285	1,243.72	347	782.32	456	2,071.02	326	634.02

Now, we calculate the total mean square using Equation 10.9.

$$\text{Total mean square} = \frac{\text{Total sum of squares}}{\text{Total degrees of freedom}}$$

$$= \frac{\sum_{j=1}^{m} \sum_{i=1}^{n_j} (\Upsilon_{ij} - \overline{\Upsilon})^2}{\left(\sum_{j=1}^{m} n_j\right) - 1} = \frac{1,243.72 + 782.32 + 2,071.02 + 634.02}{(10 + 10 + 10 + 10) - 1}$$

$$= \frac{4,731.08}{39} = 121.31 \ (\text{units/ml})^2$$

Next, we want to calculate the within mean square. To prepare for that calculation, we estimate the mean AST for each of the groups (stages).

$$\overline{\Upsilon}_1 = \frac{\sum_{i=1}^{n_1} \Upsilon_{i1}}{n_1} = \frac{285}{10} = 28.5 \ \text{units/ml}$$

$$\overline{\Upsilon}_2 = \frac{\sum_{i=1}^{n_2} \Upsilon_{i2}}{n_2} = \frac{347}{10} = 34.7 \ \text{units/ml}$$

$$\overline{\Upsilon}_3 = \frac{\sum_{i=1}^{n_3} \Upsilon_{i3}}{n_3} = \frac{456}{10} = 45.6 \ \text{units/ml}$$

$$\overline{\Upsilon}_4 = \frac{\sum_{i=1}^{n_4} \Upsilon_{i4}}{n_4} = \frac{326}{10} = 32.6 \ \text{units/ml}$$

Then, we calculate the squared differences between each of the observations and its corresponding group mean (i.e., the mean for that particular stage of disease) as shown in the following table:

Stage I	$(Y_{i1} - \overline{Y}_1)^2$	Stage II	$(Y_{i2} - \overline{Y}_2)^2$	Stage III	$(Y_{i3} - \overline{Y}_3)^2$	Stage IV	$(Y_{i4} - \overline{Y}_4)^2$
38	90.25	23	136.89	57	129.96	30	6.76
22	42.25	36	1.69	42	12.96	26	43.56
41	156.25	44	86.49	36	92.16	42	88.36
12	272.25	33	2.89	39	43.56	23	92.16
37	72.25	42	53.29	42	12.96	21	134.56
29	0.25	48	176.89	43	6.76	43	108.16
32	12.25	19	246.49	29	275.56	39	40.96
18	110.25	28	44.89	52	40.96	32	0.36
25	12.25	34	0.49	65	376.36	39	40.96
31	6.25	40	28.09	51	29.16	31	2.56
285	774.50	347	778.10	456	1,020.40	326	558.40

Then, we use Equation 10.10 to calculate the within mean square.

$$\text{Within mean square} = \frac{\text{Within sum of squares}}{\text{Within degrees of freedom}} = \frac{\sum_{j=1}^{m} \sum_{i=1}^{n_j} (Y_{ij} - \overline{Y}_j)^2}{\sum_{j=1}^{m} (n_j - 1)}$$

$$= \frac{774.50 + 778.10 + 1,020.40 + 558.40}{9 + 9 + 9 + 9} = \frac{3,131.40}{36} = 86.98 \; (\text{units}/\text{ml})^2$$

Next, we find the between sum of squares and the between degrees of freedom by subtraction and calculate the between mean square using Equation 10.11.

$$\text{Between mean square} = \frac{\text{Between sum of squares}}{\text{Between degrees of freedom}} = \frac{\sum_{j=1}^{m} \sum_{i=1}^{n_j} (\overline{Y}_j - \overline{Y})^2}{m - 1}$$

$$= \frac{\text{Total sum of squares} - \text{Within sum of squares}}{\text{Total degrees of freedom} - \text{Within degrees of freedom}}$$

$$= \frac{4,731.08 - 3,131.40}{39 - 36} = \frac{1,599.68}{3} = 533.23 \; (\text{units}/\text{ml})^2$$

To test the null hypothesis that the mean AST values for all the stages of disease are equal in the population that was sampled, we calculate an F ratio using Equation 10.12.

$$F = \frac{\text{Between mean square}}{\text{Within mean square}} = \frac{\dfrac{\displaystyle\sum_{j=1}^{m}\sum_{i=1}^{n_j} (\overline{Y}_j - \overline{Y})^2}{m - 1}}{\dfrac{\displaystyle\sum_{j=1}^{m}\sum_{i=1}^{n_j} (Y_{ij} - \overline{Y}_j)^2}{\displaystyle\sum_{j=1}^{m}(n_j - 1)}} = \frac{533.23}{86.98} = 6.13$$

From Table B.4, we find that an F value of 2.87 is associated with 3 degrees of freedom in the numerator and 35 (36 does not appear in the table) degrees of freedom in the denominator, and an α of 0.05. Since 6.13 is larger than 2.87, we reject the null hypothesis.

10.5 We begin this problem by arranging the means in order of magnitude.

Stage I	Stage IV	Stage II	Stage III
28.5	32.6	34.7	45.6

Since all four groups (stages) have the same number of observations, the standard error for the differences between means will be the same for all comparisons. That standard error is calculated using Equation 10.13.

$$SE_{\overline{Y}_1 - \overline{Y}_2} = \sqrt{\frac{s_p^2}{2}\cdot\left(\frac{1}{n_1} + \frac{1}{n_2}\right)} = \sqrt{\frac{86.98}{2}\cdot\left(\frac{1}{10} + \frac{1}{10}\right)} = 2.95$$

To compare means among the four stages, we calculate Student-Newman-Keuls statistics using Equation 10.14 and compare those calculated values to values from Table B.8. The order in which those means are compared is specified by the protocol for the Student-Newman-Keuls procedure. That protocol requires that we first examine the most extreme means. Therefore, we begin by comparing the means for Stage I (28.5) and Stage III (45.6). Then, if and only if we can reject the null hypothesis that those means are equal in the population can we compare less extreme means. The next means that can be compared are Stage I versus Stage II and Stage IV versus Stage III. That process is summarized in the following table:

Compare Stages	Difference	SE	q	k	$q_{0.05, 36, k}$	Reject H_0?
I and III	17.1	2.95	5.798	4	3.813	Yes
I and II	6.2	2.95	2.102	3	3.460	No
IV and III	13.0	2.95	4.408	3	3.460	Yes
I and IV		This comparison is not examined (I vs. II not rejected).				
IV and II		This comparison is not examined (I vs. II not rejected).				
II and III	10.9	2.95	3.696	2	2.870	Yes

10.6 a)   This question asks us to test the omnibus null hypothesis. That null hypothesis is tested by calculating an F ratio with the between mean square in the numerator and the within mean square in the denominator.

$$F = \frac{\text{Between mean square}}{\text{Within mean square}} = \frac{392.71}{78.98} = 4.97$$

We compare that calculated F ratio (4.97) with a value from Table B.4 that corresponds to 7 degrees of freedom in the numerator, 70 (72 does not appear in the table) degrees of freedom in the denominator, and an α of 0.05. That F ratio is equal to 2.14. Since 4.97 is larger than 2.14, we reject the omnibus null hypothesis and accept, by elimination, the alternative hypothesis that there are differences among the means in the population.

b)   To answer this question, we need to separate that part of the between variation in data represented by the dependent variable that is due to differences among the four stages of disease. That variation is summarized by the mean square for stage in the computer output. To test the null hypothesis that the means for the four stages of disease are equal in the population, we calculate an F ratio by dividing the mean square for stage of disease by the within mean square.

$$F = \frac{\text{Stage mean square}}{\text{Within mean square}} = \frac{677.67}{78.98} = 8.58$$

We compare this calculated F ratio (8.58) to the value from Table B.4 corresponding to 3 degrees of freedom in the numerator, 70 (72 does not appear) degrees of freedom in the denominator, and an α of 0.05. That value is equal to 2.74. Since 8.58 is larger than 2.74, we reject the null hypothesis and accept, by elimination, the alternative hypothesis that there are differences among the means corresponding to stages of disease in the population.

c)   To answer this question, we need to find the portion of the between variation in data represented by the dependent variable that is due to variation between the two treatments. That variation is summarized by the mean square for treatment in the computer output. To test the null hypothesis that the means from the two treatments are the same in the population, we calculate an F ratio by dividing the treatment mean square by the within mean square.

$$F = \frac{\text{Treatment mean square}}{\text{Within mean square}} = \frac{577.79}{78.89} = 7.32$$

We compare this calculated F ratio (7.32) to the value from Table B.4 corresponding to 1 degree of freedom in the numerator, 70 (72 does not appear) degrees of freedom in the denominator, and an α of 0.05. That value is equal to 3.98. Since 7.32 is larger than 3.98, we reject the null hypothesis and accept, by elimination, the alternative hypothesis that the means for the two treatments are different in the population.

d)   This question asks us to test the null hypothesis that there is no interaction between stage of disease and type of treatment. To test that null hypothesis, we calculate an F ratio by dividing the interaction mean square by the within mean square.

$$F = \frac{\text{Interaction mean square}}{\text{Within mean square}} = \frac{45.83}{78.98} = 0.58$$

Since this F ratio is less than one (the expected value for any F ratio when the null hypothesis is true), we do not need to compare it to a tabled value. We cannot reject the null hypothesis.

CHAPTER 11

11.1 To estimate Kendall's coefficient of concordance, we need to convert our observations to a scale of ranks and sum all the ranks for each individual. That process is summarized in the following table:

Age		DBP		SBP		Sum of Ranks (R_i)	R_i^2
Value	Rank	Value	Rank	Value	Rank		
41	1	85	3	123	1	5.0	25.00
56	12	90	12	137	14	38.0	1,444.00
51	8.5	87	6.5	132	11	26.0	676.00
62	15	90	12	139	15	42.0	1,764.00
48	6.5	90	12	124	2	20.5	420.25
55	11	89	9.5	125	3	23.5	552.25
46	4	86	4	127	5.5	13.5	182.25
59	13	87	6.5	130	9	28.5	812.25
43	2	91	14	128	7	23.0	529.00
60	14	93	15	130	9	38.0	1,444.00
51	8.5	89	9.5	136	13	31.0	961.00
54	10	87	6.5	130	9	25.5	650.25
47	5	84	1.5	133	12	18.5	342.25
44	3	84	1.5	127	5.5	10.0	100.00
48	6.5	87	6.5	126	4	17.0	289.00
						360.0	10,191.50

Then, we use Equation 11.1 to estimate Kendall's coefficient of concordance. The correction for tied ranks is:

$$\Sigma T = \Sigma(t_i^3 - t_i) = [5 \cdot (2^3 - 2)] + [2 \cdot (3^3 - 3)] + (4^3 - 4) = 138$$

and our estimate of Kendall's coefficient of concordance is:

$$W = \frac{\Sigma R_j^2 - \dfrac{(\Sigma R_j)^2}{n}}{\dfrac{[k^2 \cdot (n^3 - n)] - [k \cdot \Sigma T]}{12}} = \frac{10{,}191.50 - \dfrac{360^2}{15}}{\dfrac{[3^2 \cdot (15^3 - 15)] - [3 \cdot 138]}{12}} = 0.624$$

We can test the null hypothesis that this coefficient is equal to zero in the population by converting our estimate of Kendall's coefficient of concordance to a chi-square statistic with $n - 1$ degrees of freedom.

$$\chi^2 = k \cdot (n - 1) \cdot W = 3 \cdot (15 - 1) \cdot 0.624 = 26.217$$

Since the sample's size is 15, we find a chi-square value from Table B.7 associated with $15 - 1 = 14$ degrees of freedom and an α of 0.05. That chi-square value is equal to 23.658. Since our calculated chi-square value (26.217) is greater than 23.658, we reject the null hypothesis that the population's coefficient is equal to zero and accept, by elimination, the alternative hypothesis that it is not equal to zero.

11.2 To test the omnibus null hypothesis without making assumptions about the distribution of AST measurements, we use the Kruskal-Wallis procedure. In preparation for that procedure, we rank the values of the dependent variable and calculate the sums of those ranks for each group as shown in the following table.

Stage I		Stage II		Stage III		Stage IV	
Value	Rank	Value	Rank	Value	Rank	Value	Rank
38	23	23	6.5	57	39	30	13
22	5	36	20.5	42	30.5	26	9
41	28	44	35	36	20.5	42	30.5
12	1	33	18	39	25	23	6.5
37	22	42	30.5	42	30.5	21	4
29	11.5	48	36	43	33.5	43	33.5
32	16.5	19	3	29	11.5	39	25
18	2	28	10	52	38	32	16.5
25	8	34	19	65	40	39	25
31	14.5	40	27	51	37	31	14.5
	131.5		205.5		305.5		177.5

Then, we use Equation 11.3 to calculate the Kruskal-Wallis test statistic.

$$H = \left[\frac{12}{n_T \cdot (n_T + 1)} \cdot \sum \frac{R_j^2}{n_j} \right] - [3 \cdot (n_T + 1)]$$

$$= \left[\frac{12}{40 \cdot (40 + 1)} \cdot \left(\frac{131.5^2}{10} + \frac{205.5^2}{10} + \frac{305.5^2}{10} + \frac{177.5^2}{10} \right) \right] - [3 \cdot (40 + 1)]$$

$$= 11.897$$

Since some of the ranks are tied, we need to use Equation 11.4 to correct for those ties.

$$H_C = \frac{H}{1 - \frac{\sum (t_i^3 - t_i)}{n_T^3 - n_T}} = \frac{11.897}{1 - \frac{[6 \cdot (2^3 - 2)] + (3^3 - 3) + (4^3 - 4)}{40^3 - 40}} = 11.919$$

Samples with 10 observations in each group do not appear in Table B.9, so we compare this corrected Kruskal-Wallis value to a chi-square value from Table B.7 with $m - 1 = 3$ degrees of freedom and an α of 0.05. That chi-square value is 7.815. Since 11.919 is larger than 7.815, we reject the omnibus null hypothesis.

11.3 To make pairwise comparisons between all the groups of AST values without making assumptions about the distribution of that variable, we use Dunn's procedure. The first step in Dunn's procedure is arranging the means of the ranks for each group in numeric order.

Stage I	Stage IV	Stage II	Stage III
13.15	17.75	20.55	30.55

Next, we use Equation 11.5 to calculate the standard error for differences between mean ranks. This same standard error is used in all the comparisons since all the groups contain the same number of observations.

$$SE_{\bar{R}_1 - \bar{R}_2} = \sqrt{\left(\frac{n_T \cdot (n_T + 1)}{12} - \frac{\Sigma(t_i^3 - t_i)}{12 \cdot (n_T - 1)}\right) \cdot \left(\frac{1}{n_1} + \frac{1}{n_2}\right)}$$

$$= \sqrt{\left(\frac{40 \cdot (40 + 1)}{12} - \frac{[6 \cdot (2^3 - 2)] + (3^3 - 3) + (4^3 - 4)}{12 \cdot (40 - 1)}\right) \cdot \left(\frac{1}{10} + \frac{1}{10}\right)}$$

$$= 5.223$$

Then, we follow a protocol like the one for the Student-Newman-Keuls procedure in which we compare the most extreme mean of the ranks, and compare less extreme means if and only if the more extreme means are considered to be significantly different. The means of the ranks are converted to Q statistics for comparison to values from Table B.10. The entire process is summarized in the following table.

Compare Stages	Difference	SE	Q	k	$Q_{0.05,k}$	Reject H_0?
I and IIII	17.4	5.223	3.331	4	2.639	Yes
I and II	7.4	5.223	1.417	3	2.394	No
IV and III	12.8	5.223	2.451	3	2.394	Yes
I and IV	This comparison is not examined (I vs. II not rejected).					
IV and II	This comparison is not examined (I vs. II not rejected).					
II and III	10.0	5.223	1.915	2	1.960	No

11.4 The most striking difference between the results of Problems 11.2 and 11.3 and the results of Problems 10.4 and 10.5 is the failure to reject the null hypothesis that Stage II and Stage III have the same AST values when using Dunn's procedure after being able to reject that null hypothesis using the Student-Newman-Keuls procedure. The reason for this difference is probably due to the lower statistical power of Dunn's procedure. Remember that we lose statistical power when we convert continuous data to an ordinal scale.

11.5 a) To test the null hypothesis that all eight groups are the same in the population that was sampled (the omnibus null hypothesis), we calculate a Kruskal-Wallis test statistic by dividing the between sum of squares by the total mean square (Equation 11.7).

$$H_C = \frac{\text{Between sum of squares}}{\text{Total mean square}} = \frac{12{,}254.34}{538.32} = 22.764$$

That Kruskal-Wallis test statistic is then compared to a chi-square value from Table B.7 corresponding to $m - 1 = 7$ degrees of freedom and an α of 0.05. That chi-square value is equal to 14.067. Since 22.764 is larger than 14.067, we reject the null hypothesis and accept, by elimination, the alternative hypothesis that the eight groups are not the same in the population.

b) To test the null hypothesis that the ranks of AST values in the four stages of the disease are the same in the population that was sampled, we calculate a Kruskal-Wallis test statistic by dividing the stage sum of squares by the total mean square (Equation 11.7).

$$H_C = \frac{\text{Stage sum of squares}}{\text{Total mean square}} = \frac{9{,}007.26}{538.32} = 16.732$$

That Kruskal-Wallis test statistic is compared to a chi-square value from Table B.7 corresponding to $m - 1 = 3$ degrees of freedom and an α of 0.05. That chi-square value is equal to 7.815. Since 16.732 is larger than 7.815, we reject the null hypothesis and accept, by elimination, the alternative hypothesis that the four stages of disease are not the same in the population.

c) To test the null hypothesis that the ranks of AST values in the two treatments are the same in the population sampled, we calculate a Kruskal-Wallis test statistic by dividing the treatment sum of squares by the total mean square (Equation 11.7).

$$H_C = \frac{\text{Treatment sum of squares}}{\text{Total mean square}} = \frac{2{,}928.20}{538.32} = 5.439$$

That Kruskal-Wallis test statistic is compared to a chi-square value from Table B.7 corresponding to $m - 1 = 1$ degree of freedom and an α of 0.05. That chi-square value is equal to 3.841. Since 5.439 is larger than 3.841, we reject the null hypothesis and accept, by elimination, the alternative hypothesis that the treatments are not the same in the population.

To test the null hypothesis that there is no interaction between stage of disease and treatment in the population that was sampled, we calculate a Kruskal-Wallis test statistic by dividing the interaction sum of squares by the total mean square (Equation 11.7).

$$H_C = \frac{\text{Interaction sum of squares}}{\text{Total mean square}} = \frac{318.86}{538.32} = 0.592$$

That Kruskal-Wallis test statistic is compared to a chi-square value from Table B.7 corresponding to $7 - 3 - 1 = 3$ degrees of freedom and an α of 0.05. That chi-square value is equal to 7.815. Since 0.592 is smaller than 7.815, we do not reject the null hypothesis.

CHAPTER 12

12.1 To test the omnibus null hypothesis, we convert the likelihood ratio to a chi-square value using Equation 12.2.

$$\chi^2_{k df} = -2 \cdot \ln \text{LR} = -2 \cdot \ln(0.015389) = 8.348$$

Since this regression analysis includes three independent variables, the chi-square value calculated from the likelihood ratio has three degrees of freedom. From Table B.7, we find that a chi-square value of 7.815 corresponds to three degrees of freedom and an α of 0.05. Since 8.348 is larger than 7.815, we reject the omnibus null hypothesis and accept, by elimination, the alternative hypothesis that the collection of independent variables helps to estimate the occurrence of diabetes.

12.2 The estimated logistic regression equation for these data is:

$$\ln\left(\frac{p}{1-p}\right) = -3.370 + 0.0702 \text{ Age } + 0.1519 \text{ Sex} + 0.341 \text{ HBP}$$

Using Equation 12.5, we can estimate the probability that a 50-year-old man (in the population from which the sample was drawn) with hypertension will have diabetes.

$$p = \frac{1}{1 + e^{-(-3.370+[0.0702\cdot 50]+[0.1519\cdot 0]+[0.3041\cdot 1])}} = 0.61$$

To estimate the odds ratio for developing diabetes, we use the estimated coefficient for the indicator of hypertension and Equation 12.7.

$$\text{OR} = e^{b(X-X')} = e^{0.3041(1-0)} = 1.36$$

12.3 In this set of observations, pain reduction is represented by the dependent variable and the type of treatment is represented by the independent variable of main interest. The remaining independent variables represent potential confounders. Those confounders will be used to divide the observations into strata. Those confounders specify two factors: gender and age. Gender occurs naturally as nominal data, but age is continuous data that have been converted to a nominal scale and represented by two nominal variables (to specify three categories). With two gender categories and three age categories, we need to separate these observations into six strata. Each stratum is identified by a gender and an age category. We will look at these strata in a moment, but first let us think about estimation of the odds ratio.

There are two approaches that we might take to estimate the population's odds ratio. One is to estimate an individual odds ratio for each of the strata. The other is to estimate a single odds ratio over all the strata. Before we estimate a single odds ratio for the relationship between pain reduction and treatment, we should be comfortable in making the assumption that the relationship between pain reduction and treatment is the same over all the gender–age strata. Therefore, even if we are interested in a single estimate of the odds ratio to represent the relationship over all the strata, we need to examine the strata-specific odds ratios first. The strata-specific odds ratio estimates are calculated using Equation 9.10.

Gender = female, age = 50–59:

		Treatment	
		New	Standard
Pain	Reduced	18	10
Outcome	Not Reduced	42	50

$$\text{OR} = \frac{ad}{bc} = \frac{18 \cdot 50}{10 \cdot 42} = 2.14$$

Gender = female, age = 60–69:

		Treatment	
		New	Standard
Pain	Reduced	16	7
Outcome	Not Reduced	34	43

$$OR = \frac{ad}{bc} = \frac{16 \cdot 43}{7 \cdot 34} = 2.89$$

Gender = female, age = 70–79:

		Treatment	
		New	Standard
Pain	Reduced	13	7
Outcome	Not Reduced	27	33

$$OR = \frac{ad}{bc} = \frac{13 \cdot 33}{7 \cdot 27} = 2.27$$

Gender = male, age = 50–59:

		Treatment	
		New	Standard
Pain	Reduced	22	10
Outcome	Not Reduced	48	60

$$OR = \frac{ad}{bc} = \frac{22 \cdot 60}{10 \cdot 48} = 2.75$$

Gender = male, age = 60–69:

		Treatment	
		New	Standard
Pain	Reduced	17	8
Outcome	Not Reduced	43	52

$$OR = \frac{ad}{bc} = \frac{17 \cdot 52}{8 \cdot 43} = 2.57$$

Gender = male, age = 70–79:

		Treatment	
		New	Standard
Pain	Reduced	16	9
Outcome	Not Reduced	34	41

$$OR = \frac{ad}{bc} = \frac{16 \cdot 41}{9 \cdot 34} = 2.14$$

In this problem, the strata-specific odds ratios are close enough that we can be comfortable combining the information from the strata to make an overall (summary) estimate. That overall estimate of the odds ratio is calculated using Equation 12.14.

$$OR = \frac{\sum \frac{(a_i \cdot d_i)}{n_i}}{\sum \frac{(b_i \cdot c_i)}{n_i}} = \frac{\frac{18 \cdot 50}{120} + \frac{16 \cdot 43}{100} + \frac{13 \cdot 33}{80} + \frac{22 \cdot 60}{140} + \frac{17 \cdot 52}{120} + \frac{16 \cdot 41}{100}}{\frac{10 \cdot 42}{120} + \frac{7 \cdot 34}{100} + \frac{7 \cdot 27}{80} + \frac{10 \cdot 48}{140} + \frac{8 \cdot 43}{120} + \frac{9 \cdot 34}{100}} = 2.45$$

If we are willing to assume that the odds ratios in the population are the same for each of the strata, then we can use all the observations to test the null hypothesis that the overall (summary) odds ratio estimated in this problem is equal to one in the population from which the sample was drawn. To do that, we use Equation 12.19.

$$\chi_{\text{M-H}} = \frac{\sum [a_i] - \sum \left[\frac{(a_i + b_i) \cdot (a_i + c_i)}{n_i} \right]}{\sqrt{\sum \frac{(a_i + b_i) \cdot (c_i + d_i) \cdot (a_i + c_i) \cdot (b_i + d_i)}{n_i^2 \cdot (n_i - 1)}}}$$

$$= \frac{[18 + 16 + 13 + 22 + 17 + 16] - \left[\frac{28 \cdot 60}{120} + \frac{23 \cdot 50}{100} + \frac{20 \cdot 40}{80} + \frac{32 \cdot 70}{140} + \frac{25 \cdot 60}{120} + \frac{25 \cdot 50}{100} \right]}{\sqrt{\frac{28 \cdot 92 \cdot 60 \cdot 60}{120^2 \cdot 119} + \frac{23 \cdot 77 \cdot 50 \cdot 50}{100^2 \cdot 99} + \frac{20 \cdot 60 \cdot 40 \cdot 40}{80^2 \cdot 79} + \frac{32 \cdot 108 \cdot 70 \cdot 70}{140^2 \cdot 139} + \frac{25 \cdot 95 \cdot 60 \cdot 60}{120^2 \cdot 119} + \frac{25 \cdot 95 \cdot 50 \cdot 50}{100^2 \cdot 99}}}$$

$$= 4.69$$

To interpret that Mantel-Haenszel chi value, we compare it to a standard normal deviate from Table B.1 corresponding to an area of 0.05 split between the two tails of the standard normal distribution. That standard normal deviate is equal to 1.96. Since 4.69 is larger than 1.96, we reject the null hypothesis and accept, by elimination, the alternative hypothesis that the overall odds ratio is not equal to one in the population.

12.4 To organize these data into life tables, we need to specify for each time interval the number of persons at the beginning of the interval (N_t), the number of deaths during the interval (D_t), the number of withdrawals during the interval (W_t), the probability of surviving the interval (P_t), and the probability of surviving up to and through the interval (P_T). We are told how many individuals died and withdrew during each of the intervals, and we are told that there were 100 persons in each of the two treatment groups at the beginning of the first time interval. To complete the life tables, we must calculate the number of persons at the beginning of the remaining time intervals by subtracting the number that withdrew or died in the previous interval from the number at the beginning of the previous interval. Also we must calculate the probability of surviving the interval (using Equation 12.17) and the probability of surviving up to and through the interval (using Equation 12.18). Performing those calculations, we obtain the following life tables.

For persons receiving the placebo:

t	N_t	D_t	W_t	P_t	P_T
1	100	10	8	0.90	0.90
2	82	8	9	0.90	0.81
3	65	7	11	0.89	0.72
4	47	9	11	0.81	0.59
5	27	9	18	0.67	0.39

For persons receiving the treatment:

t	N_t	D_t	W_t	P_t	P_T
1	100	9	7	0.91	0.91
2	84	8	10	0.90	0.82
3	66	7	13	0.89	0.74
4	46	5	12	0.89	0.66
5	29	3	26	0.90	0.59

Thus, the five-year risk of death for persons receiving the placebo is the complement of the five-year cumulative probability of survival for those persons or $1 - 0.39 = 0.61$. The five-year risk of death for persons receiving the treatment is the complement of the five-year cumulative probability of survival for those persons or $1 - 0.59 = 0.41$. The difference between those five-year risks is $0.61 - 0.41 = 0.20$. This is nearly the same as the difference between the five-year risks for the life tables in Examples 12.9 and 12.10 (0.18).

12.5 The following are the survival curves for the two groups in Problem 12.4. The solid line represents persons receiving the treatment and the broken line represents persons receiving the placebo.

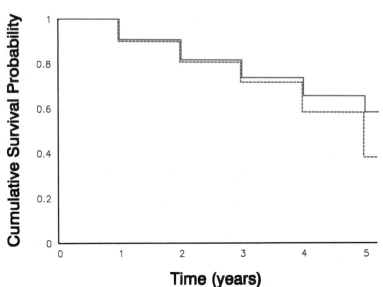

To test the null hypothesis that these two survival curves are the same in the population from which the sample was drawn, we first organize the life-table data into strata so that each stratum represents one time interval and for each stratum we have a 2 × 2 table comparing survival to treatment.

Time interval 1:

	Placebo	Treatment	
Survive	90	91	181
Die	10	9	19
	100	100	200

Time interval 2:

	Placebo	Treatment	
Survive	74	76	150
Die	8	8	16
	82	84	166

Time interval 3:

	Placebo	Treatment	
Survive	58	59	117
Die	7	7	14
	65	66	131

Time interval 4:

	Placebo	Treatment	
Survive	38	41	79
Die	9	5	14
	47	46	93

Time interval 5:

	Placebo	Treatment	
Survive	18	26	44
Die	9	3	12
	27	29	56

Next, we calculate a Mantel-Haenszel chi statistic, as we would for probabilities stratified by any confounding variable(s) (Equation 12.19).

$$\chi_{\text{M-H}} = \frac{\Sigma [a_i] - \Sigma \left[\frac{(a_i + b_i) \cdot (a_i + c_i)}{n_i} \right]}{\sqrt{\Sigma \frac{(a_i + b_i) \cdot (c_i + d_i) \cdot (a_i + c_i) \cdot (b_i + d_i)}{n_i^2 \cdot (n_i - 1)}}}$$

$$= \frac{[90 + 74 + 58 + 38 + 18] - \left[\frac{181 \cdot 100}{200} + \frac{150 \cdot 82}{166} + \frac{117 \cdot 65}{131} + \frac{79 \cdot 47}{93} + \frac{44 \cdot 27}{56} \right]}{\sqrt{\frac{181 \cdot 19 \cdot 100 \cdot 100}{200^2 \cdot 199} + \frac{150 \cdot 16 \cdot 82 \cdot 82}{166^2 \cdot 165} + \frac{117 \cdot 14 \cdot 65 \cdot 66}{131^2 \cdot 130} + \frac{79 \cdot 14 \cdot 47 \cdot 46}{93^2 \cdot 92} + \frac{44 \cdot 12 \cdot 27 \cdot 29}{56^2 \cdot 55}}}$$

$$= 1.42$$

To interpret that Mantel-Haenszel chi value, we compare it to a standard normal deviate from Table B.1 corresponding to an area of 0.05 split between the two tails of the standard normal distribution. That standard normal deviate is equal to 1.96. Since 1.42 is smaller than 1.96, we cannot reject the null hypothesis.

Even though we found, in Problem 12.4, that the difference between the five-year risks for these two (treatment and placebo) groups is nearly equal to the difference we found in five-year risks for the groups in Example 12.14, the conclusions that we draw are different. Here, we are unable to reject the null hypothesis. In Example 12.14, we were able to reject the null hypothesis. The important distinction between this problem and Example 12.14 is that the probabilities for the two groups in Example 12.14 were different for all the time intervals, whereas the probabilities for the groups were similar in early time intervals and became different in later time intervals in this problem. Remember that, when using the Mantel-Haenszel procedure in life-table analysis, differences in survival in later time intervals are less influential than are differences in survival in earlier time intervals. This is because of the decreasing number of observations in those later time intervals.

APPENDIX B

Statistical Tables

TABLE B.1 Area in one tail of the standard normal distribution* ▪

z	0	1	2	3	4	5	6	7	8	9
0.0	0.5000	0.4960	0.4920	0.4880	0.4840	0.4801	0.4761	0.4721	0.4681	0.4641
0.1	0.4602	0.4562	0.4522	0.4483	0.4443	0.4404	0.4364	0.4325	0.4286	0.4247
0.2	0.4207	0.4168	0.4129	0.4090	0.4052	0.4013	0.3974	0.3936	0.3897	0.3859
0.3	0.3821	0.3783	0.3745	0.3707	0.3669	0.3632	0.3594	0.3557	0.3520	0.3483
0.4	0.3446	0.3409	0.3372	0.3336	0.3300	0.3264	0.3228	0.3192	0.3156	0.3121
0.5	0.3085	0.3050	0.3015	0.2981	0.2946	0.2912	0.2877	0.2843	0.2810	0.2776
0.6	0.2743	0.2709	0.2676	0.2643	0.2611	0.2578	0.2546	0.2514	0.2483	0.2451
0.7	0.2420	0.2389	0.2358	0.2327	0.2297	0.2266	0.2236	0.2207	0.2177	0.2148
0.8	0.2119	0.2090	0.2061	0.2033	0.2005	0.1977	0.1949	0.1922	0.1894	0.1867
0.9	0.1841	0.1814	0.1788	0.1762	0.1736	0.1711	0.1685	0.1660	0.1635	0.1611
1.0	0.1587	0.1562	0.1539	0.1515	0.1492	0.1469	0.1446	0.1423	0.1401	0.1379
1.1	0.1357	0.1335	0.1314	0.1292	0.1271	0.1251	0.1230	0.1210	0.1190	0.1170
1.2	0.1151	0.1131	0.1112	0.1093	0.1075	0.1056	0.1038	0.1020	0.1003	0.0985
1.3	0.0968	0.0951	0.0934	0.0918	0.0901	0.0885	0.0869	0.0853	0.0838	0.0823
1.4	0.0808	0.0793	0.0778	0.0764	0.0749	0.0735	0.0721	0.0708	0.0694	0.0681
1.5	0.0668	0.0655	0.0643	0.0630	0.0618	0.0606	0.0594	0.0582	0.0571	0.0559
1.6	0.0548	0.0537	0.0526	0.0516	0.0505	0.0495	0.0485	0.0475	0.0465	0.0455
1.7	0.0446	0.0436	0.0427	0.0418	0.0409	0.0401	0.0392	0.0384	0.0375	0.0367
1.8	0.0359	0.0351	0.0344	0.0336	0.0329	0.0322	0.0314	0.0307	0.0301	0.0294
1.9	0.0287	0.0281	0.0274	0.0268	0.0262	0.0256	0.0250	0.0244	0.0239	0.0233
2.0	0.0228	0.0222	0.0217	0.0212	0.0207	0.0202	0.0197	0.0192	0.0188	0.0183
2.1	0.0179	0.0174	0.0170	0.0166	0.0162	0.0158	0.0154	0.0150	0.0146	0.0143
2.2	0.0139	0.0136	0.0132	0.0129	0.0125	0.0122	0.0119	0.0116	0.0113	0.0110
2.3	0.0107	0.0104	0.0102	0.0099	0.0096	0.0094	0.0091	0.0089	0.0087	0.0084
2.4	0.0082	0.0080	0.0078	0.0075	0.0073	0.0071	0.0069	0.0068	0.0066	0.0064
2.5	0.0062	0.0060	0.0059	0.0057	0.0055	0.0054	0.0052	0.0051	0.0049	0.0048
2.6	0.0047	0.0045	0.0044	0.0043	0.0041	0.0040	0.0039	0.0038	0.0037	0.0036
2.7	0.0035	0.0034	0.0033	0.0032	0.0031	0.0030	0.0029	0.0028	0.0027	0.0026
2.8	0.0026	0.0025	0.0024	0.0023	0.0023	0.0022	0.0021	0.0021	0.0020	0.0019
2.9	0.0019	0.0018	0.0018	0.0017	0.0016	0.0016	0.0015	0.0015	0.0014	0.0014
3.0	0.0013	0.0013	0.0013	0.0012	0.0012	0.0011	0.0011	0.0011	0.0010	0.0010
3.1	0.0010	0.0009	0.0009	0.0009	0.0008	0.0008	0.0008	0.0008	0.0007	0.0007
3.2	0.0007	0.0007	0.0006	0.0006	0.0006	0.0006	0.0006	0.0005	0.0005	0.0005
3.3	0.0005	0.0005	0.0005	0.0004	0.0004	0.0004	0.0004	0.0004	0.0004	0.0003
3.4	0.0003	0.0003	0.0003	0.0003	0.0003	0.0003	0.0003	0.0003	0.0003	0.0002
3.5	0.0002	0.0002	0.0002	0.0002	0.0002	0.0002	0.0002	0.0002	0.0002	0.0002
3.6	0.0002	0.0002	0.0001	0.0001	0.0001	0.0001	0.0001	0.0001	0.0001	0.0001
3.7	0.0001	0.0001	0.0001	0.0001	0.0001	0.0001	0.0001	0.0001	0.0001	0.0001
3.8	0.0001	0.0001	0.0001	0.0001	0.0001	0.0001	0.0001	0.0001	0.0001	0.0001

*To determine the area in one tail of the standard normal distribution, calculate a standard normal deviate (z) to two decimal places. Find the first two digits of that deviate (units and tenths) in the left-hand column. Find the third digit (hundredths) in the top row. The corresponding area is at the intersection of that column and that row.

TABLE B.2 Critical values of Student's *t* distribution*

α(2)	0.50	0.20	0.10	0.05	0.02	0.01	0.005	0.002	0.001
α(1)	0.25	0.10	0.05	0.025	0.01	0.005	0.0025	0.001	0.0005
df									
1	1.000	3.078	6.314	12.71	31.82	63.66	127.3	318.3	636.6
2	0.816	1.886	2.920	4.303	6.965	9.925	14.09	22.33	31.60
3	0.765	1.638	2.353	3.182	4.541	5.841	7.453	10.22	12.92
4	0.741	1.533	2.132	2.776	3.747	4.604	5.598	7.173	8.610
5	0.727	1.476	2.015	2.571	3.365	4.032	4.773	5.893	6.869
6	0.718	1.440	1.943	2.447	3.143	3.707	4.317	5.208	5.959
7	0.711	1.415	1.895	2.365	2.998	3.499	4.029	4.785	5.408
8	0.706	1.397	1.860	2.306	2.896	3.355	3.833	4.501	5.041
9	0.703	1.383	1.833	2.262	2.821	3.250	3.690	4.297	4.781
10	0.700	1.372	1.812	2.228	2.764	3.169	3.581	4.144	4.587
11	0.697	1.363	1.796	2.201	2.718	3.106	3.497	4.025	4.437
12	0.695	1.356	1.782	2.179	2.681	3.055	3.428	3.930	4.318
13	0.694	1.350	1.771	2.160	2.650	3.012	3.372	3.852	4.221
14	0.692	1.345	1.761	2.145	2.624	2.977	3.326	3.787	4.140
15	0.691	1.341	1.753	2.131	2.602	2.947	3.286	3.733	4.073
16	0.690	1.337	1.746	2.120	2.583	2.921	3.252	3.686	4.015
17	0.689	1.333	1.740	2.110	2.567	2.898	3.222	3.646	3.965
18	0.688	1.330	1.734	2.101	2.552	2.878	3.197	3.610	3.922
19	0.688	1.328	1.729	2.093	2.539	2.861	3.174	3.579	3.883
20	0.687	1.325	1.725	2.086	2.528	2.845	3.153	3.552	3.850
22	0.686	1.321	1.717	2.074	2.508	2.819	3.119	3.505	3.792
24	0.685	1.318	1.711	2.064	2.492	2.797	3.091	3.467	3.745
26	0.684	1.315	1.706	2.056	2.479	2.779	3.067	3.435	3.707
28	0.683	1.313	1.701	2.048	2.467	2.763	3.047	3.408	3.674
30	0.683	1.310	1.697	2.042	2.457	2.750	3.030	3.385	3.646
32	0.682	1.309	1.694	2.037	2.449	2.738	3.015	3.365	3.622
34	0.682	1.307	1.691	2.032	2.441	2.728	3.002	3.348	3.601
36	0.681	1.306	1.688	2.028	2.434	2.719	2.990	3.333	3.582
38	0.681	1.304	1.686	2.024	2.429	2.712	2.980	3.319	3.566
40	0.681	1.303	1.684	2.021	2.423	2.704	2.971	3.307	3.551
45	0.680	1.301	1.679	2.014	2.412	2.690	2.952	3.281	3.520
50	0.679	1.299	1.676	2.009	2.403	2.678	2.937	3.261	3.496
55	0.679	1.297	1.674	2.004	2.396	2.668	2.925	3.245	3.477
60	0.679	1.296	1.671	2.000	2.390	2.660	2.915	3.232	3.460
65	0.678	1.295	1.669	1.997	2.385	2.654	2.906	3.221	3.447
70	0.678	1.294	1.667	1.994	2.381	2.648	2.899	3.211	3.435
75	0.678	1.293	1.665	1.992	2.377	2.643	2.893	3.203	3.425
80	0.678	1.292	1.664	1.990	2.374	2.639	2.887	3.195	3.416
85	0.677	1.291	1.663	1.988	2.371	2.635	2.882	3.189	3.409
90	0.677	1.291	1.662	1.987	2.368	2.632	2.878	3.183	3.402
100	0.677	1.290	1.660	1.984	2.364	2.626	2.871	3.174	3.390
150	0.676	1.287	1.655	1.976	2.351	2.609	2.849	3.145	3.357
200	0.676	1.286	1.653	1.972	2.345	2.601	2.839	3.131	3.340
500	0.675	1.283	1.648	1.965	2.334	2.586	2.820	3.107	3.310
∞	0.674	1.282	1.645	1.960	2.326	2.576	2.807	3.090	3.290

*To locate a Student's *t* value, find the degrees of freedom in the leftmost column and the appropriate α at the top of the table (α(2) indicates a two-tailed value and α(1) indicates a one-tailed value). The number in the body of the table where this row and column intersect is the Student's *t* value from a distribution with that number of degrees of freedom and that corresponds to an area equal to α.

TABLE B.3 Critical values of Wilcoxon's *T* statistic*

α(2)	0.50	0.20	0.10	0.05	0.02	0.01	0.005	0.001
α(1)	0.25	0.10	0.05	0.025	0.01	0.005	0.0025	0.0005
n								
4	2	0						
5	4	2	0					
6	6	3	2	0				
7	9	5	3	2	0			
8	12	8	5	3	1	0		
9	16	10	8	5	3	1	0	
10	20	14	10	8	5	3	1	
11	24	17	13	10	7	5	3	0
12	29	21	17	13	9	7	5	1
13	35	26	21	17	12	9	7	2
14	40	31	25	21	15	12	9	4
15	47	36	30	25	19	15	12	6
16	54	42	35	29	23	19	15	8
17	61	48	41	34	27	23	19	11
18	69	55	47	40	32	27	23	14
19	77	62	53	46	37	32	27	18
20	86	69	60	52	43	37	32	21
21	95	77	67	58	49	42	37	25
22	104	86	75	65	55	48	42	30
23	114	94	83	73	62	54	48	35
24	125	104	91	81	69	61	54	40
25	136	113	100	89	76	68	60	45
26	148	124	110	98	84	75	67	51
27	160	134	119	107	92	83	74	57
28	172	145	130	116	101	91	82	64
29	185	157	140	126	110	100	90	71
30	198	169	151	137	120	109	98	78
32	226	194	175	159	140	128	116	94
34	257	221	200	182	162	148	136	111
36	289	250	227	208	185	171	157	130
38	323	281	256	235	211	194	180	150
40	358	313	286	264	238	220	204	172
42	396	348	319	294	266	247	230	195
44	436	384	353	327	296	276	258	220
46	477	422	389	361	328	307	287	246
48	521	462	426	396	362	339	318	274
50	566	503	466	434	397	373	350	304
55	688	615	573	536	493	465	438	385
60	822	739	690	648	600	567	537	476
65	968	875	820	772	718	681	647	577
70	1126	1022	960	907	846	805	767	689
75	1296	1181	1112	1053	986	940	898	811
80	1478	1351	1276	1211	1136	1086	1039	943
85	1672	1533	1451	1380	1298	1242	1191	1086
90	1878	1727	1638	1560	1471	1410	1355	1240
95	2097	1933	1836	1752	1655	1589	1529	1404
100	2327	2151	2045	1955	1850	1779	1714	1578

*To locate a Wilcoxon's *T* value, find the sample's size in the leftmost column and the appropriate α at the top of the table (α(2) indicates a two-tailed value and α(1) indicates a one-tailed value). A calculated *T* value is statistically significant (i.e., the null hypothesis can be rejected) if it is *less* than the value in the table.

TABLE B.4 Critical values of the F distribution*

α(1)	0.25	0.10	0.05	0.025	0.01	0.005	0.0025	0.001	0.0005
				Numerator df = 1					
Denom df									
1	5.83	39.9	161.	648.	4050.	16200.	64800.	$4 \cdot 10^5$	$2 \cdot 10^6$
2	2.57	8.53	18.5	38.5	98.5	199.	399.	999.0	2000.
3	2.02	5.54	10.1	17.4	34.1	55.6	89.6	167.	267
4	1.81	4.54	7.71	12.2	21.2	31.3	45.7	74.1	106.
5	1.69	4.06	6.61	10.0	16.3	22.8	31.4	47.2	63.6
6	1.62	3.78	5.99	8.81	13.7	18.6	24.8	35.5	46.1
7	1.57	3.59	5.59	8.07	12.2	16.2	21.1	29.2	37.0
8	1.54	3.46	5.32	7.57	11.3	14.7	18.8	25.4	31.6
9	1.51	3.36	5.12	7.21	10.6	13.6	17.2	22.9	28.0
10	1.49	3.29	4.96	6.94	10.0	12.8	16.0	21.0	25.5
11	1.47	3.23	4.84	6.72	9.65	12.2	15.2	19.7	23.7
12	1.46	3.18	4.75	6.55	9.33	11.8	14.5	18.6	22.2
13	1.45	3.14	4.67	6.41	9.07	11.4	13.9	17.8	21.1
14	1.44	3.10	4.60	6.30	8.86	11.1	13.5	17.1	20.2
15	1.43	3.07	4.54	6.20	8.68	10.8	13.1	16.6	19.5
16	1.42	3.05	4.49	6.12	8.53	10.6	12.8	16.1	18.9
17	1.42	3.03	4.45	6.04	8.40	10.4	12.6	15.7	18.4
18	1.41	3.01	4.41	5.98	8.29	10.2	12.3	15.4	17.9
19	1.41	2.99	4.38	5.92	8.18	10.1	12.1	15.1	17.5
20	1.40	2.97	4.35	5.87	8.10	9.94	11.9	14.8	17.2
21	1.40	2.96	4.32	5.83	8.02	9.83	11.8	14.6	16.9
22	1.40	2.95	4.30	5.79	7.95	9.73	11.6	14.4	16.6
23	1.39	2.94	4.28	5.75	7.88	9.63	11.5	14.2	16.4
24	1.39	2.93	4.26	5.72	7.82	9.55	11.4	14.0	16.2
25	1.39	2.92	4.24	5.69	7.77	9.48	11.3	13.9	16.0
26	1.38	2.91	4.23	5.66	7.72	9.41	11.2	13.7	15.8
27	1.38	2.90	4.21	5.63	7.68	9.34	11.1	13.6	15.6
28	1.38	2.89	4.20	5.61	7.64	9.28	11.0	13.5	15.5
29	1.38	2.89	4.18	5.59	7.60	9.23	11.0	13.4	15.3
30	1.38	2.88	4.17	5.57	7.56	9.18	10.9	13.3	15.2
35	1.37	2.85	4.12	5.48	7.42	8.98	10.6	12.9	14.7
40	1.36	2.84	4.08	5.42	7.31	8.83	10.4	12.6	14.4
45	1.36	2.82	4.06	5.38	7.23	8.71	10.3	12.4	14.1
50	1.35	2.81	4.03	5.34	7.17	8.63	10.1	12.2	13.9
60	1.35	2.79	4.00	5.29	7.08	8.49	9.96	12.0	13.5
70	1.35	2.78	3.98	5.25	7.01	8.40	9.84	11.8	13.3
80	1.34	2.77	3.96	5.22	6.96	8.33	9.75	11.7	13.2
90	1.34	2.76	3.95	5.20	6.93	8.28	9.68	11.6	13.0
100	1.34	2.76	3.94	5.18	6.90	8.24	9.62	11.5	12.9
200	1.33	2.73	3.89	5.10	6.76	8.06	9.38	11.2	12.6
500	1.33	2.72	3.86	5.05	6.69	7.95	9.23	11.0	12.3
∞	1.32	2.71	3.84	5.02	6.64	7.88	9.14	10.8	12.1

*To locate an F value, first find the table that is headed by the degrees of freedom in the numerator of your F ratio. Then, find the degrees of freedom in the denominator of your F ratio in the leftmost column. Finally, find the appropriate α at the top of the table. The number in the body of the table where this row and column intersect is the F statistic from a distribution with those numerator and denominator degrees of freedom and that corresponds to an area equal to α in one tail of the F distribution.

TABLE B.4 *Continued*

α(1)	0.25	0.10	0.05	0.025	0.01	0.005	0.0025	0.001	0.0005

Numerator df = 2

Denom df	0.25	0.10	0.05	0.025	0.01	0.005	0.0025	0.001	0.0005
1	7.50	49.5	200.	800.	5000.	20000.	80000.	$5 \cdot 10^5$	$2 \cdot 10^6$
2	3.00	9.00	19.0	39.0	99.0	199.	399.	999.	2000.
3	2.28	5.46	9.55	16.0	30.8	49.8	79.9	149.	237.
4	2.00	4.32	6.94	10.6	18.0	26.3	38.0	61.2	87.4
5	1.85	3.78	5.79	8.43	13.3	18.3	25.0	37.1	49.8
6	1.76	3.46	5.14	7.26	10.9	14.5	19.1	27.0	34.8
7	1.70	3.26	4.74	6.54	9.55	12.4	15.9	21.7	27.2
8	1.66	3.11	4.46	6.06	8.65	11.0	13.9	18.5	22.7
9	1.62	3.01	4.26	5.71	8.02	10.1	12.5	16.4	19.9
10	1.60	2.92	4.10	5.46	7.56	9.43	11.6	14.9	17.9
11	1.58	2.86	3.98	5.26	7.21	8.91	10.8	13.8	16.4
12	1.56	2.81	3.89	5.10	6.93	8.51	10.3	13.0	15.3
13	1.55	2.76	3.81	4.97	6.70	8.19	9.84	12.3	14.4
14	1.53	2.73	3.74	4.86	6.51	7.92	9.47	11.8	13.7
15	1.52	2.70	3.68	4.77	6.36	7.70	9.17	11.3	13.2
16	1.51	2.67	3.63	4.69	6.23	7.51	8.92	11.0	12.7
17	1.51	2.64	3.59	4.62	6.11	7.35	8.70	10.7	12.3
18	1.50	2.62	3.55	4.56	6.01	7.21	8.51	10.4	11.9
19	1.49	2.61	3.52	4.51	5.93	7.09	8.35	10.2	11.6
20	1.49	2.59	3.49	4.46	5.85	6.99	8.21	9.95	11.4
21	1.48	2.57	3.47	4.42	5.78	6.89	8.08	9.77	11.2
22	1.48	2.56	3.44	4.38	5.72	6.81	7.96	9.61	11.0
23	1.47	2.55	3.42	4.35	5.66	6.73	7.86	9.47	10.8
24	1.47	2.54	3.40	4.32	5.61	6.66	7.77	9.34	10.6
25	1.47	2.53	3.39	4.29	5.57	6.60	7.69	9.22	10.5
26	1.46	2.52	3.37	4.27	5.53	6.54	7.61	9.12	10.3
27	1.46	2.51	3.35	4.24	5.49	6.49	7.54	9.02	10.2
28	1.46	2.50	3.34	4.22	5.45	6.44	7.48	8.93	10.1
29	1.45	2.50	3.33	4.20	5.42	6.40	7.42	8.85	9.99
30	1.45	2.49	3.32	4.18	5.39	6.35	7.36	8.77	9.90
35	1.44	2.46	3.27	4.11	5.27	6.19	7.14	8.47	9.52
40	1.44	2.44	3.23	4.05	5.18	6.07	6.99	8.25	9.25
45	1.43	2.42	3.20	4.01	5.11	5.97	6.86	8.09	9.04
50	1.43	2.41	3.18	3.97	5.06	5.90	6.77	7.96	8.88
60	1.42	2.39	3.15	3.93	4.98	5.79	6.63	7.77	8.65
70	1.41	2.38	3.13	3.89	4.92	5.72	6.53	7.64	8.49
80	1.41	2.37	3.11	3.86	4.88	5.67	6.46	7.54	8.37
90	1.41	2.36	3.10	3.84	4.85	5.62	6.41	7.47	8.28
100	1.41	2.36	3.09	3.83	4.82	5.59	6.37	7.41	8.21
200	1.40	2.33	3.04	3.76	4.71	5.44	6.17	7.15	7.90
500	1.39	2.31	3.01	3.72	4.65	5.35	6.06	7.00	7.72
∞	1.39	2.30	3.00	3.69	4.61	5.30	5.99	6.91	7.60

TABLE B.4 *Continued*

				Numerator df = 3					
α(1)	0.25	0.10	0.05	0.025	0.01	0.005	0.0025	0.001	0.0005
Denom df									
1	8.20	53.6	216.	864.	5400.	21600.	86500.	$5 \cdot 10^5$	$2 \cdot 10^6$
2	3.15	9.16	19.2	39.2	99.2	199.	399.	999.	2000.
3	2.36	5.39	9.28	15.4	29.5	47.5	76.1	141.	225.
4	2.05	4.19	6.59	9.98	16.7	24.3	35.0	56.2	80.1
5	1.88	3.62	5.41	7.76	12.1	16.5	22.4	33.2	44.4
6	1.78	3.29	4.76	6.60	9.78	12.9	16.9	23.7	30.5
7	1.72	3.07	4.35	5.89	8.45	10.9	13.8	18.8	23.5
8	1.67	2.92	4.07	5.42	7.59	9.60	12.0	15.8	19.4
9	1.63	2.81	3.86	5.08	6.99	8.72	10.7	13.9	16.8
10	1.60	2.73	3.71	4.83	6.55	8.08	9.83	12.6	15.0
11	1.58	2.66	3.59	4.63	6.22	7.60	9.17	11.6	13.7
12	1.56	2.61	3.49	4.47	5.95	7.23	8.65	10.8	12.7
13	1.55	2.56	3.41	4.35	5.74	6.93	8.24	10.2	11.9
14	1.53	2.52	3.34	4.24	5.56	6.68	7.91	9.73	11.3
15	1.52	2.49	3.29	4.15	5.42	6.48	7.63	9.34	10.8
16	1.51	2.46	3.24	4.08	5.29	6.30	7.40	9.01	10.3
17	1.50	2.44	3.20	4.01	5.19	6.16	7.21	8.73	9.99
18	1.49	2.42	3.16	3.95	5.09	6.03	7.04	8.49	9.69
19	1.49	2.40	3.13	3.90	5.01	5.92	6.89	8.28	9.42
20	1.48	2.38	3.10	3.86	4.94	5.82	6.76	8.10	9.20
21	1.48	2.36	3.07	3.82	4.87	5.73	6.64	7.94	8.99
22	1.47	2.35	3.05	3.78	4.82	5.65	6.54	7.80	8.82
23	1.47	2.34	3.03	3.75	4.76	5.58	6.45	7.67	8.66
24	1.46	2.33	3.01	3.72	4.72	5.52	6.36	7.55	8.51
25	1.46	2.32	2.99	3.69	4.68	5.46	6.29	7.45	8.39
26	1.45	2.31	2.98	3.67	4.64	5.41	6.22	7.36	8.27
27	1.45	2.30	2.96	3.65	4.60	5.36	6.16	7.27	8.16
28	1.45	2.29	2.95	3.63	4.57	5.32	6.10	7.19	8.07
29	1.45	2.28	2.93	3.61	4.54	5.28	6.05	7.12	7.98
30	1.44	2.28	2.92	3.59	4.51	5.24	6.00	7.05	7.89
35	1.43	2.25	2.87	3.52	4.40	5.09	5.80	6.79	7.56
40	1.42	2.23	2.84	3.46	4.31	4.98	5.66	6.59	7.33
45	1.42	2.21	2.81	3.42	4.25	4.89	5.55	6.45	7.15
50	1.41	2.20	2.79	3.39	4.20	4.83	5.47	6.34	7.01
60	1.41	2.18	2.76	3.34	4.13	4.73	5.34	6.17	6.81
70	1.40	2.16	2.74	3.31	4.07	4.66	5.26	6.06	6.67
80	1.40	2.15	2.72	3.28	4.04	4.61	5.19	5.97	6.57
90	1.39	2.15	2.71	3.26	4.01	4.57	5.14	5.91	6.49
100	1.39	2.14	2.70	3.25	3.98	4.54	5.11	5.86	6.43
200	1.38	2.11	2.65	3.18	3.88	4.41	4.94	5.63	6.16
500	1.37	2.09	2.62	3.14	3.82	4.33	4.64	5.51	6.01
∞	1.37	2.08	2.61	3.12	3.78	4.28	4.77	5.42	5.91

TABLE B.4 *Continued* ■

				Numerator df = 4					
α(1)	0.25	0.10	0.05	0.025	0.01	0.005	0.0025	0.001	0.0005
Denom df									
1	8.58	55.8	225.	900.	5620.	22500.	90000.	$6 \cdot 10^5$	$2 \cdot 10^6$
2	3.23	9.24	19.2	39.2	99.2	199.	399.	999.	2000.
3	2.39	5.34	9.12	15.1	28.7	46.2	73.9	137.	218.
4	2.06	4.11	6.39	9.60	16.0	23.2	33.3	53.4	76.1
5	1.89	3.52	5.19	7.39	11.4	15.6	21.0	31.1	41.5
6	1.79	3.18	4.53	6.23	9.15	12.0	15.7	21.9	28.1
7	1.72	2.96	4.12	5.52	7.85	10.1	12.7	17.2	21.4
8	1.66	2.81	3.84	5.05	7.01	8.81	10.9	14.4	17.6
9	1.63	2.69	3.63	4.72	6.42	7.96	9.74	12.6	15.1
10	1.59	2.61	3.48	4.47	5.99	7.34	8.89	11.3	13.4
11	1.57	2.54	3.36	4.28	5.67	6.88	8.25	10.3	12.2
12	1.55	2.48	3.26	4.12	5.41	6.52	7.76	9.63	11.2
13	1.53	2.43	3.18	4.00	5.21	6.23	7.37	9.07	10.5
14	1.52	2.39	3.11	3.89	5.04	6.00	7.06	8.62	9.95
15	1.51	2.36	3.06	3.80	4.89	5.80	6.80	8.25	9.48
16	1.50	2.33	3.01	3.73	4.77	5.64	6.58	7.94	9.08
17	1.49	2.31	2.96	3.66	4.67	5.50	6.39	7.68	8.75
18	1.48	2.29	2.93	3.61	4.58	5.37	6.23	7.46	8.47
19	1.47	2.27	2.90	3.56	4.50	5.27	6.09	7.27	8.23
20	1.47	2.25	2.87	3.51	4.43	5.17	5.97	7.10	8.02
21	1.46	2.23	2.84	3.48	4.37	5.09	5.86	6.95	7.83
22	1.45	2.22	2.82	3.44	4.31	5.02	5.76	6.81	7.67
23	1.45	2.21	2.80	3.41	4.26	4.95	5.67	6.70	7.52
24	1.44	2.19	2.78	3.38	4.22	4.89	5.60	6.59	7.39
25	1.44	2.18	2.76	3.35	4.18	4.84	5.53	6.49	7.27
26	1.44	2.17	2.74	3.33	4.14	4.79	5.46	6.41	7.16
27	1.43	2.17	2.73	3.31	4.11	4.74	5.40	6.33	7.06
28	1.43	2.16	2.71	3.29	4.07	4.70	5.35	6.25	6.97
29	1.43	2.15	2.70	3.27	4.04	4.66	5.30	6.19	6.89
30	1.42	2.14	2.69	3.25	4.02	4.62	5.25	6.12	6.82
35	1.41	2.11	2.64	3.18	3.91	4.48	5.07	5.88	6.51
40	1.40	2.09	2.61	3.13	3.83	4.37	4.93	5.70	6.30
45	1.40	2.07	2.58	3.09	3.77	4.29	4.83	5.56	6.13
50	1.39	2.06	2.56	3.05	3.72	4.23	4.75	5.46	6.01
60	1.38	2.04	2.53	3.01	3.65	4.14	4.64	5.31	5.82
70	1.38	2.03	2.50	2.97	3.60	4.08	4.56	5.20	5.70
80	1.38	2.02	2.49	2.95	3.56	4.03	4.50	5.12	5.60
90	1.37	2.01	2.47	2.93	3.53	3.99	4.45	5.06	5.53
100	1.37	2.00	2.46	2.92	3.51	3.96	4.42	5.02	5.48
200	1.36	1.97	2.42	2.85	3.41	3.84	4.26	4.81	5.23
500	1.35	1.96	2.39	2.81	3.36	3.76	4.17	4.69	5.09
∞	1.35	1.94	2.37	2.79	3.32	3.72	4.11	4.62	5.00

TABLE B.4 *Continued*

					Numerator df = 5				
$\alpha(1)$	0.25	0.10	0.05	0.025	0.01	0.005	0.0025	0.001	0.0005
Denom df									
1	8.82	57.2	230.	922.	5760.	23100.	92200.	$6 \cdot 10^5$	$2 \cdot 10^6$
2	3.28	9.29	19.3	39.3	99.3	199.	399.	999.	2000.
3	2.41	5.31	9.01	14.9	28.2	45.4	72.6	135.	214.
4	2.07	4.05	6.26	9.36	15.5	22.5	32.3	51.7	73.6
5	1.89	3.45	5.05	7.15	11.0	14.9	20.2	29.8	39.7
6	1.79	3.11	4.39	5.99	8.75	11.5	14.9	20.8	26.6
7	1.71	2.88	3.97	5.29	7.46	9.52	12.0	16.2	20.2
8	1.66	2.73	3.69	4.82	6.63	8.30	10.3	13.5	16.4
9	1.62	2.61	3.48	4.48	6.06	7.47	9.12	11.7	14.1
10	1.59	2.52	3.33	4.24	5.64	6.87	8.29	10.5	12.4
11	1.56	2.45	3.20	4.04	5.32	6.42	7.67	9.58	11.2
12	1.54	2.39	3.11	3.89	5.06	6.07	7.20	8.89	10.4
13	1.52	2.35	3.03	3.77	4.86	5.79	6.82	8.35	9.66
14	1.51	2.31	2.96	3.66	4.69	5.56	6.51	7.92	9.11
15	1.49	2.27	2.90	3.58	4.56	5.37	6.26	7.57	8.66
16	1.48	2.24	2.85	3.50	4.44	5.21	6.05	7.27	8.29
17	1.47	2.22	2.81	3.44	4.34	5.07	5.87	7.02	7.98
18	1.46	2.20	2.77	3.38	4.25	4.96	5.72	6.81	7.71
19	1.46	2.18	2.74	3.33	4.17	4.85	5.58	6.62	7.48
20	1.45	2.16	2.71	3.29	4.10	4.76	5.46	6.46	7.27
21	1.44	2.14	2.68	3.25	4.04	4.68	5.36	6.32	7.10
22	1.44	2.13	2.66	3.22	3.99	4.61	5.26	6.19	6.94
23	1.43	2.11	2.64	3.18	3.94	4.54	5.18	6.08	6.80
24	1.43	2.10	2.62	3.15	3.90	4.49	5.11	5.98	6.68
25	1.42	2.09	2.60	3.13	3.85	4.43	5.04	5.89	6.56
26	1.42	2.08	2.59	3.10	3.82	4.38	4.98	5.80	6.46
27	1.42	2.07	2.57	3.08	3.78	4.34	4.92	5.73	6.37
28	1.41	2.06	2.56	3.06	3.75	4.30	4.87	5.66	6.28
29	1.41	2.06	2.55	3.04	3.73	4.26	4.82	5.59	6.21
30	1.41	2.05	2.53	3.03	3.70	4.23	4.78	5.53	6.13
35	1.40	2.02	2.49	2.96	3.59	4.09	4.60	5.30	5.85
40	1.39	2.00	2.45	2.90	3.51	3.99	4.47	5.13	5.64
45	1.38	1.98	2.42	2.86	3.45	3.91	4.37	5.00	5.49
50	1.37	1.97	2.40	2.83	3.41	3.85	4.30	4.90	5.37
60	1.37	1.95	2.37	2.79	3.34	3.76	4.19	4.76	5.20
70	1.36	1.93	2.35	2.75	3.29	3.70	4.11	4.66	5.08
80	1.36	1.92	2.33	2.73	3.26	3.65	4.05	4.58	4.99
90	1.35	1.91	2.32	2.71	3.23	3.62	4.01	4.53	4.92
100	1.35	1.91	2.31	2.70	3.21	3.59	3.97	4.48	4.87
200	1.34	1.88	2.26	2.63	3.11	3.47	3.82	4.29	4.64
500	1.33	1.86	2.23	2.59	3.05	3.40	3.73	4.18	4.51
∞	1.33	1.85	2.21	2.57	3.02	3.35	3.68	4.10	4.42

TABLE B.4 *Continued*

				Numerator df = 6					
α(1)	0.25	0.10	0.05	0.025	0.01	0.005	0.0025	0.001	0.0005
Denom df									
1	8.98	58.2	234.	937.	5860.	23400.	93700.	$6 \cdot 10^5$	$2 \cdot 10^6$
2	3.31	9.33	19.3	39.3	99.3	199.	399.	999.	2000.
3	2.42	5.28	8.94	14.7	27.9	44.8	71.7	133.	211.
4	2.08	4.01	6.16	9.20	15.2	22.0	31.5	50.5	71.9
5	1.89	3.40	4.95	6.98	10.7	14.5	19.6	28.8	38.5
6	1.78	3.05	4.28	5.82	8.47	11.1	14.4	20.0	25.6
7	1.71	2.83	3.87	5.12	7.19	9.16	11.5	15.5	19.3
8	1.65	2.67	3.58	4.65	6.37	7.95	9.83	12.9	15.7
9	1.61	2.55	3.37	4.32	5.80	7.13	8.68	11.1	13.3
10	1.58	2.46	3.22	4.07	5.39	6.54	7.87	9.93	11.7
11	1.55	2.39	3.09	3.88	5.07	6.10	7.27	9.05	10.6
12	1.53	2.33	3.00	3.73	4.82	5.76	6.80	8.38	9.74
13	1.51	2.28	2.92	3.60	4.62	5.48	6.44	7.86	9.07
14	1.50	2.24	2.85	3.50	4.46	5.26	6.14	7.44	8.53
15	1.48	2.21	2.79	3.41	4.32	5.07	5.89	7.09	8.10
16	1.47	2.18	2.74	3.34	4.20	4.91	5.68	6.80	7.74
17	1.46	2.15	2.70	3.28	4.10	4.78	5.51	6.56	7.43
18	1.45	2.13	2.66	3.22	4.01	4.66	5.36	6.35	7.18
19	1.44	2.11	2.63	3.17	3.94	4.56	5.23	6.18	6.95
20	1.44	2.09	2.60	3.13	3.87	4.47	5.11	6.02	6.76
21	1.43	2.08	2.57	3.09	3.81	4.39	5.01	5.88	6.59
22	1.42	2.06	2.55	3.05	3.76	4.32	4.92	5.76	6.44
23	1.42	2.05	2.53	3.02	3.71	4.26	4.84	5.65	6.30
24	1.41	2.04	2.51	2.99	3.67	4.20	4.76	5.55	6.18
25	1.41	2.02	2.49	2.97	3.63	4.15	4.70	5.46	6.07
26	1.41	2.01	2.47	2.94	3.59	4.10	4.64	5.38	5.98
27	1.40	2.00	2.46	2.92	3.56	4.06	4.58	5.31	5.89
28	1.40	2.00	2.45	2.90	3.53	4.02	4.53	5.24	5.80
29	1.40	1.99	2.43	2.88	3.50	3.98	4.48	5.18	5.73
30	1.39	1.98	2.42	2.87	3.47	3.95	4.44	5.12	5.66
35	1.38	1.95	2.37	2.80	3.37	3.81	4.27	4.89	5.39
40	1.37	1.93	2.34	2.74	3.29	3.71	4.14	4.73	5.19
45	1.36	1.91	2.31	2.70	3.23	3.64	4.05	4.61	5.04
50	1.36	1.90	2.29	2.67	3.19	3.58	3.98	4.51	4.93
60	1.35	1.87	2.25	2.63	3.12	3.49	3.87	4.37	4.76
70	1.34	1.86	2.23	2.59	3.07	3.43	3.79	4.28	4.64
80	1.34	1.85	2.21	2.57	3.04	3.39	3.74	4.20	4.56
90	1.33	1.84	2.20	2.55	3.01	3.35	3.70	4.15	4.50
100	1.33	1.83	2.19	2.54	2.99	3.33	3.66	4.11	4.45
200	1.32	1.80	2.14	2.47	2.89	3.21	3.52	3.92	4.22
500	1.31	1.79	2.12	2.43	2.84	3.14	3.43	3.81	4.10
∞	1.31	1.77	2.10	2.41	2.80	3.09	3.37	3.74	4.02

TABLE B.4 *Continued*

	Numerator df = 7								
α(1)	0.25	0.10	0.05	0.025	0.01	0.005	0.0025	0.001	0.0005
Denom df									
1	9.10	58.9	237.	948.	5930.	23700.	94900.	$6 \cdot 10^5$	$2 \cdot 10^6$
2	3.34	9.35	19.4	39.4	99.4	199.	399.	999.	2000.
3	2.43	5.27	8.89	14.6	27.7	44.4	71.0	132.	209.
4	2.08	3.98	6.09	9.07	15.0	21.6	31.0	49.7	70.7
5	1.89	3.37	4.88	6.85	10.5	14.2	19.1	28.2	37.6
6	1.78	3.01	4.21	5.70	8.26	10.8	14.0	19.5	24.9
7	1.70	2.78	3.79	4.99	6.99	8.89	11.2	15.0	18.7
8	1.64	2.62	3.50	4.53	6.18	7.69	9.49	12.4	15.1
9	1.60	2.51	3.29	4.20	5.61	6.88	8.36	10.7	12.8
10	1.57	2.41	3.14	3.95	5.20	6.30	7.56	9.52	11.2
11	1.54	2.34	3.01	3.76	4.89	5.86	6.97	8.66	10.1
12	1.52	2.28	2.91	3.61	4.64	5.52	6.51	8.00	9.28
13	1.50	2.23	2.83	3.48	4.44	5.25	6.15	7.49	8.63
14	1.49	2.19	2.76	3.38	4.28	5.03	5.86	7.08	8.11
15	1.47	2.16	2.71	3.29	4.14	4.85	5.62	6.74	7.68
16	1.46	2.13	2.66	3.22	4.03	4.69	5.41	6.46	7.33
17	1.45	2.10	2.61	3.16	3.93	4.56	5.24	6.22	7.04
18	1.44	2.08	2.58	3.10	3.84	4.44	5.09	6.02	6.78
19	1.43	2.06	2.54	3.05	3.77	4.34	4.96	5.85	6.57
20	1.43	2.04	2.51	3.01	3.70	4.26	4.85	5.69	6.38
21	1.42	2.02	2.49	2.97	3.64	4.18	4.75	5.56	6.21
22	1.41	2.01	2.46	2.93	3.59	4.11	4.66	5.44	6.07
23	1.41	1.99	2.44	2.90	3.54	4.05	4.58	5.33	5.94
24	1.40	1.98	2.42	2.87	3.50	3.99	4.51	5.23	5.82
25	1.40	1.97	2.40	2.85	3.46	3.94	4.44	5.15	5.71
26	1.39	1.96	2.39	2.82	3.42	3.89	4.38	5.07	5.62
27	1.39	1.95	2.37	2.80	3.39	3.85	4.33	5.00	5.53
28	1.39	1.94	2.36	2.78	3.36	3.81	4.28	4.93	5.45
29	1.38	1.93	2.35	2.76	3.33	3.77	4.24	4.87	5.38
30	1.38	1.93	2.33	2.75	3.30	3.74	4.19	4.82	5.31
35	1.37	1.90	2.29	2.68	3.20	3.61	4.02	4.59	5.04
40	1.36	1.87	2.25	2.62	3.12	3.51	3.90	4.44	4.85
45	1.35	1.85	2.22	2.58	3.07	3.43	3.81	4.32	4.71
50	1.34	1.84	2.20	2.55	3.02	3.38	3.74	4.22	4.60
60	1.33	1.82	2.17	2.51	2.95	3.29	3.63	4.09	4.44
70	1.33	1.80	2.14	2.47	2.91	3.23	3.56	3.99	4.32
80	1.32	1.79	2.13	2.45	2.87	3.19	3.50	3.92	4.24
90	1.32	1.78	2.11	2.43	2.84	3.15	3.46	3.87	4.18
100	1.32	1.78	2.10	2.42	2.82	3.13	3.43	3.83	4.13
200	1.30	1.75	2.06	2.35	2.73	3.01	3.29	3.65	3.92
500	1.30	1.73	2.03	2.31	2.68	2.94	3.20	3.54	3.80
∞	1.29	1.72	2.01	2.29	2.64	2.90	3.15	3.47	3.72

TABLE B.4 *Continued*   ■

					Numerator df = 8				
α(1)	0.25	0.10	0.05	0.025	0.01	0.005	0.0025	0.001	0.0005
Denom df									
1	9.19	59.4	239.	957.	5980.	23900.	95700.	$6 \cdot 10^5$	$2 \cdot 10^6$
2	3.35	9.37	19.4	39.4	99.4	199.	399.	999.	2000.
3	2.44	5.25	8.85	14.5	27.5	44.1	70.5	131.	208.
4	2.08	3.95	6.04	8.98	14.8	21.4	30.6	49.0	69.7
5	1.89	3.34	4.82	6.76	10.3	14.0	18.8	27.6	36.9
6	1.78	2.98	4.15	5.60	8.10	10.6	13.7	19.0	24.3
7	1.70	2.75	3.73	4.90	6.84	8.68	10.9	14.6	18.2
8	1.64	2.59	3.44	4.43	6.03	7.50	9.24	12.0	14.6
9	1.60	2.47	3.23	4.10	5.47	6.69	8.12	10.4	12.4
10	1.56	2.38	3.07	3.85	5.06	6.12	7.33	9.20	10.9
11	1.53	2.30	2.95	3.66	4.74	5.68	6.74	8.35	9.76
12	1.51	2.24	2.85	3.51	4.50	5.35	6.29	7.71	8.94
13	1.49	2.20	2.77	3.39	4.30	5.08	5.93	7.21	8.29
14	1.48	2.15	2.70	3.29	4.14	4.86	5.64	6.80	7.78
15	1.46	2.12	2.64	3.20	4.00	4.67	5.40	6.47	7.37
16	1.45	2.09	2.59	3.12	3.89	4.52	5.20	6.19	7.02
17	1.44	2.06	2.55	3.06	3.79	4.39	5.03	5.96	6.73
18	1.43	2.04	2.51	3.01	3.71	4.28	4.89	5.76	6.48
19	1.42	2.02	2.48	2.96	3.63	4.18	4.76	5.59	6.27
20	1.42	2.00	2.45	2.91	3.56	4.09	4.65	5.44	6.09
21	1.41	1.98	2.42	2.87	3.51	4.01	4.55	5.31	5.92
22	1.40	1.97	2.40	2.84	3.45	3.94	4.46	5.19	5.78
23	1.40	1.95	2.37	2.81	3.41	3.88	4.38	5.09	5.65
24	1.39	1.94	2.36	2.78	3.36	3.83	4.31	4.99	5.54
25	1.39	1.93	2.34	2.75	3.32	3.78	4.25	4.91	5.43
26	1.38	1.92	2.32	2.73	3.29	3.73	4.19	4.83	5.34
27	1.38	1.91	2.31	2.71	3.26	3.69	4.14	4.76	5.25
28	1.38	1.90	2.29	2.69	3.23	3.65	4.09	4.69	5.18
29	1.37	1.89	2.28	2.67	3.20	3.61	4.04	4.64	5.11
30	1.37	1.88	2.27	2.65	3.17	3.58	4.00	4.58	5.04
35	1.36	1.85	2.22	2.58	3.07	3.45	3.83	4.36	4.78
40	1.35	1.83	2.18	2.53	2.99	3.35	3.71	4.21	4.59
45	1.34	1.81	2.15	2.49	2.94	3.28	3.62	4.09	4.45
50	1.33	1.80	2.13	2.46	2.89	3.22	3.55	4.00	4.34
60	1.32	1.77	2.10	2.41	2.82	3.13	3.45	3.86	4.19
70	1.32	1.76	2.07	2.38	2.78	3.08	3.37	3.77	4.08
80	1.31	1.75	2.06	2.35	2.74	3.03	3.32	3.70	4.00
90	1.31	1.74	2.04	2.34	2.72	3.00	3.28	3.65	3.94
100	1.30	1.73	2.03	2.32	2.69	2.97	3.25	3.61	3.89
200	1.29	1.70	1.98	2.26	2.60	2.86	3.11	3.43	3.68
500	1.28	1.68	1.96	2.22	2.55	2.79	3.03	3.33	3.56
∞	1.28	1.67	1.94	2.19	2.51	2.74	2.97	3.27	3.48

TABLE B.4 *Continued*   ■

	Numerator df = 9								
α(1)	0.25	0.10	0.05	0.025	0.01	0.005	0.0025	0.001	0.0005
Denom df									
1	9.26	59.9	241.	963.	6020.	24100.	96400.	$6 \cdot 10^5$	$2 \cdot 10^6$
2	3.37	9.38	19.4	39.4	99.4	199.	399.	999.	2000.
3	2.44	5.24	8.81	14.5	27.3	43.9	70.1	130.	207.
4	2.08	3.94	6.00	8.90	14.7	21.1	30.3	48.5	69.0
5	1.89	3.32	4.77	6.68	10.2	13.8	18.5	27.2	36.3
6	1.77	2.96	4.10	5.52	7.98	10.4	13.4	18.7	23.9
7	1.69	2.72	3.68	4.82	6.72	8.51	10.7	14.3	17.8
8	1.63	2.56	3.39	4.36	5.91	7.34	9.03	11.8	14.3
9	1.59	2.44	3.18	4.03	5.35	6.54	7.92	10.1	12.1
10	1.56	2.35	3.02	3.78	4.94	5.97	7.14	8.96	10.6
11	1.53	2.27	2.90	3.59	4.63	5.54	6.56	8.12	9.48
12	1.51	2.21	2.80	3.44	4.39	5.20	6.11	7.48	8.66
13	1.49	2.16	2.71	3.31	4.19	4.94	5.76	6.98	8.03
14	1.47	2.12	2.65	3.21	4.03	4.72	5.47	6.58	7.52
15	1.46	2.09	2.59	3.12	3.89	4.54	5.23	6.26	7.11
16	1.44	2.06	2.54	3.05	3.78	4.38	5.04	5.98	6.77
17	1.43	2.03	2.49	2.98	3.68	4.25	4.87	5.75	6.49
18	1.42	2.00	2.46	2.93	3.60	4.14	4.72	5.56	6.24
19	1.41	1.98	2.42	2.88	3.52	4.04	4.60	5.39	6.03
20	1.41	1.96	2.39	2.84	3.46	3.96	4.49	5.24	5.85
21	1.40	1.95	2.37	2.80	3.40	3.88	4.39	5.11	5.69
22	1.39	1.93	2.34	2.76	3.35	3.81	4.30	4.99	5.55
23	1.39	1.92	2.32	2.73	3.30	3.75	4.22	4.89	5.43
24	1.38	1.91	2.30	2.70	3.26	3.69	4.15	4.80	5.31
25	1.38	1.89	2.28	2.68	3.22	3.64	4.09	4.71	5.21
26	1.37	1.88	2.27	2.65	3.18	3.60	4.03	4.64	5.12
27	1.37	1.87	2.25	2.63	3.15	3.56	3.98	4.57	5.04
28	1.37	1.87	2.24	2.61	3.12	3.52	3.93	4.50	4.96
29	1.36	1.86	2.22	2.59	3.09	3.48	3.89	4.45	4.89
30	1.36	1.85	2.21	2.57	3.07	3.45	3.85	4.39	4.82
35	1.35	1.82	2.16	2.50	2.96	3.32	3.68	4.18	4.57
40	1.34	1.79	2.12	2.45	2.89	3.22	3.56	4.02	4.38
45	1.33	1.77	2.10	2.41	2.83	3.15	3.47	3.91	4.25
50	1.32	1.76	2.07	2.38	2.78	3.09	3.40	3.82	4.14
60	1.31	1.74	2.04	2.33	2.72	3.01	3.30	3.69	3.98
70	1.31	1.72	2.02	2.30	2.67	2.95	3.23	3.60	3.88
80	1.30	1.71	2.00	2.28	2.64	2.91	3.17	3.53	3.80
90	1.30	1.70	1.99	2.26	2.61	2.87	3.13	3.48	3.74
100	1.29	1.69	1.97	2.24	2.59	2.85	3.10	3.44	3.69
200	1.28	1.66	1.93	2.18	2.50	2.73	2.96	3.26	3.49
500	1.27	1.64	1.90	2.14	2.44	2.66	2.88	3.16	3.37
∞	1.27	1.63	1.88	2.11	2.41	2.62	2.83	3.10	3.30

TABLE B.4 *Continued*

					Numerator df = 10				
α(1)	0.25	0.10	0.05	0.025	0.01	0.005	0.0025	0.001	0.0005
Denom df									
1	9.32	60.2	242.	969.	6060.	24200.	96900.	$6 \cdot 10^5$	$2 \cdot 10^6$
2	3.38	9.39	19.4	39.4	99.4	199.	399.	999.	2000.
3	2.44	5.23	8.79	14.4	27.2	43.7	69.8	129.	206.
4	2.08	3.92	5.96	8.84	14.5	21.0	30.0	48.1	68.3
5	1.89	3.30	4.74	6.62	10.1	13.6	18.3	26.9	35.9
6	1.77	2.94	4.06	5.46	7.87	10.3	13.2	18.4	23.5
7	1.69	2.70	3.64	4.76	6.62	8.38	10.5	14.1	17.5
8	1.63	2.54	3.35	4.30	5.81	7.21	8.87	11.5	14.0
9	1.59	2.42	3.14	3.96	5.26	6.42	7.77	9.89	11.8
10	1.55	2.32	2.98	3.72	4.85	5.85	6.99	8.75	10.3
11	1.52	2.25	2.85	3.53	4.54	5.42	6.41	7.92	9.24
12	1.50	2.19	2.75	3.37	4.30	5.09	5.97	7.29	8.43
13	1.48	2.14	2.67	3.25	4.10	4.82	5.62	6.80	7.81
14	1.46	2.10	2.60	3.15	3.94	4.60	5.33	6.40	7.31
15	1.45	2.06	2.54	3.06	3.80	4.42	5.10	6.08	6.91
16	1.44	2.03	2.49	2.99	3.69	4.27	4.90	5.81	6.57
17	1.43	2.00	2.45	2.92	3.59	4.14	4.73	5.58	6.29
18	1.42	1.98	2.41	2.87	3.51	4.03	4.59	5.39	6.05
19	1.41	1.96	2.38	2.82	3.43	3.93	4.46	5.22	5.84
20	1.40	1.94	2.35	2.77	3.37	3.85	4.35	5.08	5.66
21	1.39	1.92	2.32	2.73	3.31	3.77	4.26	4.95	5.50
22	1.39	1.90	2.30	2.70	3.26	3.70	4.17	4.83	5.36
23	1.38	1.89	2.27	2.67	3.21	3.64	4.09	4.73	5.24
24	1.38	1.88	2.25	2.64	3.17	3.59	4.03	4.64	5.13
25	1.37	1.87	2.24	2.61	3.13	3.54	3.96	4.56	5.03
26	1.37	1.86	2.22	2.59	3.09	3.49	3.91	4.48	4.94
27	1.36	1.85	2.20	2.57	3.06	3.45	3.85	4.41	4.86
28	1.36	1.84	2.19	2.55	3.03	3.41	3.81	4.35	4.78
29	1.35	1.83	2.18	2.53	3.00	3.38	3.76	4.29	4.71
30	1.35	1.82	2.16	2.51	2.98	3.34	3.72	4.24	4.65
35	1.34	1.79	2.11	2.44	2.88	3.21	3.56	4.03	4.39
40	1.33	1.76	2.08	2.39	2.80	3.12	3.44	3.87	4.21
45	1.32	1.74	2.05	2.35	2.74	3.04	3.35	3.76	4.08
50	1.31	1.73	2.03	2.32	2.70	2.99	3.28	3.67	3.97
60	1.30	1.71	1.99	2.27	2.63	2.90	3.18	3.54	3.82
70	1.30	1.69	1.97	2.24	2.59	2.85	3.11	3.45	3.71
80	1.29	1.68	1.95	2.21	2.55	2.80	3.05	3.39	3.64
90	1.29	1.67	1.94	2.19	2.52	2.77	3.01	3.34	3.58
100	1.28	1.66	1.93	2.18	2.50	2.74	2.98	3.30	3.53
200	1.27	1.63	1.88	2.11	2.41	2.63	2.84	3.12	3.33
500	1.26	1.61	1.85	2.07	2.36	2.56	2.76	3.02	3.22
∞	1.25	1.60	1.83	2.05	2.32	2.52	2.71	2.96	3.14

TABLE B.4 *Continued*

				Numerator df = 12					
α(1)	0.25	0.10	0.05	0.025	0.01	0.005	0.0025	0.001	0.0005
Denom df									
1	9.41	60.7	244.	977.	6110.	24400.	97700.	$6 \cdot 10^5$	$2 \cdot 10^6$
2	3.39	9.41	19.4	39.4	99.4	199.	399.	999.	2000.
3	2.45	5.22	8.74	14.3	27.1	43.4	69.3	128.	204.
4	2.08	3.90	5.91	8.75	14.4	20.7	29.7	47.4	67.4
5	1.89	3.27	4.68	6.52	9.89	13.4	18.0	26.4	35.2
6	1.77	2.90	4.00	5.37	7.72	10.0	12.9	18.0	23.0
7	1.68	2.67	3.57	4.67	6.47	8.18	10.3	13.7	17.0
8	1.62	2.50	3.28	4.20	5.67	7.01	8.61	11.2	13.6
9	1.58	2.38	3.07	3.87	5.11	6.23	7.52	9.57	11.4
10	1.54	2.28	2.91	3.62	4.71	5.66	6.75	8.45	9.94
11	1.51	2.21	2.79	3.43	4.40	5.24	6.18	7.63	8.88
12	1.49	2.15	2.69	3.28	4.16	4.91	5.74	7.00	8.09
13	1.47	2.10	2.60	3.15	3.96	4.64	5.40	6.52	7.48
14	1.45	2.05	2.53	3.05	3.80	4.43	5.12	6.13	6.99
15	1.44	2.02	2.48	2.96	3.67	4.25	4.88	5.81	6.59
16	1.43	1.99	2.42	2.89	3.55	4.10	4.69	5.55	6.26
17	1.41	1.96	2.38	2.82	3.46	3.97	4.52	5.32	5.98
18	1.40	1.93	2.34	2.77	3.37	3.86	4.38	5.13	5.75
19	1.40	1.91	2.31	2.72	3.30	3.76	4.26	4.97	5.55
20	1.39	1.89	2.28	2.68	3.23	3.68	4.15	4.82	5.37
21	1.38	1.87	2.25	2.64	3.17	3.60	4.06	4.70	5.21
22	1.37	1.86	2.23	2.60	3.12	3.54	3.97	4.58	5.08
23	1.37	1.84	2.20	2.57	3.07	3.47	3.89	4.48	4.96
24	1.36	1.83	2.18	2.54	3.03	3.42	3.83	4.39	4.85
25	1.36	1.82	2.16	2.51	2.99	3.37	3.76	4.31	4.75
26	1.35	1.81	2.15	2.49	2.96	3.33	3.71	4.24	4.66
27	1.35	1.80	2.13	2.47	2.93	3.28	3.66	4.17	4.58
28	1.34	1.79	2.12	2.45	2.90	3.25	3.61	4.11	4.51
29	1.34	1.78	2.10	2.43	2.87	3.21	3.56	4.05	4.44
30	1.34	1.77	2.09	2.41	2.84	3.18	3.52	4.00	4.38
35	1.32	1.74	2.04	2.34	2.74	3.05	3.36	3.79	4.13
40	1.31	1.71	2.00	2.29	2.66	2.95	3.25	3.64	3.95
45	1.30	1.70	1.97	2.25	2.61	2.88	3.16	3.53	3.82
50	1.30	1.68	1.95	2.22	2.56	2.82	3.09	3.44	3.71
60	1.29	1.66	1.92	2.17	2.50	2.74	2.99	3.32	3.57
70	1.28	1.64	1.89	2.14	2.45	2.68	2.92	3.23	3.46
80	1.27	1.63	1.88	2.11	2.42	2.64	2.87	3.16	3.39
90	1.27	1.62	1.86	2.09	2.39	2.61	2.83	3.11	3.33
100	1.27	1.61	1.85	2.08	2.37	2.58	2.80	3.07	3.28
200	1.25	1.58	1.80	2.01	2.27	2.47	2.66	2.90	3.09
500	1.24	1.56	1.77	1.97	2.22	2.40	2.58	2.81	2.97
∞	1.24	1.55	1.75	1.94	2.18	2.36	2.53	2.74	2.90

TABLE B.4 *Continued*   ■

					Numerator df = 14				
α(1)	0.25	0.10	0.05	0.025	0.01	0.005	0.0025	0.001	0.0005
Denom df									
1	9.47	61.1	245.	983.	6140.	24600.	98300.	$6 \cdot 10^5$	$2 \cdot 10^6$
2	3.41	9.42	19.4	39.4	99.4	199.	399.	999.	2000.
3	2.45	5.20	8.71	14.3	26.9	43.2	69.0	128.	203.
4	2.08	3.88	5.87	8.68	14.2	20.5	29.4	46.9	66.8
5	1.89	3.25	4.64	6.46	9.77	13.2	17.8	26.1	34.7
6	1.76	2.88	3.96	5.30	7.60	9.88	12.7	17.7	22.6
7	1.68	2.64	3.53	4.60	6.36	8.03	10.1	13.4	16.6
8	1.62	2.48	3.24	4.13	5.56	6.87	8.43	10.9	13.3
9	1.57	2.35	3.03	3.80	5.01	6.09	7.35	9.33	11.1
10	1.54	2.26	2.86	3.55	4.60	5.53	6.58	8.22	9.67
11	1.51	2.18	2.74	3.36	4.29	5.10	6.02	7.41	8.62
12	1.48	2.12	2.64	3.21	4.05	4.77	5.58	6.79	7.84
13	1.46	2.07	2.55	3.08	3.86	4.51	5.24	6.31	7.23
14	1.44	2.02	2.48	2.98	3.70	4.30	4.96	5.93	6.75
15	1.43	1.99	2.42	2.89	3.56	4.12	4.73	5.62	6.36
16	1.42	1.95	2.37	2.82	3.45	3.97	4.54	5.35	6.03
17	1.41	1.93	2.33	2.75	3.35	3.84	4.37	5.13	5.76
18	1.40	1.90	2.29	2.70	3.27	3.73	4.23	4.94	5.53
19	1.39	1.88	2.26	2.65	3.19	3.64	4.11	4.78	5.33
20	1.38	1.86	2.22	2.60	3.13	3.55	4.00	4.64	5.15
21	1.37	1.84	2.20	2.56	3.07	3.48	3.91	4.51	5.00
22	1.36	1.83	2.17	2.53	3.02	3.41	3.82	4.40	4.87
23	1.36	1.81	2.15	2.50	2.97	3.35	3.75	4.30	4.75
24	1.35	1.80	2.13	2.47	2.93	3.30	3.68	4.21	4.64
25	1.35	1.79	2.11	2.44	2.89	3.25	3.62	4.13	4.54
26	1.34	1.77	2.09	2.42	2.86	3.20	3.56	4.06	4.46
27	1.34	1.76	2.08	2.39	2.82	3.16	3.51	3.99	4.38
28	1.33	1.75	2.06	2.37	2.79	3.12	3.46	3.93	4.30
29	1.33	1.75	2.05	2.36	2.77	3.09	3.42	3.88	4.24
30	1.33	1.74	2.04	2.34	2.74	3.06	3.38	3.82	4.18
35	1.31	1.70	1.99	2.27	2.64	2.93	3.22	3.62	3.93
40	1.30	1.68	1.95	2.21	2.56	2.83	3.10	3.47	3.76
45	1.29	1.66	1.92	2.17	2.51	2.76	3.02	3.36	3.63
50	1.28	1.64	1.89	2.14	2.46	2.70	2.95	3.27	3.52
60	1.27	1.62	1.86	2.09	2.39	2.62	2.85	3.15	3.38
70	1.27	1.60	1.84	2.06	2.35	2.56	2.78	3.06	3.28
80	1.26	1.59	1.82	2.03	2.31	2.52	2.73	3.00	3.20
90	1.26	1.58	1.80	2.02	2.29	2.49	2.69	2.95	3.14
100	1.25	1.57	1.79	2.00	2.27	2.46	2.65	2.91	3.10
200	1.24	1.54	1.74	1.93	2.17	2.35	2.52	2.74	2.91
500	1.23	1.52	1.71	1.89	2.12	2.28	2.44	2.64	2.79
∞	1.22	1.50	1.69	1.87	2.08	2.24	2.39	2.58	2.72

TABLE B.4 *Continued* ■

					Numerator df = 16				
α(1)	0.25	0.10	0.05	0.025	0.01	0.005	0.0025	0.001	0.0005
Denom df									
1	9.52	61.3	246.	987.	6170.	24700.	98700.	$6 \cdot 10^5$	$2 \cdot 10^6$
2	3.41	9.43	19.4	39.4	99.4	199.	399.	999.	2000.
3	2.46	5.20	8.69	14.2	26.8	43.0	68.7	127.	202.
4	2.08	3.86	5.84	8.63	14.2	20.4	29.2	46.6	66.2
5	1.88	3.23	4.60	6.40	9.68	13.1	17.6	25.8	34.3
6	1.76	2.86	3.92	5.24	7.52	9.76	12.6	17.4	22.3
7	1.68	2.62	3.49	4.54	6.28	7.91	9.91	13.2	16.4
8	1.62	2.45	3.20	4.08	5.48	6.76	8.29	10.8	13.0
9	1.57	2.33	2.99	3.74	4.92	5.98	7.21	9.15	10.9
10	1.53	2.23	2.83	3.50	4.52	5.42	6.45	8.05	9.46
11	1.50	2.16	2.70	3.30	4.21	5.00	5.89	7.24	8.43
12	1.48	2.09	2.60	3.15	3.97	4.67	5.46	6.63	7.65
13	1.46	2.04	2.51	3.03	3.78	4.41	5.11	6.16	7.05
14	1.44	2.00	2.44	2.92	3.62	4.20	4.84	5.78	6.57
15	1.42	1.96	2.38	2.84	3.49	4.02	4.61	5.46	6.18
16	1.41	1.93	2.33	2.76	3.37	3.87	4.42	5.20	5.86
17	1.40	1.90	2.29	2.70	3.27	3.75	4.25	4.99	5.59
18	1.39	1.87	2.25	2.64	3.19	3.64	4.11	4.80	5.36
19	1.38	1.85	2.21	2.59	3.12	3.54	3.99	4.64	5.16
20	1.37	1.83	2.18	2.55	3.05	3.46	3.89	4.49	4.99
21	1.36	1.81	2.16	2.51	2.99	3.38	3.79	4.37	4.84
22	1.36	1.80	2.13	2.47	2.94	3.31	3.71	4.26	4.71
23	1.35	1.78	2.11	2.44	2.89	3.25	3.63	4.16	4.59
24	1.34	1.77	2.09	2.41	2.85	3.20	3.56	4.07	4.48
25	1.34	1.76	2.07	2.38	2.81	3.15	3.50	3.99	4.39
26	1.33	1.75	2.05	2.36	2.78	3.11	3.45	3.92	4.30
27	1.33	1.74	2.04	2.34	2.75	3.07	3.40	3.86	4.22
28	1.32	1.73	2.02	2.32	2.72	3.03	3.35	3.80	4.15
29	1.32	1.72	2.01	2.30	2.69	2.99	3.31	3.74	4.08
30	1.32	1.71	1.99	2.28	2.66	2.96	3.27	3.69	4.02
35	1.30	1.67	1.94	2.21	2.56	2.83	3.11	3.48	3.78
40	1.29	1.65	1.90	2.15	2.48	2.74	2.99	3.34	3.61
45	1.28	1.63	1.87	2.11	2.43	2.66	2.90	3.23	3.48
50	1.27	1.61	1.85	2.08	2.38	2.61	2.84	3.14	3.38
60	1.26	1.59	1.82	2.03	2.31	2.53	2.74	3.02	3.23
70	1.26	1.57	1.79	2.00	2.27	2.47	2.67	2.93	3.13
80	1.25	1.56	1.77	1.97	2.23	2.43	2.62	2.87	3.06
90	1.25	1.55	1.76	1.95	2.21	2.39	2.58	2.82	3.00
100	1.24	1.54	1.75	1.94	2.19	2.37	2.55	2.78	2.96
200	1.23	1.51	1.69	1.87	2.09	2.25	2.41	2.61	2.76
500	1.22	1.49	1.66	1.83	2.04	2.19	2.33	2.52	2.65
∞	1.21	1.47	1.64	1.80	2.00	2.14	2.28	2.45	2.58

TABLE B.4 *Continued*   ▬

					Numerator df = 18				
α(1)	0.25	0.10	0.05	0.025	0.01	0.005	0.0025	0.001	0.0005
Denom df									
1	9.55	61.6	247.	990.	6190.	24800.	99100.	$6 \cdot 10^5$	$2 \cdot 10^6$
2	3.42	9.44	19.4	39.4	99.4	199.	399.	999.	2000.
3	2.46	5.19	8.67	14.2	26.8	42.9	68.5	127.	202.
4	2.08	3.85	5.82	8.59	14.1	20.3	29.0	46.3	65.8
5	1.88	3.22	4.58	6.36	9.61	13.0	17.4	25.6	34.0
6	1.76	2.85	3.90	5.20	7.45	9.66	12.4	17.3	22.0
7	1.67	2.61	3.47	4.50	6.21	7.83	9.79	13.1	16.2
8	1.61	2.44	3.17	4.03	5.41	6.68	8.18	10.6	12.8
9	1.56	2.31	2.96	3.70	4.86	5.90	7.11	9.01	10.7
10	1.53	2.22	2.80	3.45	4.46	5.34	6.35	7.91	9.30
11	1.50	2.14	2.67	3.26	4.15	4.92	5.79	7.11	8.27
12	1.47	2.08	2.57	3.11	3.91	4.59	5.36	6.51	7.50
13	1.45	2.02	2.48	2.98	3.72	4.33	5.02	6.03	6.90
14	1.43	1.98	2.41	2.88	3.56	4.12	4.74	5.66	6.43
15	1.42	1.94	2.35	2.79	3.42	3.95	4.51	5.35	6.04
16	1.40	1.91	2.30	2.72	3.31	3.80	4.32	5.09	5.72
17	1.39	1.88	2.26	2.65	3.21	3.67	4.16	4.87	5.45
18	1.38	1.85	2.22	2.60	3.13	3.56	4.02	4.68	5.23
19	1.37	1.83	2.18	2.55	3.05	3.46	3.90	4.52	5.03
20	1.36	1.81	2.15	2.50	2.99	3.38	3.79	4.38	4.86
21	1.36	1.79	2.12	2.46	2.93	3.31	3.70	4.26	4.71
22	1.35	1.78	2.10	2.43	2.88	3.24	3.62	4.15	4.58
23	1.34	1.76	2.08	2.39	2.83	3.18	3.54	4.05	4.46
24	1.34	1.75	2.05	2.36	2.79	3.12	3.47	3.96	4.35
25	1.33	1.74	2.04	2.34	2.75	3.08	3.41	3.88	4.26
26	1.33	1.72	2.02	2.31	2.72	3.03	3.36	3.81	4.17
27	1.32	1.71	2.00	2.29	2.68	2.99	3.31	3.75	4.10
28	1.32	1.70	1.99	2.27	2.65	2.95	3.26	3.69	4.02
29	1.31	1.69	1.97	2.25	2.63	2.92	3.22	3.63	3.96
30	1.31	1.69	1.96	2.23	2.60	2.89	3.18	3.58	3.90
35	1.29	1.65	1.91	2.16	2.50	2.76	3.02	3.38	3.66
40	1.28	1.62	1.87	2.11	2.42	2.66	2.90	3.23	3.49
45	1.27	1.60	1.84	2.07	2.36	2.59	2.82	3.12	3.36
50	1.27	1.59	1.81	2.03	2.32	2.53	2.75	3.04	3.26
60	1.26	1.56	1.78	1.98	2.25	2.45	2.65	2.91	3.11
70	1.25	1.55	1.75	1.95	2.20	2.39	2.58	2.83	3.01
80	1.24	1.53	1.73	1.92	2.17	2.35	2.53	2.76	2.94
90	1.24	1.52	1.72	1.91	2.14	2.32	2.49	2.71	2.88
100	1.23	1.52	1.71	1.89	2.12	2.29	2.46	2.68	2.84
200	1.22	1.48	1.66	1.82	2.03	2.18	2.32	2.51	2.65
500	1.21	1.46	1.62	1.78	1.97	2.11	2.24	2.41	2.54
∞	1.20	1.44	1.60	1.75	1.93	2.06	2.19	2.35	2.47

TABLE B.4 *Continued*   ■

				Numerator df = 20					
α(1)	**0.25**	**0.10**	**0.05**	**0.025**	**0.01**	**0.005**	**0.0025**	**0.001**	**0.0005**
Denom df									
1	9.58	61.7	248.	993.	6210.	24800.	99300.	$6 \cdot 10^5$	$2 \cdot 10^6$
2	3.43	9.44	19.4	39.4	99.4	199.	399.	999.	2000.
3	2.46	5.18	8.66	14.2	26.7	42.8	68.3	126.	201.
4	2.08	3.84	5.80	8.56	14.0	20.2	28.9	46.1	65.5
5	1.88	3.21	4.56	6.33	9.55	12.9	17.3	25.4	33.8
6	1.76	2.84	3.87	5.17	7.40	9.59	12.3	17.1	21.8
7	1.67	2.59	3.44	4.47	6.16	7.75	9.70	12.9	16.0
8	1.61	2.42	3.15	4.00	5.36	6.61	8.09	10.5	12.7
9	1.56	2.30	2.94	3.67	4.81	5.83	7.02	8.90	10.6
10	1.52	2.20	2.77	3.42	4.41	5.27	6.27	7.80	9.17
11	1.49	2.12	2.65	3.23	4.10	4.86	5.71	7.01	8.14
12	1.47	2.06	2.54	3.07	3.86	4.53	5.28	6.40	7.37
13	1.45	2.01	2.46	2.95	3.66	4.27	4.94	5.93	6.78
14	1.43	1.96	2.39	2.84	3.51	4.06	4.66	5.56	6.31
15	1.41	1.92	2.33	2.76	3.37	3.88	4.44	5.25	5.93
16	1.40	1.89	2.28	2.68	3.26	3.73	4.25	4.99	5.61
17	1.39	1.86	2.23	2.62	3.16	3.61	4.09	4.78	5.34
18	1.38	1.84	2.19	2.56	3.08	3.50	3.95	4.59	5.12
19	1.37	1.81	2.16	2.51	3.00	3.40	3.83	4.43	4.92
20	1.36	1.79	2.12	2.46	2.94	3.32	3.72	4.29	4.75
21	1.35	1.78	2.10	2.42	2.88	3.24	3.63	4.17	4.60
22	1.34	1.76	2.07	2.39	2.83	3.18	3.54	4.06	4.47
23	1.34	1.74	2.05	2.36	2.78	3.12	3.47	3.96	4.36
24	1.33	1.73	2.03	2.33	2.74	3.06	3.40	3.87	4.25
25	1.33	1.72	2.01	2.30	2.70	3.01	3.34	3.79	4.16
26	1.32	1.71	1.99	2.28	2.66	2.97	3.28	3.72	4.07
27	1.32	1.70	1.97	2.25	2.63	2.93	3.23	3.66	3.99
28	1.31	1.69	1.96	2.23	2.60	2.89	3.19	3.60	3.92
29	1.31	1.68	1.94	2.21	2.57	2.86	3.14	3.54	3.86
30	1.30	1.67	1.93	2.20	2.55	2.82	3.11	3.49	3.80
35	1.29	1.63	1.88	2.12	2.44	2.69	2.95	3.29	3.56
40	1.28	1.61	1.84	2.07	2.37	2.60	2.83	3.14	3.39
45	1.27	1.58	1.81	2.03	2.31	2.53	2.74	3.04	3.26
50	1.26	1.57	1.78	1.99	2.27	2.47	2.68	2.95	3.16
60	1.25	1.54	1.75	1.94	2.20	2.39	2.58	2.83	3.02
70	1.24	1.53	1.72	1.91	2.15	2.33	2.51	2.74	2.92
80	1.23	1.51	1.70	1.88	2.12	2.29	2.46	2.68	2.85
90	1.23	1.50	1.69	1.86	2.09	2.25	2.42	2.63	2.79
100	1.23	1.49	1.68	1.85	2.07	2.23	2.38	2.59	2.75
200	1.21	1.46	1.62	1.78	1.97	2.11	2.25	2.42	2.56
500	1.20	1.44	1.59	1.74	1.92	2.04	2.17	2.33	2.45
∞	1.19	1.42	1.57	1.71	1.88	2.00	2.12	2.27	2.37

TABLE B.4 *Continued*

				Numerator df = ∞					
α(1)	0.25	0.10	0.05	0.025	0.01	0.005	0.0025	0.001	0.0005
Denom df									
1	9.85	63.3	254.	1020.	6370.	25500.	$1 \cdot 10^5$	$6 \cdot 10^5$	$3 \cdot 10^6$
2	3.48	9.49	19.5	39.5	99.5	199.	399.	999.	2000.
3	2.47	5.13	8.53	13.9	26.1	41.8	66.8	123.	196.
4	2.08	3.76	5.63	8.26	13.5	19.3	27.6	44.0	62.6
5	1.87	3.11	4.37	6.02	9.02	12.1	16.3	23.8	31.6
6	1.74	2.72	3.67	4.85	6.88	8.88	11.4	15.7	20.0
7	1.65	2.47	3.23	4.14	5.65	7.08	8.81	11.7	14.4
8	1.58	2.29	2.93	3.67	4.86	5.95	7.25	9.33	11.3
9	1.53	2.16	2.71	3.33	4.31	5.19	6.21	7.81	9.26
10	1.48	2.06	2.54	3.08	3.91	4.64	5.47	6.76	7.91
11	1.45	1.97	2.40	2.88	3.60	4.23	4.93	6.00	6.93
12	1.42	1.90	2.30	2.72	3.36	3.90	4.51	5.42	6.20
13	1.40	1.85	2.21	2.60	3.17	3.65	4.18	4.97	5.64
14	1.38	1.80	2.13	2.49	3.00	3.44	3.91	4.60	5.19
15	1.36	1.76	2.07	2.40	2.87	3.26	3.69	4.31	4.83
16	1.34	1.72	2.01	2.32	2.75	3.11	3.50	4.06	4.52
17	1.33	1.69	1.96	2.25	2.65	2.98	3.34	3.85	4.27
18	1.32	1.66	1.92	2.19	2.57	2.87	3.20	3.67	4.05
19	1.30	1.63	1.88	2.13	2.49	2.78	3.08	3.51	3.87
20	1.29	1.61	1.84	2.09	2.42	2.69	2.97	3.38	3.71
21	1.28	1.59	1.81	2.04	2.36	2.61	2.88	3.26	3.56
22	1.28	1.57	1.78	2.00	2.31	2.55	2.80	3.15	3.43
23	1.27	1.55	1.76	1.97	2.26	2.48	2.72	3.05	3.32
24	1.26	1.53	1.73	1.94	2.21	2.43	2.65	2.97	3.22
25	1.25	1.52	1.71	1.91	2.17	2.38	2.59	2.89	3.13
26	1.25	1.50	1.69	1.88	2.13	2.33	2.54	2.82	3.05
27	1.24	1.49	1.67	1.85	2.10	2.29	2.48	2.75	2.97
28	1.24	1.48	1.65	1.83	2.06	2.25	2.44	2.69	2.90
29	1.23	1.47	1.64	1.81	2.03	2.21	2.39	2.64	2.84
30	1.23	1.46	1.62	1.79	2.01	2.18	2.35	2.59	2.78
35	1.20	1.41	1.56	1.70	1.89	2.04	2.18	2.38	2.54
40	1.19	1.38	1.51	1.64	1.80	1.93	2.06	2.23	2.37
45	1.18	1.35	1.47	1.59	1.74	1.85	1.97	2.12	2.23
50	1.16	1.33	1.44	1.55	1.68	1.79	1.89	2.03	2.13
60	1.15	1.29	1.39	1.48	1.60	1.69	1.78	1.89	1.98
70	1.13	1.27	1.35	1.44	1.54	1.62	1.69	1.79	1.87
80	1.12	1.24	1.32	1.40	1.49	1.56	1.63	1.72	1.79
90	1.12	1.23	1.30	1.37	1.46	1.52	1.58	1.66	1.72
100	1.11	1.21	1.28	1.35	1.43	1.49	1.54	1.62	1.67
200	1.07	1.14	1.19	1.23	1.28	1.31	1.35	1.39	1.42
500	1.05	1.09	1.11	1.14	1.16	1.18	1.20	1.23	1.24
∞	1.00	1.00	1.00	1.00	1.00	1.00	1.00	1.00	1.00

TABLE B.5 Critical values of Spearman's correlation coefficient*

α(2)	0.50	0.20	0.10	0.05	0.02	0.01	0.005	0.002	0.001
α(1)	0.25	0.10	0.05	0.025	0.01	0.005	0.0025	0.001	0.0005
n									
4	0.600	1.000	1.000						
5	0.500	0.800	0.900	1.000	1.000				
6	0.371	0.657	0.829	0.886	0.943	1.000	1.000		
7	0.321	0.571	0.714	0.786	0.893	0.929	0.964	1.000	1.000
8	0.310	0.524	0.643	0.738	0.833	0.881	0.905	0.952	0.976
9	0.267	0.483	0.600	0.700	0.783	0.833	0.867	0.917	0.933
10	0.248	0.455	0.564	0.648	0.745	0.794	0.830	0.879	0.903
11	0.236	0.427	0.536	0.618	0.709	0.755	0.800	0.845	0.873
12	0.217	0.406	0.503	0.587	0.678	0.727	0.769	0.818	0.846
13	0.209	0.385	0.484	0.560	0.648	0.703	0.747	0.791	0.824
14	0.200	0.367	0.464	0.538	0.626	0.679	0.723	0.771	0.802
15	0.189	0.354	0.446	0.521	0.604	0.654	0.700	0.750	0.779
16	0.182	0.341	0.429	0.503	0.582	0.635	0.679	0.729	0.762
17	0.176	0.328	0.414	0.485	0.566	0.615	0.662	0.713	0.748
18	0.170	0.317	0.401	0.472	0.550	0.600	0.643	0.695	0.728
19	0.165	0.309	0.391	0.460	0.535	0.584	0.628	0.677	0.712
20	0.161	0.299	0.380	0.447	0.520	0.570	0.612	0.662	0.696
21	0.156	0.292	0.370	0.435	0.508	0.556	0.599	0.648	0.681
22	0.152	0.284	0.361	0.425	0.496	0.544	0.586	0.634	0.667
23	0.148	0.278	0.353	0.415	0.486	0.532	0.573	0.622	0.654
24	0.144	0.271	0.344	0.406	0.476	0.521	0.562	0.610	0.642
25	0.142	0.265	0.337	0.398	0.466	0.511	0.551	0.598	0.630
26	0.138	0.259	0.331	0.390	0.457	0.501	0.541	0.587	0.619
27	0.136	0.255	0.324	0.382	0.448	0.491	0.531	0.577	0.608
28	0.133	0.250	0.317	0.375	0.440	0.483	0.522	0.567	0.598
29	0.130	0.245	0.312	0.368	0.433	0.475	0.513	0.558	0.589
30	0.128	0.240	0.306	0.362	0.425	0.467	0.504	0.549	0.580
35	0.118	0.222	0.283	0.335	0.394	0.433	0.468	0.510	0.539
40	0.110	0.207	0.264	0.313	0.368	0.405	0.439	0.479	0.507
45	0.103	0.194	0.248	0.294	0.347	0.382	0.414	0.453	0.479
50	0.097	0.184	0.235	0.279	0.329	0.363	0.393	0.430	0.456
55	0.093	0.175	0.224	0.266	0.314	0.346	0.375	0.411	0.435
60	0.089	0.168	0.214	0.255	0.300	0.331	0.360	0.394	0.418
65	0.085	0.161	0.206	0.244	0.289	0.318	0.346	0.379	0.402
70	0.082	0.155	0.198	0.235	0.278	0.307	0.333	0.365	0.388
75	0.079	0.150	0.191	0.227	0.269	0.297	0.322	0.353	0.375
80	0.076	0.145	0.185	0.220	0.260	0.287	0.312	0.342	0.363
85	0.074	0.140	0.180	0.213	0.252	0.279	0.303	0.332	0.353
90	0.072	0.136	0.174	0.207	0.245	0.271	0.294	0.323	0.343
95	0.070	0.133	0.170	0.202	0.239	0.264	0.287	0.314	0.334
100	0.068	0.129	0.165	0.197	0.233	0.257	0.279	0.307	0.326

*To find the Spearman's correlation coefficient that is associated with a certain chance of making a Type I error, find the column associated with that value of α at the top of the table (α(2) is a two-tailed value and α(1) is a one-tailed value) and the row associated with the sample's size in the leftmost column. The value in the body of the table where that column and row intersect is the absolute value of Spearman's correlation coefficient that is expected to occur in α of the samples from a population with Spearman's correlation coefficient equal to zero.

TABLE B.6 Critical values of Mann-Whitney U statistics*

$\alpha(2)$		0.20	0.10	0.05	0.02	0.01	0.005	0.002	0.001
$\alpha(1)$		0.10	0.05	0.025	0.01	0.005	0.0025	0.001	0.0005
n_S	n_L								
1	1	--	--	--	--	--	--	--	--
	2	--	--	--	--	--	--	--	--
	3	--	--	--	--	--	--	--	--
	4	--	--	--	--	--	--	--	--
	5	--	--	--	--	--	--	--	--
	6	--	--	--	--	--	--	--	--
	7	--	--	--	--	--	--	--	--
	8	--	--	--	--	--	--	--	--
	9	9	--	--	--	--	--	--	--
	10	10	--	--	--	--	--	--	--
	12	12	--	--	--	--	--	--	--
	14	14	--	--	--	--	--	--	--
	16	16	--	--	--	--	--	--	--
	18	18	--	--	--	--	--	--	--
	20	19	20	--	--	--	--	--	--
	22	21	22	--	--	--	--	--	--
	24	23	24	--	--	--	--	--	--
	26	25	26	--	--	--	--	--	--
	28	27	28	--	--	--	--	--	--
	30	28	30	--	--	--	--	--	--
	32	30	32	--	--	--	--	--	--
	34	32	34	--	--	--	--	--	--
	36	34	36	--	--	--	--	--	--
	38	36	38	--	--	--	--	--	--
1	40	37	39	40	--	--	--	--	--
2	2	--	--	--	--	--	--	--	--
	3	6	--	--	--	--	--	--	--
	4	8	--	--	--	--	--	--	--
	5	9	10	--	--	--	--	--	--
	6	11	12	--	--	--	--	--	--
	7	10	14	--	--	--	--	--	--
	8	14	15	16	--	--	--	--	--
	9	16	17	18	--	--	--	--	--
	10	17	19	20	--	--	--	--	--
	12	20	22	23	--	--	--	--	--
	14	23	25	27	28	--	--	--	--
	16	27	29	31	32	--	--	--	--
	18	30	32	34	36	--	--	--	--
	20	33	36	38	39	40	--	--	--
	22	36	39	41	43	44	--	--	--
	24	39	42	45	47	48	--	--	--
	26	42	46	48	51	52	--	--	--
	28	45	49	52	54	55	56	--	--
2	30	48	53	55	58	59	60	--	--

*To find the Mann-Whitney U statistic that is associated with a certain chance of making a Type I error, find the column associated with that value of α at the top of the table ($\alpha(2)$ is a two-tailed value and $\alpha(1)$ is a one-tailed value) and the row associated with the number of observations in the groups being compared in the leftmost column (n_s is the smaller of the two groups). The value in the body of the table where that column and row intersect is the value of the Mann-Whitney U statistic that is expected to occur in α of the samples from a population in which there is no association between the groups.

TABLE B.6 *Continued* ▪

$\alpha(2)$		0.20	0.10	0.05	0.02	0.01	0.005	0.002	0.001
$\alpha(1)$		0.10	0.05	0.025	0.01	0.005	0.0025	0.001	0.0005
n_S	n_L								
2	32	51	56	59	62	63	64	--	--
	34	55	59	63	65	67	68	--	--
	36	58	63	66	69	71	72	--	--
	38	61	66	70	73	75	76	--	--
2	40	64	69	73	77	78	79	--	--
3	3	8	9	--	--	--	--	--	--
	4	11	12	--	--	--	--	--	--
	5	13	14	15	--	--	--	--	--
	6	15	16	17	--	--	--	--	--
	7	15	19	20	21	--	--	--	--
	8	19	21	22	24	--	--	--	--
	9	22	23	25	26	27	--	--	--
	10	24	26	27	29	30	--	--	--
	12	28	31	32	34	35	36	--	--
	14	32	35	37	40	41	42	--	--
	16	37	40	42	45	46	47	--	--
	18	41	45	47	50	52	53	54	--
	20	45	49	52	55	57	58	60	--
	22	50	54	57	60	62	64	65	66
	24	54	59	62	66	68	69	71	72
	26	58	63	67	71	73	75	77	78
	28	63	68	72	76	79	80	82	83
	30	67	73	77	81	84	86	88	89
	32	71	77	82	87	89	91	94	95
	34	76	82	87	92	95	97	99	101
	36	80	87	92	97	100	103	105	106
	38	84	91	97	102	105	108	111	112
3	40	89	96	102	107	111	114	116	118
4	4	13	15	16	--	--	--	--	--
	5	16	18	19	20	--	--	--	--
	6	19	21	22	23	24	--	--	--
	7	20	24	25	27	28	--	--	--
	8	25	27	28	30	31	32	--	--
	9	27	30	32	33	35	36	--	--
	10	30	33	35	37	38	39	40	--
	12	36	39	41	43	45	46	48	--
	14	41	45	47	50	52	53	55	56
	16	47	50	53	57	59	60	62	63
	18	52	56	60	63	66	67	69	71
	20	58	62	66	70	72	75	77	78
	22	63	68	72	77	79	82	84	85
	24	69	74	79	83	86	89	91	93
	26	74	80	85	90	93	96	98	100
	28	80	86	91	96	100	103	106	108
4	30	85	92	97	103	107	110	113	115

TABLE B.6 *Continued*

α(2)	0.20	0.10	0.05	0.02	0.01	0.005	0.002	0.001
α(1)	0.10	0.05	0.025	0.01	0.005	0.0025	0.001	0.0005

n_S	n_L								
4	32	91	98	104	110	114	117	120	122
	34	96	104	110	116	120	124	127	130
	36	102	110	116	123	127	131	135	137
	38	107	116	122	130	134	138	142	144
4	40	113	121	129	136	141	145	149	152
5	5	20	21	23	24	25	--	--	--
	6	23	25	27	28	29	30	--	--
	7	24	29	30	32	34	35	--	--
	8	30	32	34	36	38	39	40	--
	9	33	36	38	40	42	43	44	45
	10	37	39	42	44	46	47	49	50
	12	43	47	49	52	54	56	58	59
	14	50	54	57	60	63	64	67	68
	16	57	61	65	68	71	73	75	77
	18	63	68	72	76	79	81	84	86
	20	70	75	80	84	87	90	93	95
	22	77	82	87	92	96	98	102	104
	24	84	90	95	100	104	107	110	113
	26	90	97	102	108	112	115	119	121
	28	97	104	110	116	120	124	128	130
	30	104	111	117	124	128	132	136	139
	32	110	118	125	132	137	141	145	148
	34	117	125	132	140	145	149	154	157
	36	124	132	140	148	153	158	163	166
	38	130	140	147	156	161	166	171	175
	40	137	147	155	164	169	174	180	184
6	6	27	29	31	33	34	35	--	--
	7	29	34	36	38	39	40	42	--
	8	35	38	40	42	44	45	47	48
	9	39	42	44	47	49	50	52	53
	10	43	46	49	52	54	55	57	58
	12	51	55	58	61	63	65	68	69
	14	59	63	67	71	73	75	78	79
	16	67	71	75	80	83	85	88	90
	18	74	80	84	89	92	95	98	100
	20	82	88	93	98	102	105	108	111
	22	90	96	102	108	111	115	119	121
	24	98	105	111	117	121	125	129	132
	26	106	113	119	126	131	134	139	142
	28	114	122	128	135	140	144	149	152
6	30	122	130	137	145	150	154	159	163

TABLE B.6 *Continued*

α(2)	0.20	0.10	0.05	0.02	0.01	0.005	0.002	0.001
α(1)	0.10	0.05	0.025	0.01	0.005	0.0025	0.001	0.0005

n_S	n_L								
6	32	129	138	146	154	159	164	169	173
	34	137	147	154	163	169	174	179	183
	36	145	155	163	172	178	184	190	194
	38	153	163	172	182	188	193	200	204
6	40	161	172	181	191	197	203	210	214
7	7	36	38	41	43	45	46	48	49
	8	40	43	46	49	50	52	54	55
	9	45	48	51	54	56	58	60	61
	10	49	53	56	59	61	63	65	67
	12	58	63	66	70	72	75	77	79
	14	67	72	76	81	83	86	89	91
	16	76	82	86	91	94	97	101	103
	18	85	91	96	102	105	108	112	115
	20	94	101	106	112	116	120	124	126
	22	103	110	116	123	127	131	135	138
	24	112	120	126	133	138	142	147	150
	26	121	129	136	144	149	153	158	162
	28	130	139	146	154	160	164	170	174
	30	139	149	156	165	170	176	181	185
	32	148	158	166	175	181	187	193	197
	34	157	168	176	186	192	198	204	209
	36	166	177	186	196	203	209	216	221
	38	175	187	196	207	214	220	227	232
7	40	184	196	206	217	225	231	239	244
8	8	45	49	51	55	57	58	60	62
	9	50	54	57	61	63	65	67	68
	10	56	60	63	67	69	71	74	75
	12	66	70	74	79	81	84	87	89
	14	76	81	86	90	94	96	100	102
	16	86	92	97	102	106	109	113	115
	18	96	103	108	114	118	122	126	129
	20	106	113	119	126	130	134	139	142
	22	117	124	131	138	142	147	152	155
	24	127	135	142	150	155	159	165	168
	26	137	146	153	161	167	172	177	181
	28	147	156	164	173	179	184	190	195
	30	157	167	175	185	191	197	203	208
	32	167	178	187	197	203	209	216	221
	34	177	188	198	208	215	222	229	234
	36	188	199	209	220	228	234	242	247
	38	198	210	220	232	240	247	255	260
8	40	208	221	231	244	252	259	268	273

TABLE B.6 *Continued*

α(2)	0.20	0.10	0.05	0.02	0.01	0.005	0.002	0.001
α(1)	0.10	0.05	0.025	0.01	0.005	0.0025	0.001	0.0005

n_S	n_L								
9	9	56	60	64	67	70	72	74	76
	10	62	66	70	74	77	79	82	83
	12	73	78	82	87	90	93	96	98
	14	85	90	95	100	104	107	111	113
	16	96	102	107	113	117	121	125	128
	18	107	114	120	126	131	135	139	142
	20	118	126	132	140	144	149	154	157
	22	130	138	145	153	158	162	168	172
	24	141	150	157	166	171	176	182	186
	26	152	162	170	179	185	190	196	201
	28	164	174	182	192	198	204	211	215
	30	175	185	194	205	212	218	225	230
	32	186	197	207	218	225	231	239	244
	34	197	209	219	231	238	245	253	259
	36	209	221	232	244	252	259	267	273
	38	220	233	244	257	265	273	282	288
9	40	231	245	257	270	279	286	296	302
10	10	68	73	77	81	84	87	90	92
	12	81	86	91	96	99	102	106	108
	14	93	99	104	110	114	117	121	124
	16	106	112	118	124	129	133	137	140
	18	118	125	132	139	143	148	153	156
	20	130	138	145	153	158	163	168	172
	22	143	152	159	167	173	178	184	188
	24	155	165	173	182	188	193	200	204
	26	168	178	186	196	202	208	215	220
	28	180	191	200	210	217	223	231	236
	30	192	204	213	224	232	238	246	252
	32	205	217	227	239	246	253	262	267
	34	217	230	241	253	261	268	277	283
	36	229	243	254	267	276	284	293	299
	38	242	256	268	281	290	299	308	315
10	40	254	269	281	296	305	314	324	331

TABLE B.7 Critical values of the chi-square distribution*

α(1)	0.50	0.25	0.10	0.05	0.025	0.01	0.005	0.001
df								
1	0.455	1.323	2.706	3.841	5.024	6.635	7.879	10.828
2	1.386	2.773	4.605	5.991	7.378	9.210	10.597	13.816
3	2.366	4.108	6.251	7.815	9.348	11.345	12.838	16.266
4	3.357	5.385	7.779	9.488	11.143	13.277	14.860	18.467
5	4.351	6.626	9.236	11.070	12.833	15.086	16.750	20.515
6	5.348	7.841	10.645	12.592	14.449	16.812	18.548	22.458
7	6.346	9.037	12.017	14.067	16.013	18.475	20.278	24.322
8	7.344	10.219	13.362	15.507	17.535	20.090	21.955	26.124
9	8.343	11.389	14.684	16.919	19.023	21.666	23.589	27.877
10	9.342	12.549	15.987	18.307	20.483	23.209	25.188	29.588
11	10.341	13.701	17.275	19.675	21.920	24.725	26.757	31.264
12	11.340	14.845	18.549	21.026	23.337	26.217	28.300	32.909
13	12.340	15.984	19.812	22.362	24.736	27.688	29.819	34.528
14	13.339	17.117	21.064	23.685	26.119	29.141	31.319	36.123
15	14.339	18.245	22.307	24.996	27.488	30.578	32.801	37.697
16	15.338	19.369	23.542	26.296	28.845	32.000	34.267	39.252
17	16.338	20.489	24.769	27.587	30.191	33.409	35.718	40.790
18	17.338	21.605	25.989	28.869	31.526	34.805	37.156	42.312
19	18.338	22.718	27.204	30.144	32.852	36.191	38.582	43.820
20	19.337	23.828	28.412	31.410	34.170	37.566	39.997	45.315
21	20.337	24.935	29.615	32.671	35.479	38.932	41.401	46.797
22	21.337	26.039	30.813	33.924	36.781	40.289	42.796	48.268
23	22.337	27.141	32.007	35.172	38.076	41.638	44.181	49.728
24	23.337	28.241	33.196	36.415	39.364	42.980	45.559	51.179
25	24.337	29.339	34.382	37.652	40.646	44.314	46.928	52.620
26	25.336	30.435	35.563	38.885	41.923	45.642	48.290	54.052
27	26.336	31.528	36.741	40.113	43.195	46.963	49.645	55.476
28	27.336	32.620	37.916	41.337	44.461	48.278	50.993	56.892
29	28.336	33.711	39.087	42.557	45.722	49.588	52.336	58.301
30	29.336	34.800	40.256	43.773	46.979	50.892	53.672	59.703
35	34.336	40.223	46.059	49.802	53.203	57.342	60.275	66.619
40	39.335	45.616	51.805	55.758	59.342	63.691	66.766	73.402
45	44.335	50.985	57.505	61.656	65.410	69.957	73.166	80.077
50	49.335	56.334	63.167	67.505	71.420	76.154	79.490	86.661
55	54.335	61.665	68.796	73.311	77.380	82.292	85.749	93.168
60	59.335	66.981	74.397	79.082	83.298	88.379	91.952	99.607
65	64.335	72.285	79.973	84.821	89.177	94.422	98.105	105.99
70	69.334	77.577	85.527	90.531	95.023	100.43	104.22	112.32
75	74.334	82.858	91.061	96.217	100.84	106.39	110.29	118.60
80	79.334	88.130	96.578	101.88	106.63	112.33	116.32	124.84
85	84.334	93.394	102.08	107.52	112.39	118.24	122.33	131.04
90	89.334	98.650	107.57	113.15	118.14	124.12	128.30	137.21
95	94.334	103.90	113.04	118.75	123.86	129.97	134.25	143.34
100	99.334	109.14	118.50	124.34	129.56	135.81	140.17	149.45

*To locate a chi-square value, find the degrees of freedom in the leftmost column and the appropriate α at the top of the table (only one-tailed α values are appropriate in the chi-square distribution). The number in the body of the table where this row and column intersect is the chi-square value from a distribution with that number of degrees of freedom and that corresponds to an area equal to α in one tail.

TABLE B.8 Critical values of the q distribution*

$\alpha(2) = 0.10$									
k	2	3	4	5	6	7	8	9	10
df									
1	8.929	13.44	16.36	18.49	20.15	21.51	22.64	23.62	24.48
2	4.130	5.733	6.773	7.538	8.139	8.633	9.049	9.409	9.725
3	3.328	4.467	5.199	5.738	6.162	6.511	6.806	7.062	7.287
4	3.015	3.976	4.586	5.035	5.388	5.679	5.926	6.139	6.327
5	2.850	3.717	4.264	4.664	4.979	5.238	5.458	5.648	5.816
6	2.748	3.559	4.065	4.435	4.726	4.966	5.168	5.344	5.499
7	2.680	3.451	3.931	4.280	4.555	4.780	4.972	5.137	5.283
8	2.630	3.374	3.843	4.169	4.431	4.646	4.829	4.987	5.126
9	2.592	3.316	3.761	4.084	4.337	4.545	4.721	4.873	5.007
10	2.563	3.270	3.704	4.018	4.264	4.465	4.636	4.783	4.913
11	2.540	3.234	3.658	3.965	4.205	4.401	4.568	4.711	4.838
12	2.521	3.204	3.621	3.922	4.156	4.349	4.511	4.652	4.776
13	2.505	3.179	3.589	3.885	4.116	4.305	4.464	4.602	4.724
14	2.491	3.158	3.563	3.854	4.081	4.267	4.424	4.560	4.680
15	2.479	3.140	3.540	3.828	4.052	4.235	4.390	4.524	4.641
16	2.469	3.124	3.520	3.804	4.026	4.207	4.360	4.492	4.608
17	2.460	3.110	3.503	3.784	4.004	4.183	4.334	4.464	4.579
18	2.452	3.098	3.488	3.767	3.984	4.161	4.311	4.440	4.554
19	2.445	3.087	3.474	3.751	3.966	4.142	4.290	4.418	4.531
20	2.439	3.078	3.462	3.736	3.950	4.124	4.271	4.398	4.510
30	2.400	3.017	3.386	3.648	3.851	4.016	4.155	4.275	4.381
40	2.381	2.988	3.349	3.605	3.803	3.963	4.099	4.215	4.317
60	2.363	2.959	3.312	3.562	3.755	3.911	4.042	4.155	4.254
∞	2.326	2.902	3.240	3.478	3.661	3.808	3.931	4.037	4.129

k	11	12	13	14	15	16	17	18	19
df									
1	25.24	25.92	26.54	27.10	27.62	28.10	28.54	28.96	29.35
2	10.01	10.26	10.49	10.70	10.89	11.07	11.24	11.39	11.54
3	7.487	7.667	7.832	7.982	8.120	8.249	8.368	8.479	8.584
4	6.495	6.645	6.783	6.909	7.025	7.133	7.233	7.327	7.414
5	5.966	6.101	6.223	6.336	6.440	6.536	6.626	6.710	6.789
6	5.637	5.762	5.875	5.979	6.075	6.164	6.247	6.325	6.398
7	5.413	5.530	5.637	5.735	5.826	5.910	5.988	6.061	6.130
8	5.250	5.362	5.464	5.558	5.644	5.724	5.799	5.869	5.935
9	5.127	5.234	5.333	5.423	5.506	5.583	5.655	5.723	5.786
10	5.029	5.134	5.229	5.317	5.397	5.472	5.542	5.607	5.668
11	4.951	5.053	5.146	5.231	5.309	5.382	5.450	5.514	5.573
12	4.886	4.986	5.077	5.160	5.236	5.308	5.374	5.436	5.495
13	4.832	4.930	5.019	5.100	5.176	5.245	5.311	5.372	5.429
14	4.786	4.882	4.970	5.050	5.124	5.192	5.256	5.316	5.373
15	4.746	4.841	4.927	5.006	5.079	5.147	5.209	5.269	5.324
16	4.712	4.805	4.890	4.968	5.040	5.107	5.169	5.227	5.282
17	4.682	4.774	4.858	4.935	5.005	5.071	5.133	5.190	5.244
18	4.655	4.746	4.829	4.905	4.975	5.040	5.101	5.158	5.211
19	4.631	4.721	4.803	4.879	4.948	5.012	5.073	5.129	5.182
20	4.609	4.699	4.780	4.855	4.924	4.987	5.047	5.103	5.155
30	4.474	4.559	4.635	4.706	4.770	4.830	4.886	4.939	4.988
40	4.408	4.490	4.564	4.632	4.695	4.752	4.807	4.857	4.905
60	4.342	4.421	4.493	4.558	4.619	4.675	4.727	4.775	4.821
∞	4.211	4.285	4.351	4.412	4.468	4.519	4.568	4.612	4.654

*To find a value of q, first locate the table headed by the appropriate value of α. Then, find the degrees of freedom in the leftmost column and the number of means involved in the comparison (k) in the top row of the table. Where this row and column intersect is the value of q corresponding to an area of α in the q distribution with that number of degrees of freedom and k means.

TABLE B.8 *Continued*

				α(2) = 0.05					
k	**2**	**3**	**4**	**5**	**6**	**7**	**8**	**9**	**10**
df									
1	17.97	26.98	32.82	37.08	40.41	43.12	45.40	47.36	49.07
2	6.085	8.331	9.798	10.88	11.74	12.44	13.03	13.54	13.99
3	4.501	5.910	6.825	7.502	8.037	8.478	8.853	9.177	9.462
4	3.927	5.040	5.757	6.287	6.707	7.053	7.347	7.602	7.826
5	3.635	4.602	5.218	5.673	6.033	6.330	6.582	6.802	6.995
6	3.461	4.339	4.896	5.305	5.628	5.895	6.122	6.319	6.493
7	3.344	4.165	4.681	5.060	5.359	5.606	5.815	5.998	6.158
8	3.261	4.041	4.529	4.886	5.167	5.399	5.597	5.767	5.918
9	3.199	3.949	4.415	4.756	5.024	5.244	5.432	5.595	5.739
10	3.151	3.877	4.327	4.654	4.912	5.124	5.305	5.461	5.599
11	3.113	3.820	4.256	4.574	4.823	5.028	5.202	5.353	5.487
12	3.082	3.773	4.199	4.508	4.751	4.950	5.119	5.265	5.395
13	3.055	3.735	4.151	4.453	4.690	4.885	5.049	5.192	5.318
14	3.033	3.702	4.111	4.407	4.639	4.829	4.990	5.131	5.254
15	3.014	3.674	4.076	4.367	4.595	4.782	4.940	5.077	5.198
16	2.998	3.649	4.046	4.333	4.557	4.741	4.897	5.031	5.150
17	2.984	3.628	4.020	4.303	4.524	4.705	4.858	4.991	5.108
18	2.971	3.609	3.997	4.277	4.495	4.673	4.824	4.956	5.071
19	2.960	3.593	3.977	4.253	4.469	4.645	4.794	4.924	5.038
20	2.950	3.578	3.958	4.232	4.445	4.620	4.768	4.896	5.008
30	2.888	3.486	3.845	4.102	4.302	4.464	4.602	4.720	4.824
40	2.858	3.442	3.791	4.039	4.232	4.389	4.521	4.635	4.735
60	2.829	3.399	3.737	3.977	4.163	4.314	4.441	4.550	4.646
∞	2.772	3.314	3.633	3.858	4.030	4.170	4.286	4.387	4.474

k	**11**	**12**	**13**	**14**	**15**	**16**	**17**	**18**	**19**
df									
1	50.59	51.96	53.20	54.33	55.36	56.32	57.22	58.04	58.83
2	14.39	14.75	15.08	15.38	15.65	15.91	16.14	16.37	16.57
3	9.717	9.946	10.15	10.35	10.53	10.69	10.84	10.98	11.11
4	8.027	8.208	8.373	8.525	8.664	8.794	8.914	9.028	9.134
5	7.168	7.324	7.466	7.596	7.717	7.828	7.932	8.030	8.122
6	6.649	6.789	6.917	7.034	7.143	7.244	7.338	7.426	7.508
7	6.302	6.431	6.550	6.658	6.759	6.852	6.939	7.020	7.097
8	6.054	6.175	6.287	6.389	6.483	6.571	6.653	6.729	6.802
9	5.867	5.983	6.089	6.186	6.276	6.359	6.437	6.510	6.579
10	5.722	5.833	5.935	6.028	6.114	6.194	6.269	6.339	6.405
11	5.605	5.713	5.811	5.901	6.984	6.062	6.134	6.202	6.265
12	5.511	5.615	5.710	5.798	5.878	5.953	6.023	6.089	6.151
13	5.431	5.533	5.625	5.711	5.789	5.862	5.931	5.995	6.055
14	5.364	5.463	5.554	5.637	5.714	5.786	5.852	5.915	5.974
15	5.306	5.404	5.493	5.574	5.649	5.720	5.785	5.846	5.904
16	5.256	5.352	5.439	5.520	5.593	5.662	5.727	5.786	5.843
17	5.212	5.307	5.392	5.471	5.544	5.612	5.675	5.734	5.790
18	5.174	5.267	5.352	5.429	5.501	5.568	5.630	5.688	5.743
19	5.140	5.231	5.315	5.391	5.462	5.528	5.589	5.647	5.701
20	5.108	5.199	5.282	5.357	5.427	5.493	5.553	5.610	5.663
30	4.917	5.001	5.077	5.147	5.211	5.271	5.327	5.379	5.429
40	4.824	4.904	4.977	5.044	5.106	5.163	5.216	5.266	5.313
60	4.732	4.808	4.878	4.942	5.001	5.056	5.107	5.154	5.199
∞	4.552	4.622	4.685	4.743	4.796	4.845	4.891	4.934	4.974

TABLE B.8 *Continued*   ■

				$\alpha(2) = 0.01$					
k	**2**	**3**	**4**	**5**	**6**	**7**	**8**	**9**	**10**
df									
1	90.03	135.0	164.3	185.6	202.2	215.8	227.2	237.0	245.6
2	14.04	19.02	22.29	24.72	26.63	28.20	29.53	30.68	31.69
3	8.261	10.62	12.17	13.33	14.24	15.00	15.64	16.20	16.69
4	6.512	8.120	9.173	9.958	10.58	11.10	11.55	11.93	12.27
5	5.702	6.976	7.804	8.421	8.913	9.321	9.669	9.972	10.24
6	5.243	6.331	7.033	7.556	7.973	8.318	8.613	8.869	9.097
7	4.949	5.919	6.543	7.005	7.373	7.679	7.939	8.166	8.368
8	4.746	5.635	6.204	6.625	6.960	7.237	7.474	7.681	7.863
9	4.596	5.428	5.957	6.348	6.658	6.915	7.134	7.325	7.495
10	4.482	5.270	5.769	6.163	6.428	6.669	6.875	7.055	7.213
11	4.392	5.146	5.621	5.970	6.247	6.476	6.672	6.842	6.992
12	4.320	5.046	5.502	5.836	6.101	6.321	6.507	6.670	6.814
13	4.260	4.964	5.404	5.727	5.981	6.192	6.372	6.528	6.667
14	4.210	4.895	5.322	5.634	5.881	6.085	6.258	6.409	6.543
15	4.168	4.836	5.252	5.556	5.796	5.994	6.162	6.309	6.439
16	4.131	4.786	5.192	5.489	5.722	5.915	6.079	6.222	6.349
17	4.099	4.742	5.140	5.430	5.659	5.847	6.007	6.147	6.270
18	4.071	4.703	5.094	5.379	5.603	5.788	5.944	6.081	6.201
19	4.046	4.670	5.054	5.334	5.554	5.735	5.889	6.022	6.141
20	4.024	4.639	5.018	5.294	5.510	5.688	5.839	5.970	6.087
30	3.889	4.455	4.799	5.048	5.242	5.401	5.536	5.653	5.756
40	3.825	4.367	4.696	4.931	5.114	5.265	5.392	5.502	5.559
60	3.762	4.282	4.595	4.818	4.991	5.133	5.253	5.356	5.447
∞	3.643	4.120	4.403	4.603	4.757	4.882	4.987	5.078	5.157

k	**11**	**12**	**13**	**14**	**15**	**16**	**17**	**18**	**19**
df									
1	253.2	260.0	266.2	271.8	277.0	281.8	286.3	290.4	294.3
2	32.59	33.40	34.13	34.81	35.43	36.00	36.53	37.03	37.50
3	17.13	17.53	17.89	18.22	18.52	18.81	19.07	19.32	19.55
4	12.57	12.84	13.09	13.32	13.53	13.73	13.91	14.08	14.24
5	10.48	10.70	10.89	11.08	11.24	11.40	11.55	11.68	11.81
6	9.301	9.485	9.653	9.808	9.951	10.08	10.21	10.32	10.43
7	8.548	8.711	8.860	8.997	9.124	9.242	9.353	9.456	9.554
8	8.027	8.176	8.312	8.436	8.552	8.659	8.760	8.854	8.943
9	7.647	7.784	7.910	8.025	8.132	8.232	8.325	8.412	8.495
10	7.356	7.485	7.603	7.712	7.812	7.906	7.993	8.076	8.153
11	7.128	7.250	7.362	7.465	7.560	7.649	7.732	7.809	7.883
12	6.943	7.060	7.167	7.265	7.356	7.441	7.520	7.594	7.665
13	6.791	6.903	7.006	7.101	7.188	7.269	7.345	7.417	7.485
14	6.664	6.772	6.871	6.962	7.047	7.126	7.199	7.268	7.333
15	6.555	6.660	6.757	6.845	6.927	7.003	7.074	7.142	7.204
16	6.462	6.564	6.658	6.744	6.823	6.898	6.967	7.032	7.093
17	6.381	6.480	6.572	6.656	6.734	6.806	6.873	6.937	6.997
18	6.310	6.407	6.497	6.579	6.655	6.725	6.792	6.854	6.912
19	6.247	6.342	6.430	6.510	6.585	6.654	6.719	6.780	6.837
20	6.191	6.285	6.371	6.450	6.523	6.591	6.654	6.714	6.771
30	5.849	5.932	6.008	6.078	6.143	6.203	6.259	6.311	6.361
40	5.686	5.764	5.835	5.900	5.961	6.017	6.069	6.119	6.165
60	5.528	5.601	5.667	5.728	5.785	5.837	5.886	5.931	5.974
∞	5.227	5.290	5.348	5.400	5.448	5.493	5.535	5.574	5.611

TABLE B.8 *Continued*

				$\alpha(2) = 0.001$					
k	2	3	4	5	6	7	8	9	10
df									
1	900.3	1351.	1643.	1856.	2022.	2158.	2272.	2370.	2455.
2	44.69	60.42	70.77	78.43	84.49	89.46	93.67	97.30	100.5
3	18.28	23.32	26.65	29.13	31.11	32.74	34.12	35.33	36.39
4	12.18	14.99	16.84	18.23	19.34	20.26	21.04	21.73	22.33
5	9.714	11.67	12.96	13.93	14.71	15.35	15.90	16.38	16.81
6	8.427	9.960	10.97	11.72	12.32	12.83	13.26	13.63	13.97
7	7.648	8.930	9.763	10.40	10.90	11.32	11.68	11.99	12.27
8	7.130	8.250	8.978	9.522	9.958	10.32	10.64	10.91	11.15
9	6.762	7.768	8.419	8.906	9.295	9.619	9.897	10.14	10.36
10	6.487	7.411	8.006	8.450	8.804	9.099	9.352	9.573	9.769
11	6.275	7.136	7.687	8.098	8.426	8.699	8.933	9.138	9.319
12	6.106	6.917	7.436	7.821	8.127	8.383	8.601	8.793	8.962
13	5.970	6.740	7.231	7.595	7.885	8.126	8.333	8.513	8.673
14	5.856	6.594	7.062	7.409	7.685	7.915	8.110	8.282	8.434
15	5.760	6.470	6.920	7.252	7.517	7.736	7.925	8.088	8.234
16	5.678	6.365	6.799	7.119	7.374	7.585	7.766	7.923	8.063
17	5.608	6.275	6.695	7.005	7.250	7.454	7.629	7.781	7.916
18	5.546	6.196	6.604	6.905	7.143	7.341	7.510	7.657	7.788
19	5.492	6.127	6.525	6.817	7.049	7.242	7.405	7.549	7.676
20	5.444	6.065	6.454	6.740	6.966	7.154	7.313	7.453	7.577
30	5.156	5.698	6.033	6.278	6.470	6.628	6.763	6.880	6.984
40	5.022	5.528	5.838	6.063	6.240	6.386	6.509	6.616	6.711
60	4.894	5.365	5.653	5.860	6.022	6.155	6.268	6.366	6.451
∞	4.654	5.063	5.309	5.484	5.619	5.730	5.823	5.903	5.973

k	11	12	13	14	15	16	17	18	19
df									
1	2532.	2600.	2662.	2718.	2770.	2818.	2863.	2904.	2943.
2	103.3	105.9	108.2	110.4	112.3	114.2	115.9	117.4	118.9
3	37.34	38.20	38.98	39.69	40.35	40.97	41.54	42.07	42.58
4	22.87	23.36	23.81	24.21	24.59	24.94	25.27	25.58	25.87
5	17.18	17.53	17.85	18.13	18.41	18.66	18.89	19.10	19.31
6	14.27	14.54	14.79	15.01	15.22	15.42	15.60	15.78	15.94
7	12.52	12.74	12.95	13.14	13.32	13.48	13.64	13.78	13.92
8	11.36	11.56	11.74	11.91	12.06	12.21	12.34	12.47	12.59
9	10.55	10.73	10.89	11.03	11.18	11.30	11.42	11.54	11.64
10	9.946	10.11	10.25	10.39	10.52	10.64	10.75	10.85	10.95
11	9.482	9.630	9.766	9.892	10.01	10.12	10.22	10.31	10.41
12	9.115	9.254	9.381	9.489	9.606	9.707	9.802	9.891	9.975
13	8.817	8.948	9.068	9.178	9.281	9.376	9.466	9.550	9.629
14	8.571	8.696	8.809	8.914	9.012	9.103	9.188	9.267	9.343
15	8.365	8.483	8.592	8.693	8.786	8.872	8.954	9.030	9.102
16	8.189	8.303	8.407	8.504	8.593	8.676	8.755	8.828	8.897
17	8.037	8.148	8.248	8.342	8.427	8.508	8.583	8.654	8.720
18	7.906	8.012	8.110	8.199	8.283	8.361	8.434	8.502	8.567
19	7.790	7.893	7.988	8.075	8.156	8.232	8.303	8.369	8.432
20	7.688	7.788	7.880	7.966	8.044	8.118	8.186	8.251	8.312
30	7.077	7.162	7.239	7.310	7.375	7.437	7.494	7.548	7.599
40	6.796	6.872	6.942	7.007	7.067	7.122	7.174	7.223	7.269
60	6.528	6.598	6.661	6.720	6.774	6.824	6.871	6.914	6.956
∞	6.036	6.092	6.144	6.191	6.234	6.274	6.312	6.347	6.380

TABLE B.9 Critical values of Kruskal-Wallis H statistics*

n_1	n_2	n_3	n_4	n_5	$\alpha(2)$ 0.10	0.05	0.02	0.01	0.005	0.002	0.001
2	2	2			4.571						
3	2	1			4.286						
3	2	2			4.500	4.714					
3	3	1			4.571	5.143					
3	3	2			4.556	5.361	6.250				
3	3	3			4.622	5.600	6.489	(7.200)	7.200		
4	2	1			4.500						
4	2	2			4.458	5.333	6.000				
4	3	1			4.056	5.208					
4	3	2			4.511	5.444	6.144	6.444	7.000		
4	3	3			4.709	5.791	6.564	6.745	7.318	8.018	
4	4	1			4.167	4.967	(6.667)	6.667			
4	4	2			4.555	5.455	6.600	7.036	7.282	7.855	
4	4	3			4.545	5.598	6.712	7.144	7.598	8.227	8.909
4	4	4			4.654	5.692	6.962	7.654	8.000	8.654	9.269
5	2	1			4.200	5.000					
5	2	2			4.373	5.160	6.000	6.533			
5	3	1			4.018	4.960	6.044				
5	3	2			4.651	5.251	6.124	6.909	7.182		
5	3	3			4.533	5.648	6.533	7.079	7.636	8.048	8.727
5	4	1			3.987	4.985	6.431	6.955	7.364		
5	4	2			4.541	5.273	6.505	7.205	7.573	8.114	8.591
5	4	3			4.549	5.656	6.676	7.445	7.927	8.481	8.795
5	4	4			4.619	5.657	6.953	7.760	8.189	8.868	9.168
5	5	1			4.109	5.127	6.145	7.309	8.182		
5	5	2			4.623	5.338	6.446	7.338	8.131	6.446	7.338
5	5	3			4.545	5.705	6.866	7.578	8.316	8.809	9.521
5	5	4			4.523	5.666	7.000	7.823	8.523	9.163	9.606
5	5	5			4.940	5.780	7.220	8.000	8.780	9.620	9.920
6	1	1			-----						
6	2	1			4.200	4.822					
6	2	2			4.545	5.345	6.182	6.982			
6	3	1			3.909	4.855	6.236				
6	3	2			4.682	5.348	6.227	6.970	7.515	8.182	
6	3	3			4.538	5.615	6.590	7.410	7.872	8.628	9.346
6	4	1			4.038	4.947	6.174	7.106	7.614		
6	4	2			4.494	5.340	6.571	7.340	7.846	8.494	8.827
6	4	3			4.604	5.610	6.725	7.500	8.033	8.918	9.170
6	4	4			4.595	5.681	6.900	7.795	8.381	9.167	9.861
6	5	1			4.128	4.990	6.138	7.182	8.077	8.515	

*To find a value of H, find the numbers of observations in the groups of dependent variable values in the leftmost column. It does not matter which of the groups is considered to be group 1, etc. Then locate the desired α value in the top row of the table. Where this row and column intersect is the value of the H statistic that is expected to occur in α of the samples from a population in which there is no association among groups with those numbers of observations. Numbers in parentheses indicate where H statistics cannot be calculated for a given α and a certain number of observations. Here, we recommend using the H statistic corresponding to the next lower value of α.

TABLE B.9 *Continued*   ■

n_1	n_2	n_3	n_4	n_5	$\alpha(2)$ 0.10	0.05	0.02	0.01	0.005	0.002	0.001
6	5	2			4.596	5.338	6.585	7.376	8.196	8.967	9.189
6	5	3			4.535	5.602	6.829	7.590	8.314	9.150	9.669
6	5	4			4.522	5.661	7.018	7.936	8.643	9.458	9.960
6	5	5			4.547	5.729	7.110	8.028	8.859	9.771	10.271
6	6	1			4.000	4.945	6.286	7.121	8.165	9.077	9.692
6	6	2			4.438	5.410	6.667	7.467	8.210	9.219	9.752
6	6	3			4.558	5.625	6.900	7.725	8.458	9.458	10.150
6	6	4			4.548	5.724	7.107	8.000	8.754	9.662	10.342
6	6	5			4.542	5.765	7.152	8.124	8.987	9.948	10.524
6	6	6			4.643	5.801	7.240	8.222	9.170	10.187	10.889
7	7	7			4.594	5.819	7.332	8.378	9.373	10.516	11.310
8	8	8			4.595	5.805	7.355	8.465	9.495	10.805	11.705
2	2	1	1		-----						
2	2	2	1		5.357	5.679					
2	2	2	2		5.667	6.167	(6.667)	6.667			
3	1	1	1		-----						
3	2	1	1		5.143						
3	2	2	1		5.556	5.833	6.500				
3	2	2	2		5.644	6.333	6.978	7.133	7.533		
3	3	1	1		5.333	6.333					
3	3	2	1		5.689	6.244	6.689	7.200	7.400		
3	3	2	2		5.745	6.527	7.182	7.636	7.873	8.018	8.455
3	3	3	1		5.655	6.600	7.109	7.400	8.055	8.345	
3	3	3	2		5.879	6.727	7.636	8.105	8.379	8.803	9.030
3	3	3	3		6.026	7.000	7.872	8.538	8.897	9.462	9.513
4	1	1	1		-----						
4	2	1	1		5.250	5.833					
4	2	2	1		5.533	6.133	6.667	7.000			
4	2	2	2		5.755	6.545	7.091	7.391	7.964	8.291	
4	3	1	1		5.067	6.178	6.711	7.067			
4	3	2	1		5.591	6.309	7.018	7.455	7.773	8.182	
4	3	2	2		5.750	6.621	7.530	7.871	8.273	8.689	8.909
4	3	3	1		5.689	6.545	7.485	7.758	8.212	8.697	9.182
4	3	3	2		5.872	6.795	7.763	8.333	8.718	9.167	8.455
4	3	3	3		6.016	6.984	7.995	8.659	9.253	9.709	10.016
4	4	1	1		5.182	5.945	7.091	7.909	7.909		
4	4	2	1		5.568	6.386	7.364	7.886	8.341	8.591	8.909
4	4	2	2		5.808	6.731	7.750	8.346	8.692	9.269	9.462
4	4	3	1		5.692	6.635	7.660	8.231	8.583	9.038	9.327
4	4	3	2		5.901	6.874	7.951	8.621	9.165	9.615	9.945

TABLE B.9 *Continued*   ■

					α(2)	0.10	0.05	0.02	0.01	0.005	0.002	0.001
n_1	n_2	n_3	n_4	n_5								
4	4	3	3		6.019	7.038	8.181	8.876	9.495	10.105	10.467
4	4	4	1		5.564	6.725	7.879	8.588	9.000	9.478	9.758
4	4	4	2		5.914	6.957	8.157	8.871	9.486	10.043	10.429
4	4	4	3		6.042	7.142	8.350	9.075	9.742	10.542	10.929
4	4	4	4		6.088	7.235	8.515	9.287	9.971	10.809	11.338
2	1	1	1	1	-----						
2	2	1	1	1	5.786						
2	2	2	1	1	6.250	6.750					
2	2	2	2	1	6.600	7.133	(7.533)	7.533			
2	2	2	2	2	6.982	7.418	8.073	8.291	(8.727)	8.727	
3	1	1	1	1	-----						
3	2	1	1	1	6.139	6.583					
3	2	2	1	1	6.511	6.800	7.400	7.600			
3	2	2	2	1	6.709	7.309	7.836	8.127	8.327	8.618	
3	2	2	2	2	6.955	7.682	8.303	8.682	8.985	9.273	9.364
3	3	1	1	1	6.311	7.111	7.467				
3	3	2	1	1	6.600	7.200	7.892	8.073	8.345		
3	3	2	2	1	6.788	7.591	8.258	8.576	8.924	9.167	9.303
3	3	2	2	2	7.026	7.910	8.667	9.115	9.474	9.769	10.026
3	3	3	1	1	6.788	7.576	8.242	8.424	8.848	(9.455)	9.455
3	3	3	2	1	6.910	7.769	8.590	9.051	9.410	9.769	9.974
3	3	3	2	2	7.121	8.044	9.011	9.505	9.890	10.330	10.637
3	3	3	3	1	7.077	8.000	8.879	9.451	9.846	10.286	10.549
3	3	3	3	2	7.210	8.200	9.267	9.876	10.333	10.838	11.171
3	3	3	3	3	7.333	8.333	9.467	10.200	10.733	10.267	11.667

TABLE B.10   Critical values of Dunn's Q statistics*

α(2)	0.50	0.20	0.10	0.05	0.02	0.01	0.005	0.002	0.001
k									
2	0.674	1.282	1.645	1.960	2.327	2.576	2.807	3.091	3.291
3	1.383	1.834	2.128	2.394	2.713	2.936	3.144	3.403	3.588
4	1.732	2.128	2.394	2.639	2.936	3.144	3.342	3.588	3.765
5	1.960	2.327	2.576	2.807	3.091	3.291	3.481	3.719	3.891
6	2.128	2.475	2.713	2.936	3.209	3.403	3.588	3.820	3.988
7	2.261	2.593	2.823	3.038	3.304	3.494	3.675	3.902	4.067
8	2.369	2.690	2.914	3.124	3.384	3.570	3.748	3.972	4.134
9	2.461	2.773	2.992	3.197	3.453	3.635	3.810	4.031	4.191
10	2.540	2.845	3.059	3.261	3.512	3.692	3.865	4.083	4.241
11	2.609	2.908	3.119	3.317	3.565	3.743	3.914	4.129	4.286
12	2.671	2.965	3.172	3.368	3.613	3.789	3.957	4.171	4.326
13	2.726	3.016	3.220	3.414	3.656	3.830	3.997	4.209	4.363
14	2.777	3.062	3.264	3.456	3.695	3.868	4.034	4.244	4.397
15	2.823	3.105	3.304	3.494	3.731	3.902	4.067	4.276	4.428
16	2.866	3.144	3.342	3.529	3.765	3.935	4.098	4.305	4.456
17	2.905	3.181	3.376	3.562	3.796	3.965	4.127	4.333	4.483
18	2.942	3.215	3.409	3.593	3.825	3.993	4.154	4.359	4.508
19	2.976	3.246	3.439	3.622	3.852	4.019	4.179	4.383	4.532
20	3.008	3.276	3.467	3.649	3.878	4.044	4.203	4.406	4.554
21	3.038	3.304	3.494	3.675	3.902	4.067	4.226	4.428	4.575
22	3.067	3.331	3.519	3.699	3.925	4.089	4.247	4.448	4.595
23	3.094	3.356	3.543	3.722	3.947	4.110	4.268	4.468	4.614
24	3.120	3.380	3.566	3.744	3.968	4.130	4.287	4.486	4.632
25	3.144	3.403	3.588	3.765	3.988	4.149	4.305	4.504	4.649

*To find a value of Q, find the number of means of ranks included in the comparison interval in the leftmost column, then locate the desired α value in the top row of the table. Where this row and column intersect is the value of Q that is expected to occur in α of the samples from a population in which there is no association between the groups.

APPENDIX C
Flowchart of Statistics

   Chapters 4 through 12 in *Statistical First Aid* are structured to reflect the thinking process of the statistician when choosing a statistical procedure to analyze a particular set of data. At the beginning of each of those chapters, the procedures discussed in that particular chapter appear in a flowchart that summarizes the statistician's thinking process. In this appendix, we have brought those flowcharts together so that they are easier to use. As explained in the text of *Statistical First Aid*, you should start by using the master flowchart that appears below. Following this flowchart will lead to the chapter that discusses the types of statistical procedures that might be used to analyze a particular set of data. The flowcharts following the master flowchart in this appendix are labeled according to the chapter in which they are discussed. Following these flowcharts will reveal the most commonly used statistical procedure to analyze a particular data set.

   In each of the following flowcharts, point estimates are indicated in color, statistical procedures are indicated in color and underlined, and common names for a general class of statistical procedures appear in boxes.

MASTER FLOWCHART

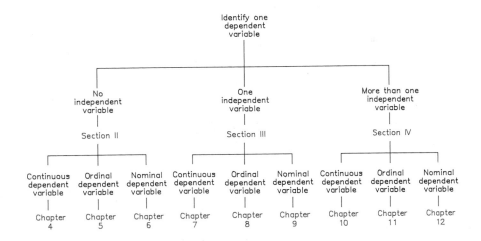

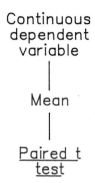

Continuous
dependent
variable

|

Mean

|

Paired t
test

CHAPTER 4 Univariable analysis of continuous dependent
variables.

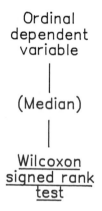

Ordinal
dependent
variable

CHAPTER 5 Univariable analysis of ordinal dependent variables.

|

(Median)

|

Wilcoxon
signed rank
test

CHAPTER 6 Univariable analysis of nominal dependent variables.

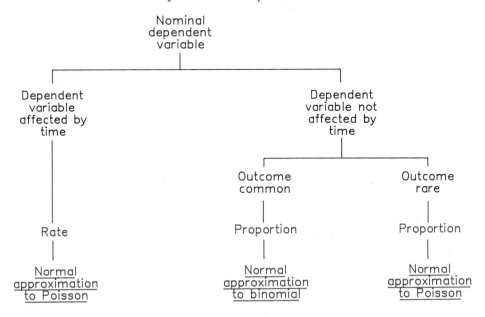

CHAPTER 7 Bivariable analysis of continuous dependent variables.

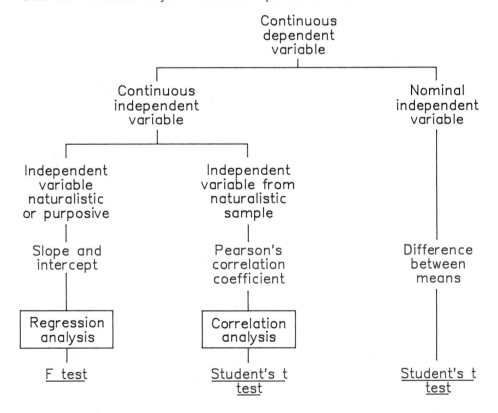

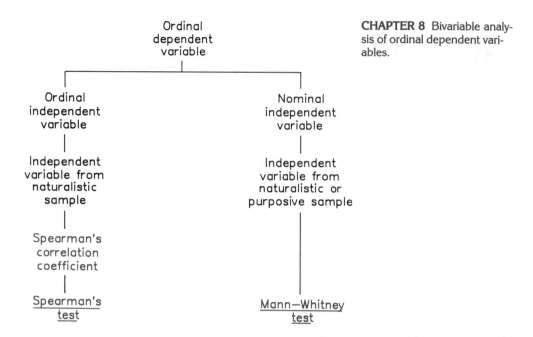

CHAPTER 8 Bivariable analysis of ordinal dependent variables.

CHAPTER 9 Bivariable analysis of nominal dependent variables.

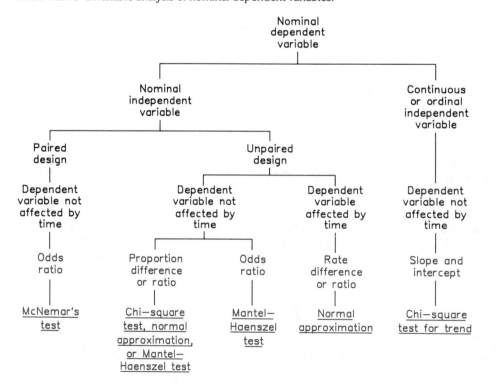

CHAPTER 10 Multivariable analysis of continuous dependent variables.

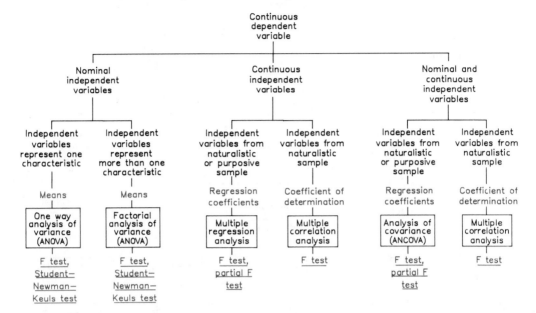

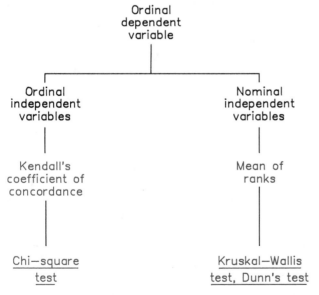

CHAPTER 11 Multivariable analysis of ordinal dependent variables.

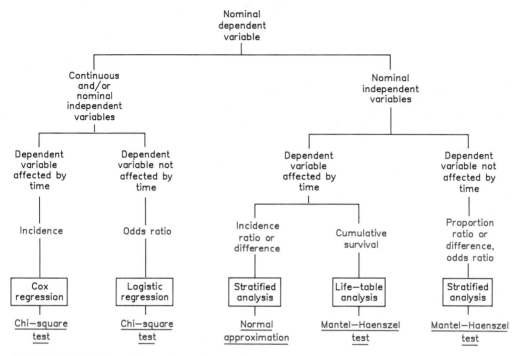

CHAPTER 12 Multivariable analysis of nominal dependent variables.

Index